T0133261

Medical Protestants

Medical Protestants

The Eclectics in American Medicine,
1825–1939

John S. Haller, Jr.

Southern Illinois University Press
Carbondale and Edwardsville

Copyright © 1994 by the Board of Trustees,
Southern Illinois University
Paperback edition 2013
All rights reserved
Printed in the United States of America
16   15   14   13   4   3   2   1

The Library of Congress has cataloged the hardcover edition as follows:

Haller, John S.
    Medical protestants : the eclectics in American medicine,
    1825–1939 / John S. Haller, Jr.
        p.   cm. — (Medical humanities series)
    Includes bibliographical references and index.
    1. Medicine, Eclectic—United States—History. I. Title.
    II. Series
    [DNLM: 1. History of Medicine, 19th Cent.—United States.
    2. History of Medicine, 20th Cent.—United States. 3. Eclecticism.
    WZ70 AA1 H18m   1994]
    RV61.H35   1994
    615.5'3—dc20   93-7389
    ISBN 0-8093-1894-6   CIP
    ISBN-13: 978-0-8093-1894-0 (cloth)

    ISBN-13: 978-0-8093-3142-0 (pbk. : alk. paper)
    ISBN-10: 0-8093-3142-X (pbk. : alk. paper)
    ISBN-13: 978-0-8093-8106-7 (ebook)
    ISBN-10: 0-8093-8106-0 (ebook)

The paper used in this publication meets the minimum requirements of
American National Standard for Information Sciences—Permanence
of Paper for Printed Library Materials, ANSI z39.48-1992. ∞

for JONATHAN

Eclecticism is as much a protest in the field of medicine as was Luther's Reformation in the domain of religion. We are protestants against the old dogmas of medicine, just as the disciples of Luther were protestants against the dogmas of the Papal church. Medical protestants came up spontaneously from the people, and in time were rallied together and organized under able leaders into associations which are now known as auxiliary, state and national bodies; and herein our medical protestantism differs from religious protestantism, for in the latter, the leader came first, and the people rallied to his standard. Eclecticism is, therefore, a protest against the old methods of practice, and is the direct outgrowth of the people, and we may say, of the common people.

—*Edward B. Foote*, M.D.

Contents

Illustrations

Acknowledgments

I am particularly grateful to three individuals for their advice and counsel in the preparation of this manuscript. Glen W. Davidson, chair of the Department of Medical Humanities at the Southern Illinois University School of Medicine was especially helpful in turning me to specific materials and themes. His steady counsel, as both chairman and colleague, has proven invaluable. My appreciation also goes to James Pascal Imperato, M.D., editor of the *New York State Journal of Medicine*, whose initial reading of the manuscript convinced me that I was taking the right tack in pursuing this seemingly forgotten sectarian group. His steady support of my research interests over the years has been particularly gratifying. Finally, I wish to thank Kenneth M. Ludmerer, M.D., of the Washington University School of Medicine, St. Louis. His reading of the manuscript, along with his collegial advice, gave me added assurance that I had a story to tell about the eclectics that fit into the fabric of American social and intellectual history. Others to whom I am indebted include David H. Gilbert, Richard D. DeBacher and Susan Wilson at SIU Press; freelance copyeditor Kathryn Koldehoff; and colleagues Mark Foster, Rickey Hendricks, David P. Werlich, Benjamin A. Shepherd, John H. Yopp, Glendon F. Drake, Gilbert Schmidt, Betty McDowell, William and Jo Holohan, and Barbara Parker. Most importantly, I am grateful to my wife, Robin, who, as with all of my research, offered inspiration, encouragement, criticism, and substantial assistance, including proofing numerous drafts and indexing the finished manuscript.

Like most authors of historical works, I am especially obligated to the historian-collector-librarians and their professional staffs. It was their generosity of time and experienced assistance that made it possible for me to enrich my understanding of the subject matter and to carry out the necessary research. I wish to extend my special gratitude to librarian Rebecca A. Perry, archivist and conservator William C. Black, and the staff of the Lloyd Library and Museum in Cincinnati, Ohio. They provided invaluable assistance in opening to me the resources of the Lloyd Library and its wonderful collection on the eclectics. Other librarians to whom I am indebted include Kathy Fahey, Karen Drickamer, James W. Fox, Kimbra Stout, Andrew Tax, Harry Davis, Iva McRoberts, Mary Lee Schmidt, Rose Marie Weckenmann, Kenneth G. Peterson, Carolyn Snyder, Patricia Breivik, Lori Arp, Elnora M. Mercado, Betsy Porter, Jay Schafer, Connie Whitson, Mary Lou Goodyear, Rutherford Witthus, Eveline L. Yang, Joan Fiscella, Jean Hemphill, Marilyn Mitchell, and Muriel E. Woods.

Finally, my gratitude would not be complete without noting the fine libraries whose collections I used. These include the Morris Library of Southern Illinois University, Carbondale; the Medical Library of Southern Illinois University, Springfield; Norlin Library of the University of Colorado, Boulder; Denison Library of the University of Colorado Health Sciences Center, Denver; the University of Denver Library; the University of Oregon Medical School Library, Eugene; the University of Utah Library, Salt Lake City; Kent State University Library; Indiana State University Library, Terre Haute; Drake University Library, Des Moines; the University of California at Irvine Medical Sciences Library; Indiana University Library, Bloomington; Johns Hopkins University Library, Baltimore; the National Library of Medicine, Bethesda, Maryland; and especially the Center for Research Libraries, Chicago.

Introduction

In the freshness of its youth, the eclectic school of reform medicine stood as a symbol of America's optimism, imagination, enthusiasms, and eccentricities. Of solid Yankee inheritance, the school represented a powerful statement of the fraternity that its adherents felt with the great world movements of thought. In their writings, the eclectics portrayed themselves as authentic protestants, saving therapeutics from the errors and extravagances of orthodox medicine. Along with homeopaths, they saw themselves as offering a viable alternative to those in the early decades of the nineteenth century who had wearied of allopathy's pretensions and failures. Having fostered a revolutionary challenge, they hoped to redress the shortcomings of orthodox practice with proof of their botanic successes, directing attention to a simpler and less drastic form of medicine. Although scornfully rejected by regulars, the eclectics imitated their magisterial air as, for a score of years and in two dozen colleges and more than sixty-five journals, they asserted the wisdom of their theory and the maxims of reform practice.

The eclectic school, sometimes called the American school, flourished at a time when both the art and the science of medicine were undergoing profound if not traumatic crises of faith. At the heart of these crises was not only a disillusionment with traditional therapeutics but an intense questioning of the principles and philosophy upon which it had been built. Increasingly, American physicians and their patients felt that medicine had lost the ability to cure. The originators of reform practice met this crisis by offering a therapeutics built around herbal medicines and a more empirical approach to disease. In the early decades of the nineteenth century when therapeutic nihilism, or recklessness, threatened to destroy the bond between physician and patient, eclectics offered an optimistic palliative that healed, comforted, and reassured Americans that medicine was indeed governed by rational laws. Eclectic practitioners portrayed their medicine as a unifying force, one that had salvaged the public's loss of faith in medicine. Unlike the speculative rationalism of the system builders, which forced patients into tight patterns of correct therapeutic behavior, the eclectics urged the application of any technique that worked, thus restoring faith in all medical systems while reassuring followers that order existed despite medicine's apparent disarray. They symbolized a faith in science and practical experience, the value of self-direction and dedication, and the distrust of theory as an end in itself.

I have chosen to recount the story of eclectic medicine in the same textual manner in which the eclectics viewed themselves, namely, as medical protestants existing within a pluralistic culture. Like religion, medicine should not be viewed in abstraction from its adherents. Both were led by individuals who were seen as gifted with direct, immediate, and intuitive insight into life. Both stressed the importance of voluntary association, the need for equality before civilian authority, and the justification of their peculiar doctrinal emphases. The vigor and vitality, as well as the discipline and distinctiveness, with which the eclectics pursued their beliefs and asserted their right to private judgment paralleled the religious sectarians' conflict with orthodoxy and their insistence that they be allowed to practice in their own way.

America, as G. K. Chesterton so accurately explained, was a "nation with the soul of a church." It was a nation, however, whose religious beliefs were overshadowed by the greater religion of democracy and the power of a neutral civil government, which recognized all beliefs to be of equal value. In the end, this greater secular faith determined the character of sectarian peculiarities—both religious and medical—by adopting a pluralism of beliefs, ideas, and standards that, in their diversity, provided a common identity that bound people together.[1] The democratic experience demanded a pluralistic and egalitarian tradition for both religion and medicine in nineteenth-century America; nevertheless, medical orthodoxy took a markedly different road in the early twentieth century. Although willing to accommodate various emphases (e.g., family practice, gynecology, pediatrics, orthopedics) within its family circle, regular medicine flexed its monopolistic muscles to diminish the power and prestige of sectarian medicine. As a result, few sectarians were able to win professional status. Today, only osteopathy and chiropractic hold title to America's earlier sectarian legacy.

I also recount the story of eclecticism through its institutions, including the Eclectic Medical Institute of Cincinnati, Ohio, the "mother institute" of reform medical schools. Organized in 1845, it spanned ninety-four years, closing finally in 1939 after a searching self-examination and a futile struggle to retain independence. The history of the institute and its sister schools falls within the context of nineteenth-century social and intellectual life, representative in the school's early self-assertive stance within the mainstream of protestant and voluntaristic thinking, running a course parallel with the anti-intellectual and egalitarian shibboleths of Jacksonian culture, and emerging in mid-century as an alternative to allopathic practice. If anything, the eclectics mirrored the dreams, anticipations, promises, and frustrations of American culture; they were genuine Yankees intent on establishing a role for a native and more practical system of medicine independent of Europe's medical savants.

Throughout their history, the eclectic medical schools provided an avenue into the medical profession for men—and women— who lacked the financial and educational opportunities available to those of more material means. In this sense, these schools continued a tradition that had long been a subject of debate within American medicine. From remarks made in 1846 by Professor Martyn Paine of the Medical Department of New York University, who accused the newly formed American Medical Association of playing aristocratic politics behind a masquerade of curriculum reform, to the comments in 1871 of Henry J. Bigelow of Harvard University Medical School, who was an admirer of the Horatio Alger-like determination of young men who came into medicine from impoverished circumstances, there remained a tradition within medical education that advocated more democratic access. The eclectics deliberately sided with this tradition and only grudgingly followed the lead set by regulars as they changed curriculum and tightened standards for admission.[2]

From the eighteenth century and into the early nineteenth century, medical schools in Edinburgh, Scotland, and London,

England, continued to attract American students of means; but the pre–Civil War decades also witnessed increasing numbers of young men seeking postdoctoral experience in Paris, where dissection and postmortem examinations gave France a central role in clinical-pathological studies and in the emerging science of clinical statistics. Beginning in the 1870s, the educational migration abroad showed a perceptible shift from the clinical medicine of Paris to schools in Italy and Germany, where students found ways to augment their mediocre medical education with rigorous laboratory research.

While regular schools were witnessing the birth of academic medicine as a result of these European experiences, the eclectics chose a more conservative tradition, preferring to supply American society with locally educated physicians whose cures for human ills came from the inventory of botanical medicines grown on native soil. Although ostensibly open to the world of medical ideas and discoveries, the eclectics actually became more introspective as the century progressed, choosing to rely on an increasingly parochial armamentarium of acceptable cures. Without sensing a loss of dignity or of faith in themselves, they enjoyed the fruits of European intellect but always saw themselves as free to rival—if not exceed—Old World ideas by native ability. They showed little respect in this regard for canons or traditions and held their own beliefs to be equal to those of every other school of medicine. In reading their early literature, one senses that the eclectics did not feel inferior. They were confident in their abilities and gave to their work a freshness and singularity that remains a vibrant part of American medical literature. They took upon themselves the special task of working out a therapeutic system reflective of democratic institutions. Theirs was a mental adventure, which began with an undoubting confidence in the future and identified with everything genuinely American.

Like other sectarian movements that began with irrepressible energies, the eclectics had a talent for self-promotion. They were earnest in their efforts and were successful in captivating the imaginations of many in the first half of the nineteenth century, but they failed to carry out the object of their convictions. They glimpsed the possibility of a truly reformed medical practice but dissipated their energies in acrimonious debate and controversy. Impatient with details, they often failed to maintain a sense of proportion, and what began as an imaginative search for a new therapeutics bogged down in overly simplistic panaceas. Moreover, the eclectics never overcame their distrust of ideas deemed foreign. By the late nineteenth century, they found themselves in the backwaters of modernity, no longer treated with what they felt should be the proper deference due them as exponents of scientific medicine. What began as a passionate effort to liberate medicine from speculative rationalism devolved into a school of thinking that became insulated and ineffectual, little more than a historical artifact of its Philistine past. Unable to disentangle themselves from their botanic biases and ill-equipped to accept the implications of germ theory, the financial costs of salaried faculty and staff, or the research implications of laboratory science, the eclectics emerged into the twentieth century stubborn and fundamentally perplexed by the rigor demanded in the new medical curriculum and in the expectations of research. By the time Abraham Flexner wrote his landmark *Medical Education in the United States and Canada* (1910), the school's remnants were all but forgotten in the rush of modern academic medicine.

Medical Protestants

1
The American Landscape

The antecedents of American medical practice exist not only in the richness of European science and medicine but in the ideologically murky challenges of the New World frontier. From these sources, American colonists inherited an optimism that enriched them beyond measure and expanded their lives. Europe favored scholarship and brilliance, exalted high standards, forfeited experience to logic, accentuated contemptuousness, and exuded, above all else, a certain literary flourish. The American frontier bequeathed fresh simplicity, openness, high-spiritedness, vigilance, social compassion, an assumption of innocence, and an indomitable belief in common sense and practicality. From these beginnings, American practice manifested a stubborn, unconciliatory attitude that dutifully complemented both its public and its more solitary musings. It was not British and surely not European—but neither was it simply a reflection of native abilities. Few returned from Europe without a higher opinion of its greatness, tempting many to adapt elements of Old World medicine and practice into New World surroundings. Nevertheless, for those Americans living close to the soil, unexpressed in arts and letters, there existed a widespread flowering of imagination that, while youthful in its aspirations, spoke with authority, optimism, and determination.

Medical Protestants

American Improvisation

Learned doctors were a rare commodity in the early years of the colonies. "Physicians, like the upper classes in general, did not migrate overseas," observed Richard H. Shryock, "and for a long period no American towns were large enough to train such men on their own behalf."[1] When William Douglass, M.D. (1691–1752), with his medical degree from Utrecht, the Netherlands, settled in Boston in 1718, he was the only practicing physician who could boast a university degree. Understandably then, over the course of American settlement, men and women served as general practitioners for themselves and their neighbors and obtained the status of "doctor" simply by assuming the responsibility of healer. People beyond the reach of established educational institutions and statutory regulations fended for themselves, and the lack of medical education worked as no barrier to those gifted few who could inspire confidence while serving community needs.[2] Thus, guild titles seemed not to matter as the terms *doctor, surgeon*, and *physician* entered the American lexicon without the formal distinctions understood elsewhere. In effect, the sharp delineation between surgeon and physician on the Continent did not exist in the American landscape where doctors advertised themselves as practicing both physic and surgery, as well as midwifery and pharmacy. Moreover, farmers, women, indentured servants, and even slaves acquired reputations as local healers. In addition, countless hordes of itinerant pretenders beguiled the public with promises and plied their trade unencumbered by degrees, education, or regulation.

In keeping with European tradition, many ministers assumed the dual role of healer of bodies and keeper of souls, a practice that, except for the cities, predominated until about 1750. Indeed, as Richard D. Brown explained, "even the most rational and learned individuals . . . saw no clear boundary between physical and spiritual phenomena."[3] Examples of this physician-minister tradition included Cotton Mather (1663–1728), who introduced smallpox inoculation in 1721; Henry M. Mühlenberg (1711–87) of Pennsylvania; and Jared Eliot (1685–1763) of Connecticut. In *A Letter About a Good Management Under the Distemper of the Measles, at This Time Spreading in the Country* (1713), Cotton Mather recommended moderate treatment and good nursing; his book was intended "for the benefit of the poor, and such as may want the help of able physicians."[4]

In this laissez-faire environment, do-it-yourself books abounded, as did a wide array of medical almanacs, which provided a rich source of domestic medicine, recipes, commonly employed remedies, popular herbals, patent medicines, veterinary medicine, and astrology (i.e., indications for the propitious seasons of the year for bleeding and cupping). More serious works written by Simon-André Tissot (1728–97) and William Buchan (1729–1805) became the successors to Gervase Markham, *The English House-Wife* (1636); Countess Elizabeth Kent, *A Choice Manual of Rare and Select Secrets in Physick and Chyrurgery* (1653); James Hart, *Klinekeh; Or the Diet of the Diseased* (1633); Humphrey Brooke, *A Conservatory of Health* (1650); and Thomas Cogan, *The Haven of Health* (1636), which stressed the efficacy of moderate diet and condemned violent purgings and indiscriminate bleedings.[5]

John Wesley (1703–91), the founder of Methodism, authored *Primitive Physick* (1747), which went through thirty-eight British and twenty-four American editions. For him, medical knowledge included understanding the virtues of single plants that men and women of common sense could prescribe for themselves and their neighbors. He opposed polypharmacy, took issue with rationalistic theories, denigrated anatomy, anticipated both hydrotherapy and homeopathy, encouraged knowledge through experience, and advised temperance and moderation in all things. Wesley regarded care of the sick as an integral part of Methodism, and he was as passionate in his concern to provide "plain" medicine as he was to restore apostolic Christianity. As Harold Y. Vanderpool has so well argued, Wesley "sought to rescue both medicine and the church from those who had corrupted them, to purify and revitalize them by returning them to their ancient, plain, practical, and efficacious beginnings."[6]

William Buchan's *Domestic Medicine; Or, A Treatise on the Prevention and Cure of Diseases by Regimen and Simple Medicine*, went through 143 editions after its first appearance in 1769. Read by a cross section of literate society, Buchan's book was intended for use in general household practice. At least eighty thousand copies sold in Great Britain alone during the author's lifetime. While emphasizing the importance of physicians and surgeons in treating difficult or complicated cases, Buchan set out to advise families on nonspecific remedies, advocated the importance of diet and exercise, stressed the necessary balance between intake and evacuation so critical to humoral pathology, and encouraged the natural healing power of the body. Reflecting his own generation of medical thinkers, Buchan prescribed bleeding, salivation, and polypharmic remedies. Like his seventeenth-century predecessors, he attempted to mix folk medicines, empiricism, and commonsense environmentalism with the more conventional forms of rationalistic therapeutics.[7]

Not surprisingly, medical customs acquired a different meaning under the umbrella of American colonial experience. For one thing, many parents refused to send their sons back to England for medical study—not only because of the expense and difficulty of the trip itself but because many died, succumbing to smallpox and other diseases. Alternatively, parents indentured or apprenticed young men between the ages of fourteen and eighteen to practicing physicians and chirurgeons for periods of three to seven years. Included in apprenticeship was the recruitment from within medical families, that is, either coming from or marrying into medical families. By the beginning of the eighteenth century, apprenticeship became the common route to medical practice and one that resulted incidentally in sidetracking women to the subservient role as midwife.[8]

The education of the young apprentice was based on a strict contractual arrangement. "He had access to the doctor's often meagre library, learned something of the preparation and use of drugs, and was taught how to bleed, cup, extract teeth and perform a few minor operations," wrote Wyndham B. Blanton. Later, as the apprentice advanced in knowledge and experience, he accompanied the doctor on visits, watched the art of medicine practiced at the bedside, and on occasion substituted for the doctor in cases of emergency.[9]

Physicians and their apprentices had available such books as *Commentaries* and *Aphorisms*, by Gerhard van Swieten; *Institutes of Medicine*, by Hermann Boerhaave; *Sydingham*, by John Pechey; *On Fevers*, by Edward Strother; *Aphorisms*, by Hippocrates; *First Lines*, by William Cullen; *On Inoculation*, by Benjamin Rush; *Midwifery*, by Nicholas Culpeper; *On Smallpox*, by William Hillary; *Physiology*, by Albrecht von Haller; *On Fevers*, by John Huxham; and *Midwifery*, by William Smellie. American titles and reprints included William Currie, *A Dissertation on the Autumnal Remitting Fever* (1789); William Douglass, *The Practical History of a New Epidemical Eruptive Military Fever, with Anangina Ulcusculosa, Which Prevailed in Boston New-England in the Years 1735 and 1736* (1736); Thomas Cadwalader, *An Essay on the West-India Dry-Gripes* (1745); James McClurg, *Experiments Upon the Human Bile* (1772); and the *Transactions* of the American Philosophical Society (1771), the first professional journal issued before the Revolution. Except in the more settled areas, few apprentices could boast more than a single book or two as their initiation into the world of medical literature. Yet, out of this small canon of knowledge and experience emerged the system of American medical education.[10]

Although medical education in the colonies continued to mimic European medical theory, changes seemed imminent. As Shryock noted, "English professional distinctions broke down or were deliberately abandoned in the presence of the American environment." Moreover, organizations of apothecaries, surgeons, and physicians did not continue their separate existence in America. While London physicians enjoyed a status that was superior to both apothecaries and surgeons, the American environment demanded less specialization and more adjustment to the circumstances of small towns and villages, where general medical practice involved dispensing drugs, having some surgical skill, and understanding medical theory. And whether these physicians had earned degrees was less an issue than was their ability to practice medicine. The term *doctor* became a title of respect accorded these practitioners regardless of any claim to learning. At the time of the American Revolution, approximately thirty-five hundred doctors practiced in the colonies, and probably not more than four hundred had received any formal training; of that number, hardly half held a medical degree.[11]

In eighteenth-century America, pharmacy was principally in the hands of physicians who imported their goods directly from England and advertised new shipments in the newspapers. Drugs included opium, tartar emetic, rhubarb, jalap, camphor, ipecac, Glauber's salts, and various mercurials. Patent medicines included Daffy's Elixir, Bateman's Drops, Godfrey's Cordial, and Hooper's Pills. In addition, physicians compounded their own drugs (usually a responsibility turned over to apprentices) and charged for their medicines, as well as for their visits. Although the independent apothecary had begun to make a presence in the larger towns, physicians in smaller villages and rural areas continued to mix their own drugs. Drugs were also carried by preachers who sold their medicines with the same enthusiasm as they sold their bibles and religious beliefs.[12]

Of course, those young men from the American colonies in the eighteenth century who decried the apprenticeship form of learning could take formal education abroad. The early colonial doctors whose education had been obtained in the same way that other English physicians had obtained theirs—in the schools of Edinburgh, Oxford, and Cambridge in Great Britain; Padua in Italy; Montpellier in France; and Leiden and Utrecht in the Netherlands—had a medical philosophy that was based on the works of Hippocrates, Dioscorides, Galen, Ibn Sīnā (Avicenna), Andreas Vesalius, Ambroise Paré, Gabriel Fallopius, Jan Baptista van Helmont, and Sir Kenelm Digby. Such Americans as Caspar Wistar, Jr.; Benjamin Smith Barton; Philip Syng Physick; Thomas Bond; John Redman; Thomas Cadwalader; William Shippen, Jr.; Benjamin Rush; Thomas T. Hewson; John Foulke; and George Logan were among the young men who sought study beyond apprenticeship or the bachelor of medicine. They studied under William Cullen and the three generations of Alexander Monro (primus, 1697–1767, secundus, 1733–1817, and tertius, 1773–1859) of Edinburgh; brothers William and John Hunter of London; Carl von Linné at Uppsala, Sweden; they walked the wards at St. Thomas', Guy's, and St. Bartholomew's in England, Edinburgh's Royal Infirmary, and the hospitals of Paris. "So constant was the flow of American medical students to England, Scotland, and the Continent in the latter half of the eighteenth century," wrote historian Whitfield J. Bell, Jr., "that one might speak of a kind of trade in them, America exporting the raw materials for physicians and surgeons and receiving after a passage of three or four years the finished product. These colonials and young republicans filled themselves at the fountainhead of science abroad and, returning with the knowledge of the European schools and hospitals, were prepared and eager to spread their learning."[13]

By the eighteenth century, France had assumed leadership in medical education, particularly in the area of surgery. Nevertheless, the Netherlands remained a strong attraction for medical students, and students in England were acquiring a mastery of clinical and practical medicine. But by the end of the century, it was the University of Edinburgh that had become a mecca for students due to the popularity of the three Monros, who taught clinical surgery, medicine, and anatomy, and because of William Cullen, chair of the institutes of medicine, who introduced clinical lectures into medical instruction. In addition, there were such faculty as John Gregory, who held the chair of the practice of physic, John Hope in botany, and John Black in chemistry. Outside the University of Edinburgh, men like John Barclay, John Gordon, John Bell, and Robert Knox provided instruction in anatomy and vied with the Monros for medical specimens. Medical education was built principally around two chairs: the institutes of medicine and the theory and practice of medicine, with the chairs of materia medica, chemistry, and botany considered ancillary. Edinburgh's two professors of materia medica were James Home and Andrew Duncan the Younger, whose courses covered pharmacology, pharmacy, dietetics, and prescription writing. James Home later succeeded James Gregory as professor of medicine and introduced examinations into his teaching methodology. Midwifery, considered outside the standard curriculum, was chaired by Alexander and James Hamilton, father and son, from 1780 to 1840. The university organized a chair of medical jurisprudence in 1807 in response to Andrew Duncan the Younger's petition to counteract the emphasis placed on the subject in schools on the Continent.[14]

While Edinburgh had established itself as preeminent in medicine, London had become the center for surgery, with students flocking to St. Thomas', Guy's, and St. Bartholomew's hospitals for instruction. Here, the reputations of Sir Astley Cooper, William and John Hunter, and Percivall Pott held forth, and London competed with Paris as the shrine of surgical knowledge. With Oxford and Cambridge the exceptions (they were more theoretical in their curriculum and "did not recommend themselves to practical-minded colonial doctors"), American students motivated to extend their education beyond home-trained apprenticeships found in these schools a ready source of expertise. However, except for those who attended Edinburgh (139 Americans graduated from Edinburgh between 1749 and 1812) and a few other schools, nearly all colonial Americans received their medical education through apprenticeship.[15]

Herbal Medicines

Although the American colonial experience did not foster any great accomplishments in the physical sciences and was generally bare of the theoretical posturing so common among Europe's savants, colonials did add measurably to certain fields of learning, especially to medicine and natural history. "Nothing was more natural than that European-trained physicians, finding themselves in a new land with many unfamiliar plants, should seize the opportunity for botanical discoveries," wrote Daniel J. Boorstin. "Even laymen studied American flora in the hope of adding to medical knowledge."[16]

Theologians and naturalists taught that God provided each region of the world with its own medicines. Nicholas Culpeper, in *The English Physician—Enlarged* (1703), more specifically enunciated the theory that every geographic area of the world produced plants whose medicinal properties were capable of curing diseases indigenous to the region. This belief, which dates back to Paracelsus (1493–1541) and is reinforced by knowledge obtained from native American tribes, suggested that ailments striking American settlers could be treated with the local plant materia medica rather than with expensive mineral and plant drugs shipped from England.[17]

Herbal medicine received enormous impetus in the age of discovery and exploration. Although sixteenth-century medicine relied heavily on mineral drugs, the introduction of new therapeutic substances—such as guaiacum, sarsaparilla, balsam of Peru, lobelia, cascara sagrada, cocaine, curare, capsicum, arrowroot, cocillana, jalap, and tobacco—did much to turn attention to New World medicine and to the concept of drug specifics. The American Indians gave names to those plants that they believed held medicinal properties. With the coming of the Europeans, these names were either retained by the settlers or, more often, given names of the European plants that they most closely resembled. The isolation of the American frontier added to the problem of classification since settlers in distant areas of the country gave different names to identical plants.[18]

From the earliest days of settlement, observers had made note of minerals and plants whose virtues assisted in the cure of sores, wounds, and various sicknesses. Indeed, the British Crown not only ordered the Virginia colony to cultivate a garden of natural products but to determine "what kind of peculiar herbs there are, considerable either for their flower, smell, alimentary or medicinall [sic] use." The early settlers discovered sassafras, sweet gums, tobacco, and certain clays (which the native Indians ate for physic). Jamestown or jimsonweed, snakeroot, dittany (pepper-wort), turpeth, mechoacan, feverroot and ague root, lemnian earth, alum, and cancerroot abounded in Virginia. In general, Americans used sassafras for skin diseases, gout, rheumatism, and syphilis; used the pith of sassafras to form a mucilage in diseases of the eye, as well as to make a drink for relief from dysentery and nephritis; and prescribed the bark as a stimulant and astringent. Similarly, colonists took snakeroot as a tonic, diuretic, diaphoretic, and stimulant in typhoid and digestive disorders; black snakeroot for gout, rheumatism, and amenorrhea; dittany as a purge for worms; tobacco as a purge of the humors and an antidote to all poisons; jimsonweed (*Datura stramonium*) as a sedative and antispasmodic; and wild cherry bark as a specific in wounds and sores.[19]

The eighteenth-century apothecary shop contained shelves of chemical and galenical preparations—from dried roots and leaves to pills, ointments, powders, infusions, tinctures, and elixirs: Jesuit Drops, Dover's Powders, Hooper's Female Pills, Tar-Water, Huxham's Elixir, and an endless assortment of patent medicines. While the colonials continued to rely on the more expensive European mineral and vegetable drugs, increasingly they supplemented this materia medica with native plants. Except for coca, curare, and cinchona, which came from Latin America, most would later be abandoned; nevertheless, from the era of discovery through the first half of the nineteenth century, these roots and herbs provided a ready and inexpensive source of emetic, purging, and sweating drugs. Thus, when the early salubrity of the American environment turned to contagions of epidemic proportions after settlement, the colonials looked inward to the new continent for their medicinal stock.[20]

It is important to note that the regular medical profession in the United States had already established an impressive plant materia medica before botanics made their appearance. In the early days of the colonies, as well as during the nation-building years of the young republic, physicians viewed botany from a practical point of view rather than as the somnambulant pastime of the gentleman naturalist. Dr. Christopher Witt (1675–1765), a botanist and mystic, was famous for his botanical gardens at Germantown, Pennsylvania. John Bartram (1699–1777), a self-educated American botanist, spent a lifetime studying medicinally active plants unknown in Europe and introduced one hundred American plant species into Europe. Benjamin Smith Barton (1766–1815), a professor of natural history and botany at the College of Philadelphia, authored *Elements of Botany* (1803) and an unfinished *Collections for an Essay Towards a Materia Medica of the United States* (1798–1804), which was completed by his nephew William P. C. Barton as *The Vegetable Materia Medica of the United States* (1817–25). Benjamin Smith Barton also wrote articles on snakeroot and red cedar for Benjamin Franklin's *Poor Richard's Almanac* and prepared an appendix on American plants for Thomas Short's *Medicina Britannica* (1747). The same combination of talents could be claimed by Alexander Garden (ca. 1730–91); physician, naturalist, and traveler Mark Catesby (1679?–1749); John Clayton (1657–1725), who corresponded with Linné; and James Greenway, who carried on extensive correspondence with European naturalists.[21]

By the late eighteenth century, professional medicine had taken an interest in "physic gardens" for both teaching purposes and sources of medicines. Noted physicians, such as Thomas Cadwalader (1708–79), Thomas Bond, William Shippen, Sr., John Redman (1772–1808), and John Morgan (1735–89), endorsed the idea, as did Benjamin Rush.[22] Perhaps the best example of this interest came from Rush, when he wrote to the trustees of the University of Pennsylvania in Philadelphia in 1813 on the need for a botanical garden to be used by the medical schools of Boston and New York.[23] In his *Medical Inquiries and Observations* (1789), Rush encouraged the study of America's indigenous plants for their potential curing properties.

> Let me recommend to your particular attention, the indigenous medicines of our country. Cultivate or prepare as many of them as possible, and endeavor to enlarge the materia medica, by exploring the untrodden fields and forests of the United States . . . [for] the Seneka and Virginia snake-roots, the Carolina pink-root, the spice-wood, the sassafras, the butter-nut, the thoroughwort, the poke, and the stramonium are but a small part of the medicinal productions of America. I have no doubt but there are many hundred other plants which now exhale medicinal virtues. . . . Who knows but it may be reserved for

America to furnish the world, from her productions, with cures from some of those diseases which now elude the power of medicine? Who knows but that, at the foot of the Allegany mountain, there blooms a flower, that is an infallible cure for the epilepsy? Perhaps on the Monongahela, or the Potowmac, there may grow a root that shall supply, by its tonic powers, the invigorating effects of the savage or military life in the cure of consumptions.[24]

Other noted advocates of medical botany in the United States included David Hosack (1769–1835), who established the Elgin Botanic Garden in New York City; John Torrey (1796–1873) of the University of the City of New York; Charles W. Short at Transylvania University in Kentucky; Stephen Elliott (1771–1830) of Charleston, South Carolina, who authored *A Sketch of the Botany of South-Carolina and Georgia* (1821–24); Eli Ives and William Tulley at Yale College in New Haven, Connecticut; Dr. Jacob Bigelow (1786–1879) of Boston, Massachusetts, who authored *American Medical Botany* (1817–20); and Samuel Henry, author of *A New and Complete American Medical Family Herbal* (1814). Indeed, American botany received more attention in the field of natural history than did any other subject, with such authors as Andrew Michaux, Frederick Pursh, Manasseh Cutler, Henry M. Mühlenberg, and Professor Amos Eaton among the more notable.[25] The same appeal came years later from George B. Wood (1797–1879), a professor at the Philadelphia College of Pharmacy and later at the Medical Department of the University of Pennsylvania. Wood was coeditor with Franklin Bache of the *U.S. Dispensatory* and liked to remind his students of the potential benefits in indigenous plant drugs.[26]

Medical Societies and Schools

Efforts to regulate medical practice in the colonies actually preceded the establishment of medical schools. Beginning in the 1730s, more "respectable" physicians organized local societies designed to choose their membership from acceptable colleagues. Some of these societies, especially those founded by doctors educated in Europe, set educational requirements for admittance. These initial efforts, however, proved generally ineffective. "Most men seem to have believed," wrote Shryock, "that a people who entrusted their souls to all sorts of preachers, could likewise entrust their bodies to all sorts of 'doctors.'" Nevertheless, the increasing

number of European-educated physicians making their appearance in the American colonies in the late eighteenth century
brought a sense of elitism that turned, in time, to a demand for
comparable medical education of their sons without having to send
them back to Europe to get it.[27]

Informal classes and demonstrations began in Philadelphia as
early as 1750. One of the more noted teachers, William Shippen,
Jr. (1736–1808), a graduate of Edinburgh who obtained his clinical
experience in London, offered a course of lectures on anatomy
and midwifery in 1762. He also had plans to establish a school
for physic in association with Pennsylvania Hospital. His proposal
lacked the support of the trustees, who were probably not eager
to dilute the function and purpose of the hospital.[28] In 1765, his
friend John Morgan, who served as apprentice to Dr. John Redman
from 1750 to 1756 before graduating in 1763 with a medical degree
from Edinburgh, proposed to the trustees of the College of Philadelphia a chair for the theory and practice of physic—a chair he
then occupied. Approval of Morgan's proposal and professorship
was no doubt facilitated by there being five physicians among the
twenty-four trustees of the college: John Redman, Thomas Cadwalader, William Shippen, Sr., Thomas Bond, and Phineas Bond.
Thus, while medical education had actually started on this continent as early as 1538 at Santo Tomás University in Santo Domingo,
the Medical Department of the College of Philadelphia became
the first medical school in North America and became part of a
larger institution of learning, connected as well with the Pennsylvania Hospital (1751), where students started their clinical rotations
by following the house staff on rounds and by attending clinical
lectures. The instruction supplemented the system of apprenticeship by offering a two-year, graded curriculum, including clinical
lectures and hospital attendance. With the appointments of William
Shippen, Jr., to the professorship of anatomy and surgery (1765),
Adam Kuhn (who had studied under Linné) to the first professorship of materia medica and botany (1768), Benjamin Rush as professor of chemistry (1769), and Thomas Bond as professor of
clinical medicine (1767), the medical school had attained an auspicious beginning. By the close of the century, other medical colleges
had organized along similar lines, including the Medical Department of King's College (Columbia University, New York City) in
1767, which used Bridewell, the Almshouse, the Debtors' Prison,

and later the New York Hospital for its students' clinical experience; the Medical Department of Harvard College, Cambridge, Massachusetts, in 1783, where John Warren became the first professor of anatomy and surgery; and the Medical Department of Dartmouth College, Hanover, New Hampshire, in 1798. At King's College, Samuel Clossy served as professor of anatomy; Peter Middleton, physiology and pathology; John Jones, surgery; James Smith, chemistry and materia medica; Samuel Bard, theory and practice of medicine; and John V. B. Tennant, midwifery.[29]

Discontented with the prevailing laissez-faire approach of Americans to medical education, Morgan delivered a memorable inaugural address at the College of Philadelphia's commencement exercises on May 30, 1765, titled "Discourse upon the Institution of Medical Schools in America." He attacked the informality and lack of subdivisions within medicine and pleaded for separate, regular practices of physic, surgery, and pharmacy, such as he had found in his medical tours of Padua and Parma in Italy and in Edinburgh, London, and Paris. From Morgan's perspective, American medicine seemed impoverished. Yet from the vantage point of history, Morgan's opinion was by no means self-evident. As Boorstin observed, the lack of discrete subdivisions had actually benefited American medicine. "By allowing crude, fluid experience to overflow the ancient walls between departments of medical knowledge," he wrote, "men might see regulations in nature which had been obscured by guild monopolies and by the conceit of learned specialists."[30]

But Morgan's concerns did not end with a criticism of medical subdivisions. He clearly intended for Philadelphia to become the center of medical training in the colonies and to control the licensing of doctors along lines already established in London and Edinburgh. His scheme for an elite model of medical licensing, however, proved unrealistic for the American colonies and was immediately criticized as monopolistic and as being an unfair restraint on intercolonial trade. Thomas Penn, the proprietor of Pennsylvania, refused to grant Morgan a charter for a college of physicians, and the licensing scheme quickly died.[31] The matter of licensing then fell to individual colonies: New York adopted a licensing law in 1760, followed by New Jersey in 1772. With the outbreak of the Revolution, doctors established standards and qualifying examinations for those providing service to the Continental armies. Following independence, however, the authority to license reverted to the states rather than residing with national or voluntary organizations. Medical societies, which had sprung up in most of the states by 1815, advocated both testing and licensing, and some states chose a dual system of licensing, requiring either a diploma from a chartered medical school or an examination by the state medical society.[32]

By the 1830s, only Pennsylvania, Virginia, and North Carolina lacked legislative control. In some instances, state medical societies had the power to test and license; in others, state examining boards assumed this responsibility. Nevertheless, the 1780–1830 period became one of uncertainty. Having survived the colonial period with little oversight of medical practice, the new nation seemed undecided about whether the state or voluntary organizations should exercise regulatory responsibility. Equally troublesome was the nature and degree of the regulations, that is, whether penalties should be exacted; whether licensing applied only to new physicians; whether practicing physicians should be exempt or grandfathered; or whether the state should share licensing power with voluntary associations or medical schools. While many legislatures placed licensing powers in the hands of state or local medical societies, less clear were the penalizing powers of such bodies and whether they could enforce fines against quacks and empirics for practicing without a license.[33]

Despite well-structured precedents, the founding of the College of Medicine of Maryland in 1807 (later the Medical Department of the University of Maryland) by Baltimore physicians John B. Davidge, Nathaniel Potter, James Cocke, and John Shaw signaled the beginning of an indigenous American phenomenon known as the proprietary medical school, separate from any parent educational institution. Except for a smattering of anatomy, the teaching faculty (who were also the proprietors of the college) chose a substantially didactic curriculum with tuition, income, and fees divided among themselves. The school operated on a for-profit basis, and its teaching chairs, which were bought and sold as property, became valuable sources of status and income for their holders. Admission to this school and others that followed was based on the ability to pay rather than on any academic prerequisites; and, in the absence of state boards and examiners, the diploma became the license to practice.[34]

The commercialization of medical education that began with the Maryland model spread to those schools attached to universities, causing many to evolve with only a nominal affiliation with the parent institutions. By 1820, most of the older medical schools had abandoned the graded curriculum and high admission and graduation standards. Schools organized by medical societies or by private practitioners opened their doors without even a pretense of collegiate or hospital connections. From Vermont to the Piedmont and trans-Appalachian regions of the country, medical faculties organized themselves to exploit the growth of population. No fewer than 308 medical colleges had formed between 1765 and 1913, plus an additional 118 institutions of extremely questionable character.[35]

During the same period, when faculties of medical schools gained control of their own affairs and divided fees, the preceptorial system went through an equally destructive transition. Intended to supplement but not replace medical departments, it became barely visible in the education of a physician. Many students therefore had preceptorships in name only, and didactic training became the only education a student received prior to entering practice. In the absence of clinical facilities and with two ungraded school sessions lasting sixteen to twenty weeks each (the second simply a repetition of the first), the medical-education system had developed a distinctive profile that was deficient in many particulars. Bright, capable, dedicated teachers did work within this structure, but most faced an uphill struggle against a system that, in its competition for students and fees, had removed admission requirements, focused its priorities almost entirely on didacticism, and consequently lost sight of clinical and demonstrative teaching. Early efforts to establish standards and licensing requirements later fell away with the proliferation of medical colleges in the early nineteenth century. The motley collection of private institutions and proprietary colleges spawned during the Jacksonian aftermath weakened the reputations of apprenticeship and didactic learning as the logical avenues to medical practice. Affiliated neither with arts and sciences faculties nor with hospitals, these newer schools reflected the competitive nature of the young republic and, in search of students, matriculated candidates with little regard to their competence or qualifications.

Not surprisingly, legislatures soon viewed all medical schools as roughly equivalent, a situation reflecting the egalitarian nature of American culture and politics and the poor quality of medical education. That state legislatures saw little difference between proprietary and university-affiliated medical schools, between regular and irregular practitioners, and between the claims of one system and another speaks volumes about the quality and social standing of the medical profession. The spirit of democracy ran high, as did a decided aversion to monopoly, elitism, intellectualism, restraint of trade in almost every form, and orthodox intolerance. By the 1840s, most states had repealed their earlier regulatory laws on medical licensing; only New Jersey, Louisiana, Michigan, and the District of Columbia retained any semblance of licensing control.[36]

Medical Systems

As Charles E. Rosenberg has so well explained, between the physician and the patient in the seventeenth, eighteenth, and early nineteenth centuries, there existed a texture of belief and behavior, of ideas and relationships, and of cause and metaphor, which explained both health and disease. Drawing upon a cosmology and a rationalistic system founded on the Hippocratic and Galenic understanding of the humors, physicians believed the body to be a "kind of stewpot, or chemico-vital reaction, proceeding calmly only if all its elements remained appropriately balanced." Not surprisingly, physicians and patients turned to the regulation of the body's secretions in an effort to ensure this balance. Thus, bleeding, purging, vomiting (puking), and perspiring represented the mainstays of medical practice and of patient expectations. In this context, physicians prescribed drugs as a means of affecting the body's secretions and not as specifics for particular diseases; drugs advertised as disease specific were condemned as the work of quacks and empirics.[37]

At the end of the sixteenth century and into the early seventeenth century, England blossomed with such illustrious persons as William Shakespeare, John Milton, Daniel Defoe, William Harvey, John Locke, Francis Glisson, Christopher Wren, and Francis Bacon. Bacon (1561–1626), whose influence on medicine came principally through Thomas Sydenham ("the English Hippocrates"), chose not to separate clinical practice and natural science in medicine. Bacon's theoretical treatment of knowledge is in *The Novum Organum* (1620), but most of his ideas on medicine are found in *The Advancement of Learning and New Atlantis* (1605), where he urged active intervention in the restoration of health, the need for diligent recording and observation (as practiced by Hippocrates), and the importance of seeking right reasons by search and comparison rather than projecting theories of causation. "Medicine," he wrote, "is a science which hath been . . . more professed than laboured, and yet more laboured than advanced; the labour having been, in my judgement, rather in circle than in progression."[38]

Although Baconians rebelled against the ancient and medieval predilection for speculative rationalism, medical thinking in colonial America and into the early nineteenth century continued to endow empiricism with the suspicious attributes of quackery. Rationalists reduced their medicine to a system based on first principles, from which all other propositions logically arose through deductive reasoning. Galen's system, for example, rested on the concepts of *form* and *matter* derived from Aristotle's metaphysics—a deductive system similar in its logical rigor to geometry.[39] The concept of *disease*, which varied little from Galenic and medieval theory, viewed illness as a perturbation in the "state" of the constitution, with therapeutic measures directed at restoring balance through a variety of intrusive regimens. Instead of recognizing distinct diseases, doctors employed such catchall words as *flux*, *fever*, and *dropsy* to describe these perturbations. Although taxonomists had begun to identify diseases by their symptoms and to differentiate particular, specific diseases, the underlying condition of disease continued to be viewed as a morbid state of the body's humors, requiring some form of bleeding, purging, sweating, or other restorative regimen. Works by William Harvey, William Cowper, Thomas Willis, Felix Platter, James Yonge, and Thomas Sydenham represented the prevailing medical philosophy at the end of the seventeenth century.

Even Thomas Sydenham (1624–89), the London practitioner whose reputation rested on the assertion that he allowed clinical observation to prevail, relied on philosophical views that "went back via the Scholastics and Galen to Plato and Aristotle." True, Sydenham believed that there were specifics for the treatment of each disease species (e.g., quinine for malaria); but he adhered to the theory of humoral pathology, hoping to know "what humoral abnormalities different patients could have in common and how those abnormalities were caused."[40] To his credit, he advocated only those drugs that *he* found useful—iron for anemia, Jesuits' bark for fever, and laudanum for pain. Neither anatomy nor post-mortem examination substituted for the study of the living body. Sydenham also eschewed the irritants, bloodlettings, and purgings so common in his day. Moreover, he criticized the manner in which observation had been denigrated in deference to postulation. He preferred to follow Bacon in choosing the analogy of botany to study disease and to establish a nosology. Most important, however, Sydenham chose bedside observation rather than orthodox medi-cine's reliance on diathesis, state of the pulse, and inspection of blood, feces, and urine. As a clinician and true empiricist, he would venture no further than his own observations of pathological phe-nomena. As an admirer of Bacon and close friend of John Locke (the founder of empirical philosophy), Sydenham became one of the severest critics of the speculations of the iatrochemists and, according to Knud Faber, "reestablished the broken connection between ancient and modern medical science."[41]

At its best and worst, medical orthodoxy sought to compile the wisdom of Hippocrates, Galen, Celsus, and the other ancient writers and to attach to their ideas more recently discovered knowl-edge, thus giving added support and authority to the traditional systems of medicine. While humoral pathology continued to appeal to the medical profession, the ancient doctrine underwent a series of progressive elaborations based on experimental observations. Reminiscent of the epicycles used by astronomers to explain vari-ances within the Ptolemaic universe, the works of Dutch naturalist Antoni van Leeuwenhoek (1632–1723) and Dutch physician Her-mann Boerhaave (1668–1738), professor of medicine and botany (1709) and of chemistry (1718) at Leiden, did not so much over-throw the wobbling paradigm of Galenic humoral concepts as they supported the ancient edifice with more "modern" knowledge. The strength of Boerhaave's *Institutiones medicae* (1721) was that it served as a paean to the past and as a standard text for medical education and practice. A firm supporter of the iatromechanical or iatrophysi-cal way of thinking in medicine, Boerhaave viewed the body as a system of solids and fluids whose structure varied according to sex, age, constitution, and disease. His nosologic system distinguished between diseases of the humors and those of the fibers, with the latter divided into those that were weak or too lax and those that were rigid or stiff. In his role as a university teacher, Boerhaave effected a synthesis between the work of Harvey—his discovery of the circulation of the blood in 1628—and the data provided by Leeuwenhoek, the demonstration of the capillary system by Marcello Malpighi (1628–94), and the works of the ancient Greek writers.[42] Somewhat an eclectic, he claimed to accept what was good in all theories. "Boerhaave's great contribution," wrote Lester S. King,

> was to construct a polished doctrinal edifice, almost monolithic, that captured men's attention, satisfied their curiosity—and restricted their imagination. . . . Only when new data were so overwhelming in quantity and significance that old concepts no longer satisfied, only when new theories, techniques, and attitudes replaced the old, when orientation shifted from the remote past to the immediate present, and the genuine obsolescence of the ancients was accepted, only then was Boerhaave superseded.[43]

By the eighteenth century, the concept of the human constitution had transformed into a Newtonian-type machine, consisting of numerous particles of differing mass that obeyed the laws of motion as they traveled through tubes and vessels of varying diameters. The human body, within this paradigm, became little more than a system of pumps and chemical balances; and pathology emphasized the state either of the fluids or of the nervous system. As for pharmacy and therapeutic measures, these had changed little from ancient times. Physicians logically turned to bleeding, purging, cupping, warm baths, blistering, mustard plasters, and other irritating agents because they assisted in reducing the volume of fluids, released obstructing matter, diverted or drew blood away from the inflammation, and relieved congestion.

Sired by the Enlightenment's view of the universe, medical science became material, objective, orderly, and ultimately knowable. Disease represented an imbalance in the body's constitutional elements. Although the groundwork had been laid for a theory of germ contagion, no clinician emerged capable of moving the concept into the practice of medicine; and except for malaria, smallpox, and syphilis—for which physicians had found specific treatments—the medical profession continued to rely on the rationalistic systems and heroic regimens of Benjamin Rush, François Broussais, John Brown, and William Cullen. Fever, the result of a mechanical obstruction of the capillaries, demanded a therapeutic regimen based on equally mechanical principles of phlebotomy and purges intended to change the diathesis of salt, putrid, and oily temperaments.[44]

William Cullen (1712–90), one of the foremost British clinicians in the eighteenth century, was thought to have stood at the "dividing line between ancient and modern medicine."[45] Known eventually as "that shining oracle of Physic," Cullen matriculated from the University of Edinburgh in 1734 and took his medical degree from Glasgow in 1740.[46] Having a penchant for nosology, he made a study of fevers and classified them as intermittent or continued. Within each of these main categories, he then distinguished various subcategories and, from his observations and findings, concluded that the "spasm" of the arteries represented the pathogenesis of fever, which he treated with sedation and rest, bloodletting (usually in the form of leeching and wet cupping), purges and blisters, the application of cold, and the avoidance of animal food. He also prescribed a number of botanical remedies, including nutmeg, gum guaiacum, and cinnamon. Cullen held the chairs of medicine and chemistry at the University of Glasgow and at Edinburgh and was the adored teacher of many American physicians in the colonial era, including the first faculty of the University of Pennsylvania Medical School. He theorized that health and disease were a matter of the body's irritability or nervous energy as controlled by the brain. This theory, known as *solidism*, stressed the nervous origination of disease, particularly the incidence of spasm and atony, as well as the acrimony of the humors.[47]

One of Cullen's disciples, Scottish physician John Brown (1735–88), objected to the efforts of nosologists to establish classifications of disease on the basis of symptoms. Such methods, borrowed from botanists, resulted in abstract disease entities bearing little relationship to the real underlying disease mechanisms. Brown also felt the same aversion to bedside efforts to make diagnoses from symptoms and physical signs. As a radical mechanist, Brown likened himself to Isaac Newton, believing that nature was both simple and uniform in its general laws and movements. In similar fashion, he viewed health as a balance between asthenia and excitability, with the physician working to balance the two. Medicine became an exact science deducible from certain a priori principles. The conditions that led to illness were sthenia, or excessive stimulation, and asthenia, the result of deficient stimulants. In other words, there was but one disease that displayed itself in two different forms and two different treatments. All symptoms were simply manifestations of the body's particular state, with treatment requiring debilitating measures for asthenic conditions and stimulants for asthenic conditions. For the former, Brown relied on moderate bloodletting, sweating, purging, a vegetarian diet, watery drinks, and vomiting; for the latter, he chose rich soups, wines, musk, camphor, and opium as his regimens of choice. In contrast with many of his peers, Brown preferred restoratives rather than the more commonly applied depletive measures. As a consequence, alcohol and opium became the principal stimulants for his patients and for himself.[48]

Considering the views of Boerhaave, Cullen, and Brown, it is not surprising that Benjamin Rush (1745–1813) of Philadelphia espoused a similar system of therapeutics. Like Brown, Rush had been a student of Cullen at Edinburgh, influenced by many of the same concerns regarding the nature of disease. In contrast to Cullen's pathology of tension (in which brain stimuli caused spasms in the vascular system), Rush theorized that disease resulted from a predisposing debility, an external stimulus, which produced "convulsion" or "excitability" in the walls of the blood vessels. These convulsions marked the true essence of fever. Not only was there one type of fever but fever always seated itself in the blood vessels. Thus, all local affections were simply symptoms of an original nonspecific disease in the blood vessels. Fever represented a unitary disease state whose pathologic process expressed itself in different symptoms. In practice, Rush followed a modified Brunonianism; while Brown recognized two pathological states (tension and laxity of tone), Rush saw but a single state of tension.[49]

The monolithic nature of Rush's theory did not vary significantly from his contemporaries or, for that matter, from his antecedents. Where he strayed was in the heroic nature of his therapeutic regimen, which he discovered during the 1793 yellow-fever epidemic in Philadelphia. Despairing of the more popular cures, Rush chose a combination of depleting and purging to remove the excitability of the system.[50] Unlike his mentor Cullen, who had employed only moderate bleeding, Rush carried traditional humoralism to the height of therapeutic recklessness with heroic, extreme bleeding and purging, undeterred by criticism or by claims that his regimen did not reconcile with the mortality rates of his patients. According to Rush, a fever depended "upon the morbid and excessive action in the blood-vessels. It is connected . . . with preternatural sensibility in their muscle fibres. The blood is the most powerful irritant which acts upon them. By abstracting a part of it, we lessen the principal cause of the fever. The effect of bloodletting is as immediate and natural . . . as the abstraction of sand is, to cure an inflammation of the eye."[51]

Rush's subsequent influence on physicians in the West and South resulted in a period of American therapeutics that seemed to know few bounds. Known as "Old Ten and Ten," Rush considered bleeding his panacea and followed it with ten grains each of calomel and jalap. In reaction to Rush's bleeding and purging regimen during the Philadelphia epidemic, critic William Cobbett remarked that Rush's practice was "one of those great discoveries which are made from time to time for the depopulation of the earth."[52] Critics had, for good reason, dubbed these heroic practitioners "Knights of the Lancet."[53]

A word of caution: it is important when using the terms *rationalism* and *empiricism* to avoid comfortable conclusions. Depending on one's angle of vision, the words become quite elastic, if not wholly confusing. Rationalistic systems, which on the surface expressed a universal principle and uniformity in treatment, became on closer scrutiny flexible systems tempered by therapeutic specificity. Indeed, with the expanse of territory in the young nation and with its variability in climate, there was a tendency to view southerners, westerners, and easterners as constitutionally and temperamentally different, implying a willingness to see therapeutic authority as more fluid than not. It also explains, to some extent, the call for regional medical education, which could more effectively correlate medical instruction with those diseases and treatments proven most beneficial to a specific region.[54]

Jefferson's Vision

With so many learned doctors practicing their own species of rationalism, it is not surprising that the medical profession failed to attract an abiding confidence within the American culture. As Thomas Jefferson and others would attest, physicians were pitifully ignorant, drastic in their healing regimens, alarming in their pretense of understanding the keys to health and disease, and rapacious in their pecuniary interests. Medicine in the days of Jefferson failed to meet the demands of doctors and their patients. Based on erroneous philosophy, it tended to relieve patients more effectively of their pocketbooks than of their ailments. When physicians insisted upon treating patients with regimens that all but guaranteed failure, these ineffective treatments robbed physicians of their status in society and, more importantly, invited a host of reformers anxious to test their theories and skills among a desperate and willing population.

In a letter to Dr. Caspar Wistar, Jr., of Philadelphia in 1807, Jefferson inquired on behalf of his fifteen-year-old grandson about educational opportunities in the Philadelphia area. After noting various climatological factors and his fear of placing the young man in a populous city until the autumnal diseases had ceased, he focused his attention on what he perceived to be the lack of sound medical education in the United States. "The only sure foundations of medicine are an intimate knowledge of the human body, and observation on the effects of medicinal substances on that. The anatomical and clinical schools, therefore, are those in which the young physician should be formed." Unfortunately, young men who entered medicine in innocence of theory and "untainted with error" were seldom able to stand clear of the "bewitching delusions" of their instructors. Few young men were strong enough to "maintain a wise infidelity." Jefferson hoped that the young practitioner would learn to appreciate the real limits of the art of medicine and that, "when the state of his patient gets beyond these, his office is to be a watchful, but quiet spectator of the operations of nature, giving them fair play by a well-regulated regimen, and by all the aid they can derive from the excitement of good spirits and hope in the patient." All too often, however, doctors chose to treat patients on the basis of some fashionable theory, abandoning sober facts for illusionary hypotheses. These medical tyros, he wrote, destroyed "more of human life in one year, than all the Robinhoods, Cartouches, and Macheaths do in a century."

> Having been so often witness to the salutary efforts which nature makes to re-establish the disordered functions, he [the physician] should rather trust to their action, than hazard the interruption of that, and a greater derangement of the system, by conjectural experiments on a machine so complicated and so unknown as the human body, and a subject so sacred as human

life. . . . One of the most successful physicians I have ever known, has assured me, that he used more bread pills, drops of colored water, and powders of hickory ashes, than of all other medicines put together. It was certainly a pious fraud. But the adventurous physician goes on, and substitutes presumption for knowledge. From the scanty field of what is known, he launches into the boundless region of what is unknown. He establishes for his guide some fanciful theory of corpuscular attraction, of chemical agency, of chemical powers, of stimuli, of irritability accumulated or exhausted, of depletion by the lancet and repletion by mercury, or some other ingenious dream, which lets him into all nature's secrets at short hand. On the principle which he thus assumes, he forms his table of nosology, analogy, to all the cases he has thus arbitrarily marshalled together. I have lived to see the disciples of Hoffman, Boerhaave, Stahl, Cullen, Brown, succeed one another like the shifting figures of a magic lantern, and their fancies, like the dresses of the annual doll-babies from Paris, becoming, from their novelty, the vogue of the day, and yielding to the next novelty their ephemeral favor. The patient, treated on the fashionable theory, sometimes gets well in spite of the medicines.

In looking to the future, Jefferson speculated that a new practice of medicine would emerge. "I hope and believe," he wrote to Wistar, "that it is from this side of the Atlantic that Europe, which has taught us so many other things, will be led into sound principles in this branch of Science, the most important of all, being that to which we commit the care of health and life."[55]

The Beginnings of Medical Change

In these early years of the republic, American society was by no means ignorant of the dissatisfaction that doctors voiced in themselves and in the sorry state of their education and medical art. Nowhere was this feeling more apparent than in the candid remarks of physicians as they viewed the "perfect chaos" of their generation's medical practices. Eminent members of the medical profession lamented the state of medical knowledge and practice, recognizing that the art and science of medicine had not kept step with the progress of scientific knowledge and that the materia medica and therapeutics were both in disarray. In the words of one early medical historian, "It was not reformation which the present state of medicine demanded, but a revolution."[56] The physician's own sense of medical dismay, combined with the public faith in the common man and an almost chiliastic belief in the body politic, culminated in peculiar forms of sectarianism and quackery that challenged medical science to listen without indignation to claims of ready cure. The causes of this increasing skepticism included an unhealthy reliance on speculative rationalism, a disbelief in the usefulness of the auxiliary sciences, the expectation of too great a therapeutic result from a given drug, the unreliable recommendations of self-proclaimed authorities, the faulty preparation of drugs, the unsystematized records of physiological drug experiments, the different views concerning primary and secondary drug effects, the growing knowledge that many cures resulted from *vis medicatrix naturae* (nature's own healing force), a fanatical faith in *and* an intolerance of the views of others, and the absence of a standard of physiological dosage.

Substantive opposition to the Galenic tradition in medicine came with the emergence of the Parisian medical school during the political and technological revolution of the 1790s. The French Revolution created new hospitals and new schools for doctors, opening opportunities for gifted students like Guillaume Dupuytren, Anthelme Richerand, Jacques Moreau, Jean Esquirol, Charles Billard, and others to practice medicine. The first twenty years of the new medicine were dominated by Philippe Pinel (1745–1826), Jean N. Corvisart des Marets (1755–1821), and Pierre J. G. Cabanis (1757–1808), who believed that there was no better place than the bedside for instruction of doctors. Empirically oriented and choosing to avoid the comforting appeal of system builders, they preferred no theory to that which contradicted facts gleaned from observation. At its best, the healing art rested upon individual case histories built on observation of phenomena at the bedside. According to Pinel, medicine demanded judgment, strict logic, and a healthy skepticism—these were the guides to proper diagnosis and prognosis.[57]

While Rush's view of medical theory prevailed in many corners of the American West and South, and while the Brunonian system had its adherents in Germany and Italy, the Paris school of medicine became the choice of those American students seeking a respite from the speculative and humoral theories of the day. In Paris, their postgraduate medical study took on a new meaning as Pierre Louis (1787–1872) and other clinical teachers demonstrated the possibility of disease identification on the basis of extensive clinical and postmortem examinations. The growth and respectability of empirical philosophy resulted in attempts to identify specific diseases in terms of localized, structural pathology. This effort, along with more careful bedside studies, the development of the stethoscope, and greater use of autopsies, meant a more focused effort on specific diseases and less interest in the body's generalized state; and with it came a skepticism of traditional therapeutics and remedies, a questioning of depletion measures, a greater interest in self-limited diseases, the need to support nature's own healing processes, and the eventual repudiation of all system builders. The works of Louis and of Gabriel Andral (1799–1876), Jean-Baptiste Bouillaud (1796–1881), Pierre-Adolphe Piorry (1794–1879), and Armand Trousseau (1801–67) dominated the period from 1830 to 1848, culminating in the beginnings of laboratory medicine with Louis Pasteur (1822–95) and Claude Bernard (1813–78). Pierre Louis's application of the numerical method became the means by which the newer school of clinicians refuted the speculative rationalism of traditional medicine. His methodology, while short on experimental research, represented a triumph of medical empiricism over metaphysical concepts of disease that for centuries had reigned unchallenged.[58]

American practitioners in the early part of the nineteenth century continued to express their faith in a rationalistic system of medicine and systematic rules applicable to individual patients, but self-doubt had encroached into their therapeutics. This shift was best expressed in a gradual decline of rationalistic thinking and a greater dependence on experience and observation. Empiricism, which regulars had relegated to the quack, charlatan, and medical pretender, became increasingly appealing from the 1840s onward. The negative implications of the term seemed less compelling in the face of medicine's bankrupt systems approach.

In many ways, Elisha Bartlett (1804–55) of Rhode Island epitomized this new thinking among American physicians.[59] Bartlett authored two significant works, *An Essay on the Philosophy of Medical Science* (1844) and *The History, Diagnosis, and Treatment of the Fevers of the United States* (1847). In the former, Bartlett reflected the extensive influence of the Paris clinical school of Gaspard Bayle (1774–1816), René Laënnec (1781–1826), Auguste Chomel, and especially Louis, to whom he dedicated his books, on his thinking as he attacked inductive reasoning and stressed the importance of pathology in the art of diagnosis. Here, too, Bartlett demonstrated his strong adherence to approximate laws (not absolute) founded on Louis' numerical-reasoning method, or the statistics of averages. Drawing examples from such rationalistic thinkers as Rush and Cullen on the orthodox side of medicine and from Samuel Hahnemann and Samuel Thomson on the sectarian side, he explained the errors of speculative theories and doctrines and the need in the future to rely on more empirical data (i.e., the observation of facts). That is to say, doctors needed to study disease by relating the findings of clinical observations with changes discovered through autopsy. Bartlett found the medical doctrines of Thomson as curious as homeopathy. As in certain forms of religion, the greatest number of Thomson's adherents were "amongst the least educated portions of the people." Homeopathy, to the contrary, was "received with especial unction and favor, by the more intelligent and better educated classes; and particularly by persons, the tendencies of whose minds are towards ultra and abstract principles in politics and morals, and rational mysticism in religion."[60]

Until the 1801 publication of *Anatomie générale, appliquée à la physiologie et à la medécine* by Marie-François-Xavier Bichat (1771–1802), the character of medical science in America had been marked almost exclusively by the medical mind of Edinburgh, a transfusion of thought that represented, according to Bartlett, "the natural and necessary consequence of the relations of the two countries." Most of the leading medical works that had appeared in Great Britain since the days of Cullen had been republished in the United States.

> While medical relations with Great Britain are still, as they will always continue to be, numerous and intimate, they are altogether less exclusive than formerly; and they are probably now inferior, in interest, influence, and importance, to those which exist between us and France. Our young men have almost entirely ceased to visit the British capitals, in order to complete their education; and the number of those who have annually repaired to Paris, for this purpose, for many years past, has been very much greater than has ever been the case with Edinburgh and London. The leading works of Louis were earlier and more widely circulated in this country, than in Great Britain; and the principles of his school and method have taken deeper

root here, than there. There is now a pretty large and constantly increasing class of young physicians, many of them personal friends and pupils of Louis, scattered through our principal cities, mostly at the North and East, thoroughly imbued with the spirit of their distinguished master, and diligently engaged in the study of positive pathology, diagnosis, and therapeutics.[61]

Bartlett's enthusiasm for French methods represented the so-called French Period in American medicine, a period of some forty years before the Civil War, as distinguished from the previous period in which Americans had studied in Edinburgh, London, and Holland and from the subsequent period (after 1870) of German and Austrian influence.[62] Bartlett gave full praise to the labors of Jean N. Corvisart des Marets, René Laënnec, and Jean-Baptiste Bouillaud in their research of pathology, diagnosis, and treatment of diseases of the lungs and heart; those of Marc Petit and Etienne Serres on fever; those of Léon Rostan, J. A. Rochoux, Claude François Lallemand, Alexandre Parent-Duchâtelet, and Raymond Durand-Fardel on diseases of the brain; those of Martin Solon and Pierre Rayer on diseases of the kidneys; those of François Valleix on neuralgia; those of Augustin Grissole on pneumonia; those of Frederic Rilliet and Paul-Joseph Barthez on diseases of children; and those of Gabriel Andral and Jules Gavarret on the blood. Above all, Bartlett praised the work of Louis, who demonstrated through his numerical method the calculation of probabilities and their application to the different branches of medical science.

The numerical method was not a new system of medicine, for it had no analogy to medical doctrines. Rather, it was a method "for the statement, analysis and appreciation of ascertained and positive phenomena and relationships. . . . It consists upon the necessity, in science, of calling things by their right names; and of stating all facts and relationships, fully, entirely, rigorously. It insists upon the necessity of accurately enumerating all phenomena that are numerable." The numerical method implied that there were no principles in medicine that "were not the aggregate result, or in other words the simple expression, of facts and their relationships." The method proved particularly relevant when comparing various methods of treatment and when demonstrating the relative superiority or weakness of one method of treatment over another.[63]

Other attacks on the system builders came from John D. God-man (1794–1830) of Annapolis, Maryland, the editor of the *Journal of Foreign Medical Science*, who introduced American physicians to the work of the Parisian school; from Samuel Jackson, in *Principles of Medicine, Founded on the Structure and Functions of the Animal Organism* (1832); and most notably from Jacob Bigelow, whose *Discourse On Self-Limited Diseases* (1835) rested on the assumption that the body ultimately expelled certain diseases that were cured by nature alone. Influenced by Pierre Louis and his numerical method, Bigelow challenged the full mettle of speculative rationalism and, with it, the value of the existing materia medica. Although once a student of Rush, he seemed not to have been tarnished by his mentor's medical recklessness. Bigelow was one of America's leading botanists. His *American Medical Botany* (1817–20) became a work of international importance. A visiting physician to Massachusetts General Hospital in Boston and professor of materia medica at Harvard, he exerted a powerful influence on the treatment of cholera during the epidemic of 1832 and on medical practice in general with his calling into question traditional therapeutics.[64]

The suggestion by such men as Nathaniel Chapman (1780–1853), Worthington Hooker (1806–67), Oliver W. Holmes (1809–94), James Jackson, Sr. (1777–1868), and Bigelow of *vis medicatrix naturae* imparted an unsettling if not outright threatening challenge to the practitioner's identity in the nineteenth century. Indeed, the possibility that *nature*, not the physician, cured the patient was as much a problem for the sectarian as it was for the regular.[65] These "internal" reformers of regular medicine tended to come from the Northeast, although a scattered few lived in the Midwest. Morally and intellectually, they were the heirs of New England, carrying a reverence for education and a passion for public duty and reform. They also reflected the Yankee attributes of self-confidence and self-righteousness. While not necessarily wealthy, they invariably came from established families, and their education was above the ordinary. A great number received their education at Harvard and at other similarly fine schools; many went abroad for their schooling; and those with religious affiliations tended to come from the upper-class denominations: the Congregationalist, Unitarian, and Episcopalian churches. These genteel reformers found themselves facing a native mentality that opposed their representations, resented their associations, and worked to deny them a stake in medicine's future. Their social position seemed as much a liability as their education. Aware that their support among regulars was too small to admit a frontal attack against sectarianism, they adopted a strategy that worked at the margins, attempting to narrow the impact of sectarians by keeping them independent of each other and off balance. For the most part, these reformers had to content themselves with limited victories.

2

Every Man His Own Physician

By the opening decades of the nineteenth century, America's optimism about its future seemed limitless.[1] From orators and poets to immigrants and frontiersmen, the United States had become a crucible of opportunity. In New England, hopes ran high that cotton manufacturing would absorb the full measure of America's domestic and foreign markets; similarly, the South saw in the cotton gin the potential for processing and marketing greater amounts of its staple crop. And throughout the vast West, which by the 1840s had become tied by telegraph lines, canal systems, and railroad networks to eastern markets, farmers, blue-collar laborers, merchants, and manufacturers, people there shared equally in the belief in material prosperity. Reflecting this unbounded faith in the future, the American political scene threw off the last vestiges of privilege and of checks on democracy by vesting the common man with a voice in governmental affairs. Democracy was no longer a "problem" to be watched and contained; it had been transformed into a "faith" that energized the nation. With the election of Andrew Jackson as president in 1828, the last barriers to an unrestricted franchise for free, white males fell as qualifications of property and religion were discarded for a broadened electorate. The election heralded the triumph of the common man over aristocratic and federalist principles in government. The rewards for this new democracy came by way of the spoils system, two-party politics, and equal access to the public purse.[2]

In culture, the nation had become a storehouse of energy, establishing a public school system, embarking on any number of fads and isms, publishing magazines and newspapers, embracing manifest destiny, fostering sentiments of nationalism, and expecting concrete evidence of individual material advancement to accompany each aspiration attained by human will and effort. Progress was no philosophical theory defined only in the context of intellectual posturing by academics; rather, it had become a demonstrable fact exemplified by experience and achievement. Americans enjoyed a faith in the efficacy of their own achievements and universalized their material advances into a theory that accounted for Europe's decay and a belief that the United States had become the true repository of Protestant reform. From individuals as diverse in their thinking as clergyman and teacher Timothy Dwight, legislator and diplomat Joel R. Poinsett, ethnologist Lewis Henry Morgan, and poet Walt Whitman emerged a literature and a frame of mind that suggested the flowering of a truly Christian civilization on the shores of the American continent—a civilization and a people destined for greatness and material achievement.

Medical Sectarianism

As early as the 1820s and 1830s, medical orthodoxy in the United States lost its privileged position as the claims and aspirations of medical sectarians demanded the liberalization of therapeutic options for the public. Allopathy faced wave after wave of irregular practitioners—herbalists, Indian and root doctors, botanics, hydropaths, homeopaths, reform, and other assorted groups—all demanding equal access to the public and equal rights before the law. The spirit of sectarian medicine ranked high among the irrepressible energies of early-nineteenth-century America. Like the religious revivalists intent on elevating the moral condition of humanity, the proponents of sectarian medicine promised to improve the species' physical condition by overthrowing existing dogmas and by encouraging people to trust in voluntarism and free choice.

Just as religious deviationists emerged from the revival possessed more of spirited protest than of theological training, so too sectarian medicine exuded a vitality short on intellectual propositions but strong on emotion. It invoked a rebellious rather than a submissive course of action, exaggerated the momentousness of its confrontation with medical orthodoxy, and proposed a disjunction with medical theory that at times verged on the outrageous in its claims and freedoms. Condemnation by regulars had not the slightest effect on these exponents of true medical protestantism, for theirs was a belief of the heart, not of doctrinal definition. The sectarians passionately believed in their touted triumphs and cures and, despite personal differences, were staunch allies in their fight against the corrupt medical practices regulars had brought with them from an even more corrupt orthodoxy in Europe. Medical sectarians drew their strength from a communal consciousness that focused on anti-intellectualism, anti-institutionalism, defiance of regular medicine, self-adulation, and rhetoric. Medical reformers knew their audience; their language was direct and simple and their appeal, cogent and powerful.

"Prior to the placing of medicine on a scientific basis, sectarianism was, of course, inevitable," wrote Abraham Flexner. "Every one started with some sort of preconceived notion; and from a logical point of view, one preconception is as good as another. Allopathy was just as sectarian as homeopathy."[3] In fact, what medical orthodoxy viewed as correct medicine was simply a relic of an extinct science, a dead husk that had taken on the form of dogma. The absolute rigidity of its tenets made it less and less credible to modern minds, which were too well aware of the relativity of their knowledge to accept a doctrine purporting to be unchangeable and infallible. Sectarians saw medical orthodoxy as languishing internally as well, attacked by a creeping paralysis, which made it unfit for the contemporary world.

The term *sect* in medicine has typically been applied to people and groups both inside and outside orthodox tradition who, as Norman Gevitz explained, "challenged the legitimacy and value of accepted therapeutic principles and practices." The advocates of such sects championed the use of alternative modes of healing based on doctrines regarded as laws. "Given their radical beliefs and approaches," noted Gevitz, "sectarians have had to form separate institutions and associations to support their continued existence and growth." Unlike folk and religious healing, sectarian beliefs rested on principles espoused as being universal *and* scientific. Many sectarians regarded themselves as having the same type and quality of education as regulars, differing only in their conclusions. In other words, although often educated in anatomy, physiology, pathology, and chemistry, they came to different conclusions about "what the knowledge derived from these fields has for overall patient treatment."[4]

Medical sectarians in the early years of the nineteenth century chose to identify themselves with such sobriquets as *reformed* or *new school* while using *old school, majority school, regular, allopathic,* and *orthodox* to depict the dominant group. In response to these descriptions, mainstream medicine applied the terms *sectarian, cultist, quack, pretender, irregular,* and *unorthodox* to differentiate themselves from these self-proclaimed apostates. The success of sectarianism can be explained in part by medical orthodoxy's misuse of bloodletting, mercury, tartar emetic, and other heroic techniques and medicines, as well as by internal dissension, which colored their public and private communications. Their popularity reflects an appeal for gentler therapeutics and reflects the public's rejection of medical orthodoxy's rigidity in the face of new ideas and practices. The reasons for the rise of sectarianism can also be found in the inability of regulars to cope with the cholera epidemics of 1832 and 1849, the American penchant for rugged individualism, the lack of a book-centered culture, the poor level of medical education, the conceit with which regulars treated irregulars, and the inability of the common man to differentiate the competing claims of medicine.

At the heart of sectarian medicine was its refusal to submit to the beliefs and pretenses of allopathy. Its message, clear and genuinely American in its mission and purpose, contended that medical therapeutics had been falsely constructed by those who had worshiped at the shrines of Europe's quixotic medical schools and who, basking in their acquired elitism, yielded to the speculative rationalism of outmoded dogma. Europe, the sectarians had argued, had lost the rigor and plain style of its medical protestant heritage; misguided, it had settled down with false hopes and had then become petrified in its own self-righteousness. Despite sincere efforts to reform itself, medicine in Europe (and presumably in the American East) had been unable to declare its independence from the past.

The dialectic of American sectarians sought to diminish if possible the status differences perceived between regular and irregular practitioners. This meant subordinating the education and the socioeconomic status claimed by medical orthodoxy. If the common man's right to voluntarism was to prevail and if the common man wished to get along with as little leadership as possible from the regulars, then guidance for that decision making had to be generated from within. As popular democracy gained in strength and confidence, it reinforced the widespread belief in the superiority of inborn, intuitive, folk wisdom over the ratiocinations of orthodoxy. Here was a medicine of the heart that dispensed with trained leadership in favor of the native practical sense of the ordinary man, with his direct access to truth. This preference for the wisdom of the common man flowered into a militant sectarianism that expressed the quintessence of the democratic creed. Here could be found a distrust of expertise, a dislike for monopoly, a desire to uproot the entrenched order of medical orthodoxy, and the concomitant repudiation of its European inheritance. Here, too, the population paired education with sterile intellect and democracy with native intuition and the power to act.

As sectarian medicine gathered momentum, its leaders enjoyed a common bond in denouncing the tightly strung metaphysics of orthodoxy. They reveled in their radical simplification of Galen and the medical ancients and in the provincialism of the American intellect. Many sectarian leaders vulgarized medicine as they developed their criterion of practicality. Nevertheless, out of their revolt against orthodoxy and, indeed, against many of the academic disciplines that supported orthodoxy, sectarians forged a highly developed rhetoric of unabashed Americanism. Interestingly, however, their hostility to orthodoxy did not apply to the ancient Greek and Roman physicians; they were exempt from the criticisms that befell their disciples. Like their counterparts in religion, the medical protestants hoped to return to the true and unblemished world of the ancients.

American sectarians tried to conserve the right of voluntary choice for a diversity of beliefs. Although they broke upon the scene as an upheaval, as a swell of Jacksonian passion and antielitism, they really intended to preserve the right of voluntarism, or choice, without restraint from the law. Sectarians clearly represented a frame of mind that ran counter to the monolithic dogmas of European-trained physicians. They reflected the energy and the self-reliance of Americans who willingly gave up the assurances of orthodox systems for more spontaneous declarations and promises. They were both bold and plain in their denunciation of older systems of medicine, and the key to their argument was the repeated word that condemned medical orthodoxy, espoused an indigenous American protestantism in medicine, dismissed eastern elitism, and fostered nationalism.

Despite its assertions, sectarian medicine remained inwardly divided between its dreams of success and the inner strength of its self-conscious provinciality. In the face of this contradiction, its leaders theorized that the westward course of settlement applied equally to medicine, that westward from Europe a purer and less complicated medicine had emerged. The American West salvaged what was left of Europe's imploded theories and took on the responsibility for reform. One can ridicule this nineteenth-century bombast, but the rhetoric of sectarian medicine promised hope for American communities, hope that, in its intensity and fervor, ran parallel to the spiritual revivalism of the time, anticipating the eschatological promises of women's rights and abolitionism in the 1840s and 1850s.

The medical extravagances that emerged from Jacksonian America did not so much represent a fragmentation of medicine as an effort toward national cohesion. Despite the rancor and discord among rival medical sects, their symbol of concordance remained as always the triumphant disestablishment of orthodoxy. Much jarring continued among the various sects, but their protracted feuds, many of which deteriorated into undignified namecalling, did not deflect them from remaining unified against the attacks of regulars. Notwithstanding their differences, sectarians united in believing in the unlawfulness of the interference waged by the regulars against them through the legislatures and in the concomitant belief in the right to their own practice and of the public's right of choice.

At the fountainhead of sectarian medicine stood the allopaths, or regulars, who boasted an uninterrupted link with the past and who decried the undisciplined and iconoclastic efforts of those failing to adhere to their idiosyncratic view of orthodoxy. Their vaunted broad-mindedness and claim to legitimacy appeared to be just as deliberately hypocritical as their rivals thought it to be. Eventually, they began losing ground to Thomsonians and eclectics in the countryside and newer towns in the Midwest and to homeopaths in the more settled urban areas. Allopaths ascribed this loss to their insistence upon education, their emphasis upon settled practices, and their more conservative (rationalistic) medical philosophy. Understandably, their assumption of superiority was strongly inbred. Their efforts to bring order to the practice of medicine were, however, the primary sources of the bitter sectarian warfare that broke out in the second half of the nineteenth century. To achieve their purposes, allopaths lobbied legislatures, made use of the press, and generally aroused the bitterness of those they sometimes unfairly accused.

As the debate evolved, sectarians viewed the demand for increased competence and educational requirements as a challenge to the principles upon which their systems had been based; with this threat before them, there was almost no limit to their calls for voluntarism. They suggested that admission to medical practice did not depend upon the result of a competitive examination and decried attempts to correlate formal education and practical intelligence. Indeed, sectarians succeeded for a time in creating in the public mind a conception of alternative medicine, which appealed to egalitarian sentiments. In vain did allopathy protest that there was nothing undemocratic about higher standards.

The "Steam and Puke" Doctor

The epitome of medical sectarianism during the first half of the nineteenth century was the system created by Samuel Thomson. Born in 1769 of strict Baptist parents (who later embraced Universal Salvation) in Alstead, New Hampshire, Samuel Thomson began working in the fields with his father at the age of four, driving cows to pasture and doing other chores. By his own recounting, he developed a curiosity regarding various herbs and, as a childhood hobby, accompanied a local herb doctor named Benton on her field trips to collect herbs. Although herb doctors made little pretense of education and regular medical qualifications, they were popular and respected in the rural countryside. The whole of Benton's practice consisted of roots and herbs, which she applied to patients or gave in hot drinks to produce sweating. At this time, too, Thomson began to chew plants to learn of their taste and effect on the body. One such plant was lobelia (*Lobelia inflata*), later called his Emetic Herb, which he delighted in encouraging other children to chew, "merely by way of sport, to see them vomit."[5] Lobelia was found in most areas of the United States and frequently given the name *Indian tobacco* by the early pioneers who, when chewing it, experienced a burning sensation, followed by giddiness and vomiting.[6] According to Morris Mattson, the Penobscot Indians used the herb, as did New England colonials, for gastritis, asthma, palpitations of the heart, strangury, and nervous affections.[7]

Before long, Thomson became a local expert on plants and directed neighbors to those roots and herbs that had medicinal powers. At sixteen, his parents had every intention of apprenticing him to a root doctor named Fuller in Westmoreland. Because of their poverty, however, they could not spare him from work; instead, young Thomson learned less formally from Doctors Fuller and Watts and from a man named Bliss, who studied with Watts and lived on the Thomson farm for seven years.

Thomson married in 1790 and eventually sired eight children. When his wife took sick after childbirth and despaired of regular medical treatment, Thomson dismissed her physicians and called upon local root doctors—who cured her. Around the same time, he also tested lobelia on a farm laborer and from this experience concluded that it could cure disease. When in 1796 his daughter failed to respond to the local physician's treatment of canker-rash (scarlet fever), Thomson turned to a combination of lobelia and steam cure. Following her recovery, he became convinced that his method had saved the child. "I sat myself in a chair, and held her in my lap, and put a blanket round us both; then my wife held a hot spider or shovel between my feet, and I poured on vinegar to raise a steam, and kept it as hot as I found she could bear, changing them as soon as they became cold. . . . I followed this plan, steaming her every two hours, for about a week, when she began to gain." With the birth of their third son, his wife was taken with ague fits and stomach cramps. This time, Thomson treated her with his own herbs. "I gave her some warm medicine to raise the inward heat, and then applied the steam. . . . This makes the fifth time I had applied to the mother of invention for assistance, and in all of them was completely successful."[8]

By 1802, Thomson's reputation in treating his family for canker-rash, measles, and various other infirmities brought recognition from neighbors who sought his treatment instead of those of the more fashionable practitioners in the area.

I am convinced myself that I possess a gift in healing the sick, because of the extraordinary success I have met with, and the protection and support I have been afforded, against the attacks of all my enemies. Whether I should have been more useful had it been my lot to have had an education, and learned the profession in the fashionable way, is impossible for me to say with certainty; probably I should have been deemed more honor in the world; but honor obtained by learning, without a natural gift, or capacity, can never, in my opinion, make a man very useful to his fellow-creatures. I wish my readers to understand me, that I do not mean to convey the idea, that learning is not necessary and essential in obtaining a proper knowledge of any profession or art; but that going to college will make a wise man of a fool, is what I am ready to deny; or that a man cannot be useful and even great in a profession, or in the arts and sciences, without a classical education, is what I think no one will have the hardihood to attempt to support, as it is contrary to reason and common sense.[9]

Thomson gave up farming in 1805 to become a full-time herb doctor, serving southern New Hampshire, Maine, and northeastern Massachusetts. His success placed him in demand with neighbors and friends, and he was soon devoting his energies to the practice of medicine. A year later, Thomson moved to Boston where he opened an infirmary; and in 1808, he took his first apprentice, a blacksmith's helper, into the practice. In 1810, at Portsmouth, New Hampshire, Thomson began manufacturing his special remedies and, before long, contracted with companies in other states to make his medicines.

To protect his medical discoveries and to ensure himself a steady income, Thomson decided to patent his healing technique. Although at first discouraged from filing a patent, he sought legal advice from Martin Chittenden, who assisted him in formulating acceptable specifications. In addition, he obtained help from Samuel L. Mitchell, M.D., of New York, then in the House of Representatives, who gave Thomson the botanic names of the herbs mentioned in his petition. Finally, on March 3, 1813, he succeeded in patenting his system of botanic medicine.[10]

During these early years, Thomson talked with both Benjamin Rush and physician-naturalist Benjamin Smith Barton, seeking their advice on how best to introduce his system to the world. Rush gave little of his time, but Barton advised him "to make friends of some celebrated doctors, and let them try the medicine, and give the public such recommendations of it as they should deem correct."[11] Fearing that doctors would claim the discovery for themselves, Thomson appealed to Barton to make his own trial of the patented system. Barton consented, and Thomson gave him the medicines with directions on their use. Thomson's hopes for an authoritative response were dashed when Barton died before completing the test. However, Benjamin Waterhouse, M.D. (1754–1846), professor of the theory and practice of medicine at Harvard University, openly advocated recognition of Thomson's contributions and pleaded with his critics to credit him with the discovery of lobelia. "Thomson is not a Quack," Waterhouse wrote. "He is an Experimenter, who accumulates knowledge by his own experience."[12]

After patenting his system, Thomson authorized agents to sell "family rights" to his botanic practice for twenty dollars. This allowed an individual to receive instructions on how to use Thomson's method of cure and to purchase *New Guide to Health; Or Botanic Family Physician* (1825) for an additional two dollars. It authorized the purchaser to practice Thomson's botanic medicine on himself and his family; it also entitled the purchaser to membership in the Friendly Botanic Society for purposes of sharing information with other users of his patented system. Thomson extended the sale of his patents to women as well as to men; as a consequence, he was the first to recognize women as practitioners in the United States.[13] With one hundred dollars and a sworn statement not to divulge the secrets of the system, a purchaser could practice on patients other than family members. But under no circumstances were patent holders permitted to resell Thomson's secret recipes; violators were subject to a sixty-dollar fine for each transgression.[14]

Thomson was an eminently practical man whose appeal to reason and self-interest satisfied the desire of families to achieve an orderly, intellectual formulation of their beliefs. He expected all laymen to participate as physicians. This democratic and flattering conception paralleled the religious sectarianism of western New York and contrasted pleasantly with the flamboyant oratory of the revival. Thomson presented a definitive answer to every issue of medicine, and—in an age when allopaths were beginning to express self-doubts—his philosophical peregrinations helped to build a consensus that transplanted easily into Ohio or Pennsylvania, the

South or the West. He seized opportunities and made them serve his purposes. Although his system proved amorphous as an intellectualized alternative, it nonetheless represented a system of beliefs and practices that followed a set formula and method of cure. The Friendly Botanic Societies, which were established to bridge individual experiences, permeated all parts of the South and West and became more democratic as they became more effective. In a certain sense, the societies represented the systematization of domestic or neighborhood medicine across the American landscape.

Thomson's medical beliefs resembled theories in vogue during the sixteenth and seventeenth centuries. His system contained aspects of Galen's humoral pathology, in that he held as true that all animal bodies were formed of the four elements: earth, air, fire, and water. Earth and water constituted the solids, while air and fire caused life and motion. He attributed all disease to the condition of cold, represented by the lessening of heat, and to an imbalance of the four elements.[15] Disease resulted from "clogging the system"; furthermore, all disease could be "removed by restoring the digestive powers, so that food may keep up that heat on which life depends." Thomson accused orthodox medicine of failing to support the body in disease. Bleeding, he said, lessened the heat and gave "double power to the cold"; the same was true with the allopaths' preference for opium, niter, and calomel.[16]

Relying on herbals, Thomson established an alternative system of medical treatment. He depended most heavily on lobelia (his "pukeweed"); hot botanicals, such as red pepper; and steam treatment. He prepared lobelia in three ways: as a powder of leaves and pods, as a tincture from the green herbs and spirits, and by reducing the seeds to a powder.[17] These natural remedies, in contrast to the regular profession's dependence on calomel, tartar emetic, and bloodletting, placed Thomson in opposition to the age of heroic practitioners (who bled, purged, and puked their patients to the point of collapse). Not surprisingly, Thomson's own system involved considerable unpleasantness, with his insistence on purging and vomiting; he was nevertheless able to deflect criticism regarding the harshness of his own system by touting the use of natural herbs rather than minerals. Another reason for the system's popularity stemmed from his efforts to represent botanic medicine as the people's revolt against medical elitism. Here was a truly democratic medicine, capable of being practiced by anyone (who bought his patent), thereby unlocking the secrets of medical practice for all.[18]

In an age of self-expression, one supporter, J. B. Spiers of Virginia, provided the following verse to express his loathing for calomel and his support for lobelia, the "Samson of the Vegetable Materia Medica."

Calomel

O when I shall resign my breath
Pray let me die a natural death,
And bid this world a long farewell,
Without one dose of Calomel.

Old Calomel *some* people hate,
And soon *all* should decide his fate.
With aches and pains he fills their bones,
And causes many doleful moans.

With indigestion—awful load,—
They drag along a dreary road—
With stiffened limbs and rotten teeth,
With foul and pestilential breath.

His victims writhe beneath his power,
And fondly court the dying hour,
To free them from the iron grasp
Of poison, fatal as the asp.

If any fears do still remain,
That patients should revive again,
And on the famed lobelia call,
And use a little steam withal.

The doctors then the people love,
Their bowels with compassion move,
They say, Dear neighbors, do be wise,
For your relief we'll soon devise.[19]

Thomson prescribed his botanic medicines with the same conviction that regulars prescribed arsenic, calomel, tartar emetic, and the other mineral drugs. In both, the intent to regulate the body's secretions—adjusting heat through purging, sweating, puking—remained the single-most important purpose. To be sure, botanics opposed the use of the lancet and the harsh mineral materia medica; yet, on balance, the premises on which both the botanics and the regulars based their therapeutic regimes remained roughly the same. The body, explained in the context of a rationalistic world that was material, objective, and quantifiable, required the interventionist strategies of a specialist who understood that body's disease and who could proceed with the art of correcting its essential secretions. Thus, the physiological response of a botanic's materia medica did not differ from that sought by the regular physician; both believed in the importance of modifying the body's secretions.[20]

The physician in America derived his professional identity from the success of his therapeutic practice—a practice that demanded an interventionist posture as the norm. Change in one direction affected the other. Thus, argued historian John H. Warner, traditional therapeutic regimens held a "symbolic significance that transcended and added meaning to their use at the bedside."[21] Although Warner argued that orthodox practitioners were distinguishable in this regard from their sectarian competitors, whether this was in fact the case among the more successful sectarians is questionable. With the exception of the Thomsonians' abhorrence of mineral drugs and depletion, the concept of the body and of disease did not differ to any great degree. Medical judgment for both sectarian and regular was based less on the practitioner's understanding of anatomy, pathology, and chemistry than on the metaphor of the body as an integrated whole, subject to imbalances that required medical intervention.

The Thomsonian method first involved the use of a steam bath to add heat, or life, to the "decaying spark," which, in conjunction with vegetable preparations, restored the system to its natural health. "In all cases where the heat of the body is so far exhausted as not to be rekindled by using the medicine and being shielded from the surrounding air by a blanket, or being in bed, and chills or stupor attend the patient, then applied heat by steaming becomes indispensably necessary." Thomson's method for steaming involved the use of several differently sized stones, which he placed in a fire until red-hot; then, with the patient sitting undressed on a chair and wrapped in blankets to shield the body from the air, the stones were immersed in a pan of hot water and placed under the patient.[22]

Following steam treatment, Thomson initiated his patented six-step procedure involving the use of emetics, purgatives, enemas, and sweat-producing herbs. He began by directing the administration of lobelia (again, pukeweed, sometimes called the *screw auger* by critics) in combination with red pepper and brandy to create a natural heat, to cleanse the stomach, to overpower the cold, and to promote free perspiration. After a second steam bath, he used red peppers, ginger, or black pepper to maintain the stomach's heat and to encourage free perspiration. Then, to "scour the stomach and bowels," he prescribed a choice of bayberry, the root of white pond lily, the inner bark of hemlock, the root of marsh rosemary, the leaves of witch hazel, the leaves of red raspberry, or squaw weed (cocash). His fourth step involved one of five different bitters plants (balmony, bitterroot, poplar bark, barberry, or the root of goldenseal) to correct the bile and restore digestion. The fifth step consisted of one of four tonic plants (typically peach meats or cherry stones), plus sugar and brandy, to strengthen the stomach and bowels. Finally, Thomson prescribed his famous Rheumatic Drops (known popularly as "No. 6") to remove pain, prevent mortification, and restore the body's natural heat. This last element, the sixth step in his cure, involved the use of wines or brandy, gum myrrh, and cayenne pepper. Botanic practitioners also gave external applications of turpentine or gum camphor to assist in the healing process.

Overall, Thomson's patented system utilized seventy different plants; however, the mainstays of his curative practice remained lobelia powder, bayberry root bark in powder, cayenne pepper, ginger, poplar bark, and his Rheumatic Drops.[23] He advised his followers to maintain a stock of essential medicines sufficient for a family for one year. These included one ounce of the Emetic Herb, two ounces of cayenne pepper, one-half pound of powdered bayberry root bark, one pound of poplar bark, one pound of ginger, and one pint of the Rheumatic Drops.[24] Thomson also prescribed American valerian, or lady's slipper, as a nervine, useful in all cases of nervous affection and in hysterical symptoms; spearmint to stop vomiting; peppermint to promote perspiration and relieve pain in the stomach and bowels; pennyroyal to warm and cleanse the stomach, producing perspiration and removing obstructions; horehound in treating cough; summer savory for toothache; mayweed in attacks of fever; wormwood to encourage an appetite and assist digestion; tansy for "hysterics" and other "female complaints"; chamomile for bowel difficulties; burdock to allay inflammation; skunk cabbage for asthma, cough, and all disorders of the lungs; and clivers for the stoppage of urine.[25]

Thomson's *New Guide to Health* went through thirteen editions and was even translated into German for the botanic practitioners in the Pennsylvania Dutch region. An excellent example of direct communication, the book was simple in organization, its sentences short and cogent, its manner almost colloquial, dependent upon repetition. Thomson further appealed to readers by quoting frequently from William Buchan and John Wesley regarding their desire for simple medicines and, most importantly, the need to demystify medicine.[26] He also crafted his stories of cures to illustrate the common habits of farmers, mechanics, and housewives, and his advice was in most respects unexceptional, being prone to a less sensational argument that depended upon frankness and common occurrence. As was customary in his time, he even appealed to his audience in verse.[27]

The rationalistic principles that lay behind Thomson's system of hot botanicals differed little from the pathological ideas of Benjamin Rush. For Rush, as stated earlier, excitability required a regimen of drastic purging and bloodletting. Dr. Thomas Cooke, a student of a Dr. Howell (a botanic physician from London), believed that Thomson's therapeutic theories were surprisingly similar to those in a work entitled *The State of Physick and of Diseases* by John Woodward and published in England in 1718. In other words, the pathology of the Thomson system fell within the Galenic tradition, and Thomson's therapeutic regimen was similarly part of a widespread interest in the use of indigenous plants for their curative value. Contemporaries, such as David Hosack and Benjamin Rush, took a keen interest in botany, and Thomson's use of lobelia was no more severe in its impact on the system than was the regular's use of tartar emetic, which created protracted nausea and debility. Those who gave testimony favoring Thomson's procedures included Professor William Byrd Powell of the University of Vermont; Professor William Tulley of Yale University; Professor George McClellan of the Jefferson Medical College; and Dr. William Robinson, who was a friend of Benjamin Rush. Benjamin Waterhouse, a friend of Thomson, wrote that, "had John Hunter . . . been born and bred where Samuel Thomson was, he would have been just such another man; and had Samuel Thomson been thrown into the same society and associations as John Hunter, he would, in my opinion, have been his equal, with probably a wider range of thought; but both are men of talent and originality of thought." Both, according to Waterhouse, had employed what was familiar around them, thereby constructing a distinctive method of cure.[28]

It was part of Thomson's strength and pride that he boasted his lack of education and his reliance instead on common sense and intuition. This confidence in the sufficiency of common sense became the cornerstone of his medicine. Lacking a formal education, he was acutely conscious of his limitations and, not content with being regarded as a rank amateur by traditional medical standards, transformed his educational impediment into an engine of scorn for the learned profession. He convinced himself and his followers that medical colleges spoiled physicians by giving them so-called learning without bedside practice. For Thomson, practice was everything. Moreover, he had a highly individualized conviction of himself and his system and insisted that others conform to his ways—a contention-breeding attitude, which eventually undermined the full impact of his system. Thomson led the democratic crusade against intellectualized medicine; however, he erred in imagining himself capable of committing an entire society to the realization of orthodox medicine's failures and in believing he could maintain within his alternative system a unified and commanding creed. The fairest way to assess Thomson is to measure him against his own times, the community in which he lived, and the patients he served. Despite the considerable internal strength of Thomsonianism, inherent weaknesses conspired to bring about its disintegration. Internal strains weakened the movement, dividing it into quarreling factions, and forced supporters, including many of his agents, through painful tests of orthodoxy.

Thomson's secret botanic system appealed to American society for a number of reasons. First and foremost, it provided an inexpensive system of medical security; for twenty dollars, a family could protect itself from illness and disease and avoid doctors' bills. Second, in a culture then self-conscious of its educational limitations, Thomson's system offered simple easy-to-follow rules. Third, Thomson allied himself to the reform-mindedness of the common man, striking out at privilege, elitism, and monopoly of every kind. For rural America, Thomsonianism represented an anchor against the insecurities of life and health. Finally, Thomson and his followers were not shy in advocating their botanic medicines. In an age of frontier bravado, they touted their system and cures while deprecating the regulars who, by their own admission, were beset with doubts about their heroic regimens. In addition to all these reasons, Thomson's system existed by the authority of the United States government, having been patented and approved by the administration of none other than Andrew Jackson.

Like the Bible and early Methodist hymns, both of which were carried by a largely illiterate population into the frontier and took the form of an oral tradition reflecting the poverty (intellectual and monetary) of the society, so sectarian medicine too moved through a similar transformation. Ancient doctrines on the basic elements, prejudices against bookish practices and educated experts, searches for simple solutions, and opposition to formal training combined to give botanic medicine an edge over that of regular doctors. That Andrew Jackson had signed Thomson's patent when it was renewed was symbolic of the special importance that his system had among the common folk of the South and West. Thomsonianism represented a rural and lower-socioeconomic movement, which included antiauthoritarianism, distrust of clerics, and egalitarianism. It was also no coincidence that the term *hunkers*, which Thomson applied to the members of the regular medical profession, was the same name given by political opponents to the anti–Free Soil wing of the New York Democratic party.[29]

Ralph Waldo Emerson's doctrine of self-reliance as expressed in 1832 represented America's intellectualized individualism and, despite its scholarly origins, differed in no great measure from the oral culture of the frontier and its own individualism. The heart of pre–Civil War transcendentalism asserted that every individual, once free of the restraints of social institutions, could realize his or her creative potential. Emerson's glorification of autonomy and self-sufficiency fit well the march of irregulars in the first half of the nineteenth century.[30]

The strength of the Thomsonians lay in their democratic appeal, offering to all the opportunity for cure without pretension. Here was a calling open to men and women alike, an opportunity not lost among pioneer women. Within the nineteenth century's sentimentality and its concept of the role of the mother in the home, a woman could ply the trade of medicine in an environment that was decidedly hers to rule. Thomson's system gave women the chance to demonstrate their then-assumed natural strength as healers and, just as importantly, helped patients avoid the embarrassment of being treated by a member of the opposite sex in delicate matters.[31]

According to Thomson, religion, government, and medicine had, in past ages, belonged to three classes of men: priests, lawyers, and physicians. "The priests held the things of religion in their own hands, and brought the people to their terms; kept the Scriptures in the dead languages, so that the common people could not read them." During the Reformation, however, they were translated into the native tongues, and each individual could, for the first time, read and interpret the words of God. In government, once considered the property of a few who "thought themselves born only to rule," the common people soon learned the "great secret of government" and began choosing their public servants. The same, Thomson argued, applied to medicine, which in great measure had been "concealed in a dead language" for only the physician to divine. With his alternative system, the secrets of medicine were open for mankind to choose and to minister.[32]

In the age of true democracy, every man became his own priest, lawyer, and physician. Safe from the avarice of professional leeches, the common man found security and monetary savings in the philosophy of do-it-yourself. In rural communities, where practitioners were in short supply, Thomson's system promised a modicum of confidence that families could provide for their own basic medical needs by purchasing access to his patent. The function of the physician in this construct was minimal at best. Instead of prescribing, Thomson educated families to take healing into their own hands. This do-it-yourself philosophy would change with the reform wing of Thomsonians, but it remained basic to orthodox Thomsonians who opposed medical schools, infirmaries, and medical societies—all of which implied the need for a medical monopoly. However, with the advent of botanic medical schools in the 1830s and 1840s, proponents extended a special tolerance to the sectarian physicians, if only to provide surgical assistance when necessary and to supplement the efforts of family practice. But among the old Thomsonians, even this adjunct status was antithetical to their self-contained system designed for the common man.[33]

Thomson's Agents

Samuel Thomson's agents formed the backbone of his medical system and made up in mobility, flexibility, and hard work what they lacked in training and education. They carried a simple medical system to the people. Whatever claims might be made for a professional class of educated physicians, the agents of Thomson, proud of their accomplishments, knew that their own way of doing things corresponded to the American landscape. Accordingly, they evolved a kind of crude pragmatism that was intent on the business of selling patents as quickly and as widely as possible. For this purpose, the elaborate equipment of an educated physician proved not only unnecessary but a serious handicap; the only justification needed for the agents' limited stock of knowledge was that they got results, measurable in the sale of Thomson's books and patents.

Thomson's agents reiterated their founder's antagonism for the educated highbrows in medicine, attacking them as bigoted and faithless hypocrites who held the patient in contempt as they practiced their craft. Not surprisingly, regulars viewed the agents as enemies rather than as coworkers, finding it difficult to cope with the challenge of these democratic awakeners. Obviously, too, regulars with settled practices faced the task of keeping alive the importance and authority of their own medicine when the agent was all too willing to appeal to a less sober argument and the spontaneity of direct communication. In their enthusiasm for selling patents, agents became extreme exponents of Thomsonianism, challenging every assumption of regular medicine. The more extravagant among them undermined the dignity of the healing profession by their personal conduct in that they chose to destroy the allegiance of patients to the regulars by denouncing their physicians as dogmatic and stuffy purveyors of authority and heroic practices.

Like the Methodist circuit riders or the vendors of books and patent medicines, Thomson's agents traveled widely through the newer towns and farming regions. Those who can be traced suggest an assortment of individualists rather than a specific type. Although they applied common methods and labored under similar conditions, they could scarcely be called intellectuals or original thinkers. Success lay in the agents' ability to meet people on their own terms and in a manner to which the people could familiarly respond. Not surprisingly, agents found themselves reaching toward doctrinal novelties as they explained Thomson's patented system of botanic cure. Without Thomson present to guard against error, they often took unintentional license with his system and, in their zeal for selling patents, made convenient interpretations of and extrapolations from Thomson's book. Selling required no preeminent abilities or extraordinary insights; rather, their motivation lay in the successful interplay between social and physical ills, necessitating the need for reform—and, of course, the promise of monetary gain.[34]

As the result of vigorous salesmanship, Thomson succeeded in selling his system of healing to a broad section of American society. "It must be a matter of national pride," commented Daniel Drake somewhat sarcastically, "that if Germany produced a Luther and England a Bacon, America has sent up from its humblest walks, a self-taught and gifted Thomson who has done for medicine what those eminent men achieved for religion and philosophy."[35] By the 1840s, Thomson and his agents had sold some one hundred thousand patents, and Thomson estimated that approximately three million people were practicing his botanic do-it-yourself system, an individualized, home-based, and family-type medicine that reflected his own upbringing and the poverty of rural America. But with his network of agents, Thomson had turned his botanic recipes into a powerful and popular system of practice.[36]

Agents spread the botanic message throughout New England and New York, moving south into Georgia and west into Ohio, Indiana, and Illinois, selling rights to the family practice in a promotional manner that anticipated the sewing machine, vacuum cleaner, and encyclopedia salesmen of later years. *The Thomsonian Recorder*, edited by Dr. Thomas Hersey, listed 167 authorized agents in 1833. States with the greatest numbers of agents included Ohio (41), Tennessee (29), Alabama (21), Indiana (11), New York (8), and Mississippi (8). Although many of these agents were believers in Thomson's system, some were simply entrepreneurs intent on making their commission and augmenting it with other sales. In Ohio, it has been estimated that almost half of the population adhered to Thomson's herbal medicines in 1835.[37] Eventually, Ohio became the publication center for many of botanic medicine's books and journals. The principal botanic supplier for the Ohio and Mississippi valleys opened for business in Ohio in competition with Thomson's own drug-manufacturing houses. In addition, other wholesale and retail drug companies formed to dispense botanic medicines.[38]

Thomsonians found eager adherents in the strongholds of

religious sectarianism, reflecting the analogous situations pertaining to both medicine and religion in the early nineteenth century. And many itinerant clergymen of the South and West gave
their endorsement to botanic medicines, extending the spirit of
Protestant reform to the healing of bodies, as well as of souls. The
"burned-over district" in western New York, along with sections
of Ohio and the South, were ripe for the claims of Thomson and
his agents. Equally significant, botanic medicine found adherents
among the Mormons, the Shakers, the Disciples of Christ, and
other religious sects spawned on the edges of America's expansion.[39]

Elias Smith (1769–1846), a Universalist preacher from Boston,
found solace and monetary comfort in Thomson's practice. Born in
Connecticut the same year as Thomson, Smith helped to transform
Thomson's herbal-medicine system into a mass movement. His
parents were of Baptist and New Light Congregationalist origins,
which provided young Smith with a firm footing in revivalism
and religious enthusiasm. His Christian calling was short-lived,
however, as he turned with the same level of enthusiasm to botanic
medicine after reputedly being cured of bilious colic by one of
Thomson's remedies.[40]

When Thomson decided to appoint a general agent to take
the lead in his practice and to give the essential information to
those who would purchase his patent rights, he chose Elias Smith.
As general agent, Smith made a 25 percent commission from medicines provided by Thomson and 50 percent (or ten dollars) from
every patent sold.[41] Not satisfied with his share of the revenues,
Smith organized in Boston those persons who had bought family
rights and formed them into a society whose members paid a one-
dollar entrance fee and were assessed twelve and one-half cents
per month for additional instructions and cheap medicines. Smith
then turned author and published his own book, *Medical Pocket-
Book, Family Physician, and Sick Man's Guide to Health* (1822), which
contained Thomson's whole system and sold for five dollars,
thereby undercutting Thomson by fifteen dollars. Intimating that
he was Thomson's partner and thus entitled to an equal share in
all profits, Smith forced Thomson to take him to court. Unfortunately for Thomson, the court determined that the specifications
of his patent were improperly prepared, and he could therefore
take no action against Smith. Thomson revised his patent January

23, 1823, and renewed it again in 1836. The patent eventually expired in 1852.[42]

Thomson, despite good intentions, never fully controlled the production of his botanic medicines. In fact, of the seventy plants recommended by Thomson, sixty of them were sold by business agents on behalf of the Shaker communities. This, and the known popularity of Shaker medicines, gave testimony to the place Thomson's materia medica held in the mainstream of nineteenth-century medicine.[43] He encouraged boycotts of pharmacists unlicensed to sell his herbs; however, many self-styled Thomsonian drug manufacturers advertised botanic and proprietary medicines, as well as medicines popular in regular medicine. To halt these infringements on what he viewed as his exclusive patent rights, Thomson took many to court, a situation that proved not only expensive but also made it a "risky business" for pharmacists and Thomsonian practitioners to use anything other than Thomson's own specified medicines."[44]

Horton Howard, a Columbus, Ohio, printer and another of Thomson's agents, published his own two-volume *Improved System of Botanic Medicine* in 1832. He also began his career as an agent in the West with authority to print Thomson's book. An effective salesman, Howard sold four thousand rights with the assistance of his subagents; and he kept all of his eighty thousand dollars in fees. Each time Thomson requested his share of the accounts, Howard refused. Discouraged with the prospect of controlling his rogue agent, Thomson revoked Howard's license, whereupon Howard established his own botanic cult. And, not to be outdone by Thomson, he added forty-two more plants to Thomson's original materia medica. Unfortunately, his own Cholera Syrup failed to protect him from the epidemic when it reached Columbus; he died in 1833. With Howard's death, the cult quickly disappeared.[45]

Howard's interest in Thomsonianism appears to have originated with his publication of Samuel Robinson's *Course of Fifteen Lectures, on Medical Botany* (1829), which went through six editions and became, next to Thomson's *New Guide to Health*, the most popular textbook on botanic medicine. Robinson, one of Thomson's more energetic proselytizers, delivered lectures on the botanic system of medicine across the Ohio countryside. Not much is known of him except that he began his career as a "lecturer" on philosophy and history. While presumably not a physician, he spoke with authority on the effects of mercury, arsenic, antimony, iron, and opium. Because of his frequent literary, philosophical, and metaphysical allusions, there is some reason to believe that he had been a clergyman. And although not listed in the Cincinnati directory, he lived in the city from 1829 through 1832, using it as his base of operations as he traveled around the state.[46]

Another of Thomson's agents, Alva Curtis (1797–1881), was born in New Hampshire and moved south in 1825, where he became a teacher in a girls' academy in Richmond, Virginia. Accounts vary, but he supposedly supported the abolitionist ideas of William Lloyd Garrison and, not surprisingly, found himself unemployed by the local gentry. He then joined forces with Thomson in 1832, becoming one of Thomson's more successful agents. The politics of abolitionism forced him to abandon Richmond and seek a more congenial environment in Columbus, where he settled in 1834. Not unlike many of the leaders of reform medicine, Curtis also became enamored of the ideas of health faddist Sylvester Graham, the theories of Franz Mesmer, and the promising possibilities of phrenology. Seeking a stronger position for Thomsonianism through the use of a more structured organization, Curtis found himself encouraging beliefs that Thomson had not espoused and eventually acquired a following in his own right, qualifying as a leader rather than a follower of Thomson. With his strong personality, Curtis led a number of Thomsonians into believing in the need for a more structured organization, one that would ensure permanence beyond the life of Thomson. Structure meant the establishment of botanic colleges, the publication of botanic journals, and the creation of a national association. Like most agents, Curtis symbolized, incited, and directed his followers. In effect, Thomson's anti-intellectualism and authoritarianism had become an embarrassment to the rising expectations of agents like Alva Curtis. The patent agents knew only too well this change in America's democratic culture, being closer to the people and recognizing their ambitions. Curtis did not have to engineer his split with Thomson; all he had to do was provide structure for a schism that had already occurred in the minds and hearts of the sect's more vocal adherents.[47]

In 1835, Curtis took over editorship of *The Thomsonian Recorder*, a journal that was then in its third volume and was subsidized by Thomson. A year later, while still within the Thomsonian fold,

Curtis began instructing students at his home under the name of the Botanico-Medical School of Columbus. On March 9, 1839, in a decision that would signal a break with his mentor, Curtis obtained a charter for the Literary and Botanico-Medical Institute of Ohio as a means of encouraging a more liberal botanic medicine than found in Thomson's strict patented system. The institute's medical department opened in Columbus in the autumn of 1839 as the College of Physicians and Surgeons. This effort was in direct opposition to Thomson's antiprofessional stance and quickly led to the schism in the movement. In 1841, Curtis moved his Botanico-Medical School to Cincinnati, where it became known as the American Medical Institute, with a faculty that included Joseph R. Buchanan, Harvey W. Hill, and Samuel Curtis. In an 1851 charter, the institution separated into the Scientific and Literary Institute and the Physiopathic College of Ohio. Eight years later, it became the Physio-Medical Institute, the name it kept until closing in 1880.[48]

The success of Thomson's *New Guide to Health* spurred others to seek similar popularity. As noted earlier, many who sought to rival Thomson had begun as agents of his botanic system before finding more lucrative opportunities in selling their own books and wares. Horton Howard's three-volume *An Improved System of Botanic Medicine* (1832) and John Kost's *Practice of Medicine According to the Plan Most Approved by the Reformed or Botanic Colleges* (1847) were two examples. A more thorough study of the botanic materia medica was published by Morris Mattson, *The American Vegetable Practice; Or a New and Improved Guide to Health Designed for the Use of Families* (1841). Begun with the encouragement of Samuel Thomson, Mattson eventually broke ranks with his mentor, accusing him of having borrowed his "discovery" from the Marshpee Indians in Massachusetts. Competing with Mattson's book was John Thomson's enlarged and improved edition of his father's *Thomsonian Materia Medica; Or Botanic Family Physician* (1841), intended to remove the deficiencies in the *New Guide to Health*. Like Elias Smith had done, Thomson's son provided thirty-one additional plant drugs, including some that were specifically denounced by the elder Thomson.[49]

Initially, Thomson's agents appealed to the poor and uneducated. As the system spread through the Middle West and South, its original dissent from the respectable, the schooled, and the established reflected aspects of its earlier strength. In time, however, the Thomsonians wanted respectability more than they wanted their anti-intellectual heritage. Thomson's view of education no doubt prevailed among many of his followers, but the botanic movement had matured to the degree that, by this time, many proponents had begun to consider formal education an essential component of the movement's future. The desire of the newer generation of botanics for a more educated profession and the growing need to defend their therapeutic position from critics, eventually overcame the older generation's suspicion of the educated practitioner.

The Politics of Medicine

The power of the botanics grew largely from the changes in state-level government licensing practices in the 1830s. Prior to that time, most state legislatures had incorporated their state medical societies, empowering them to pass on the qualifications of candidates for practice and allowing them to expel members. In time, many of these legislative acts were strengthened by stating that only those persons who were members of the societies could be duly licensed by the state or by the medical societies. The legislation implied that only those persons duly licensed could sue in the courts for their fees. Many of these provisions were repealed in the 1830s, resulting in medical practice being opened to those who had not received their education in regular schools, allowing these same persons to sue in the courts for their fees, and permitting them to practice on equal terms with regulars. So-called irregular schools blossomed with the new legislation, causing the same rights to be extended to their graduates as had applied to Old School graduates.[50]

In the early decades of the nineteenth century, for example, New York State authorized physicians to organize societies in all counties where they were not already established and permitted each county society to select a physician who could represent it in the state society. The delegates so chosen constituted the Medical Society of the State of New York. The New York law, passed in 1813, also stipulated that each county society had the right to examine any physician who presented himself; if found qualified, a county society could then issue a certificate, which entitled the holder to practice medicine or surgery in the county, as well as in any part of the state. The law further stated that persons attempting to practice medicine without recognition from one of these societies could not use the courts to collect debts incurred from the practice. In effect, the law required a botanic physician to become a member of the allopathic medical society or suffer potential financial consequences. An amendment to the act in 1821 further stipulated that "no person shall . . . be admitted to an examination as a candidate for the practice of physic or surgery who has not studied four years with a regular physician and surgeon." As amended, the law dealt what seemed to be a deathblow to all irregulars.[51]

The demand for equal rights under the law for what Daniel Drake called the "steamers and the steamed," and for other reform practitioners, was first fought in New York by Elisha Smith and John Thomson, who labored to repeal the virtual monopoly enjoyed by regulars. In 1830, a committee established by the New York State Assembly set forth the injustice of the existing law and asserted the right of all persons to select physicians of their own choosing. As a result, the legislature repealed the penalties and Governor Enos T. Throop signed the bill into law. Legislatures in other states soon followed by repealing their so-called Medical Black Laws, including Ohio and Alabama in 1833, Mississippi and Indiana in 1834, followed by Maryland in 1838, and Vermont in 1839.[52]

In 1834, the New York State Legislature reversed itself by repealing its liberal legislation and, once again, John Thomson went on the counterattack, calling for a state convention of medical protestants at Geddes in September 1834 to agitate for repeal of the law. In a resolution intended for public consumption, the convention stated that "we consider a free people as competent to select their physicians as to elect their legislators; and every law preventing the same charges the people with ignorance, and infringes on their rights."[53] In the election of 1834, a new group of legislators more favorably disposed to botanic and reformed medical practice were elected and, following numerous petitions, a new committee recommended a bill permitting adherents of botanic medicine to practice. As a last-minute compromise to regulars, however, the bill continued to prohibit reformers from having access to the courts for the purpose of recovering compensation. The committee also criticized the mushrooming of "patented" practitioners who, without education, demanded equal protection under the law with medical orthodoxy.[54]

In 1839, the Thomsonian Medical Society once again petitioned the legislature to repeal the oppressive medical act. This time, the Medical Society of the State of New York and its friends in the legislature successfully thwarted the efforts of the Thomsonians to revise the bill. In 1840, yet another committee of botanic supporters pressed the matter before the legislature. This second attempt also failed, as did subsequent efforts in 1841, 1842, and 1843. Fired by zealousness and indignation, Thomsonians sent petitions throughout the state and sought, as well, the influence of the press. In 1844, a wheelbarrow holding forty thousand petitions was rolled into the capitol, led by John Thomson and a company of botanic physicians who presented the thirty-one-yard-long petition to the legislature. This feat, impressive in its grass-roots appeal, forced the Medical Society of the State of New York into a defensive posture. The objectionable section in the revised statutes, which prohibited reformed physicians from recovering by suit or action due compensation for medical services rendered the sick, was finally repealed on May 6, 1844.[55]

As the Thomsonian movement gained momentum, it not only faced derision from allopathy but also underwent considerable internal tension as increasing numbers of botanic supporters sought to distance themselves from the authoritarian and anti-intellectual stance of the movement's founder and to seek more legitimate standing by establishing medical colleges and infirmaries. To be sure, elitism and popular prejudice had proved effective engines of unity in the early years, but having gained a measure of legal and popular respectability, followers of the system sought to strengthen the foundations of their botanic medicine with a more thorough grounding in medical botany, chemistry, anatomy, surgery, physiology, midwifery, and the theory and practice of medicine. Samuel Thomson found all of this completely at odds with his beliefs and strenuously objected to the aspirations of younger botanics, including his son, who were seeking respectability through education. "The moment you blend the simplicity of my discoveries with the abstruse sciences, such as chemistry and other discoveries that have nothing to do with medicine," he wrote, "that moment the benefit of my discoveries will be taken from the people generally, and, like all other crafts, monopolized by a few learned individuals."[56]

Thomson readily admitted that his system ignored formal medical education, but he remained adamantly opposed to any reconciliation of his beliefs with the demands of those who felt the movement needed to establish its own centers of learning. Nevertheless, the time had arrived for institutionalizing Thomson's beliefs in a manner that would subject his self-help medical practice to the rigors of education and subordinate his personality. Since medical schools were still suspect as fountainheads of deception, the early botanic medical schools organized under the euphemism *literary societies*. The leadership for this change came not from rural America but from urban areas, where competing educational standards were most formidable and where botanic reformers could no longer resist the pressures for an educated medical profession. Here, too, the desire for self-respect and for the respect of others went hand in hand. Yet the work to transform the original bias of old-school Thomsonians was constant.

In 1832, Thomson called for delegates of the various Friendly Botanic Societies to convene the first United States Thomsonian Convention. The convention, which met in Columbus, December 17, 1832, represented the first national meeting of medical professionals ever held in the United States and was intended as a mechanism for practitioners to share information regarding plants, remedies, and procedures and to display the general progress of botanic medicine. Those present at the convention gave testimony about their cures, particularly in the treatment of Asiatic cholera. In addition, the convention passed resolutions representing their collective opposition to proscriptive legislation in several states.[57] Perhaps the best description of the convention came from Madge E. Pickard and R. Carlyle Buley, who characterized the meeting as "a combination pep-meeting, love fest, and pressure-group midwife."[58] Yet the time had come, Thomson or no Thomson, for the anti-intellectual characteristics of the movement to take a backseat to ensure the future of botanic medical practice. The impulse that had quickened the democratic spirit in medicine by appealing to a practice congenial to the common man had now to reckon with younger botanics who stressed the feasibility of a botanic system within the context of medical colleges, associations, and journals. There is little doubt that their judgment was perceptive: by ensuring that their medical system reached beyond individual personalities, they offered American society a permanent alternative to established medicine.

A second convention met in Pittsburgh, Pennsylvania, in October 1833 and agreed to establish a permanent organization, as well as to organize a national Thomsonian infirmary in Baltimore. When the infirmary failed because of opposition from medical orthodoxy, local clinics based on principles of botanic medicine opened in Boston; Norfolk, Virginia; Montreal; Columbus; Hartford, Connecticut; Albany, Poughkeepsie, Troy, Kingston, Haverstraw, and Hudson, New York, providing welcome treatment during the cholera epidemics of 1832 and 1834.[59] These initiatives came not from Thomson but from Alva Curtis and others who attempted to wrest control from the authoritarianism of Thomson and his phobic aversion to a more learned system of colleges, infirmaries, and botanical associations.

The third United States Thomsonian Convention assembled in Baltimore in October 1834 and adopted the so-called Test Resolution, which stipulated that no member of the convention would use as medicines any animal, mineral, or vegetable poisons; nor would any member bleed, blister, or sell medicines that were kept secret; nor would they sell any article contrary to the principles established by Samuel Thomson. Despite this paean to the movement's leader, some at the convention found Thomson's views too restrictive and were disposed to broaden botanic medicine. For his part, Thomson suspected that the conventions had become the seedbed for dissension and, at the annual convention in 1838, he moved to dissolve the convention system entirely. The delegates, however, refused to adopt the motion, and Alva Curtis and his followers withdrew to organize the Independent Thomsonian Botanic Society. Thomson, in turn, organized the United States Thomsonian Society. With the emergence of the schism, most state societies announced their allegiance to either Curtis or Thomson, while a few allowed members to affiliate as they chose.[60] Although not the first revolt among the Thomsonians, this did constitute a definitive decision by the members of the Independent Thomsonian Botanic Society to develop a more professionalized form of botanic medicine. Unfortunately for Thomson, the days of his secret system were over, and the torch of botanic medicine passed to others concerned with establishing a more permanent and re-

spected system built on the foundation of botanic medical colleges.[61]

Physio-Medicals

Alva Curtis' effort to establish medical schools proved no easy
feat: his followers had neither textbooks nor scholarly accomplishments. Moreover, the lack of pharmaceutical resources comparable
to those of the more orthodox group forced these reformers to
rely on old Thomsonians, Shakers, and the more popular eclectics
for their medicines. This explains to some extent the close commercial relationship among botanical groups, even though, on a personal and institutional basis, they followed separate but parallel
lines of development.[62]

In the twenty years following the first Thomsonian journal in
1832, sixty-six medical journals advocated the practice of botanic
medicine. Most were short-lived and contributed in their own way
to the demise of the Thomsonian system by negating the founder's
desire to keep his patented system a trade secret. In addition,
having grown within an environment of external prejudice, the
acceptance of so many botanic journals reduced the creative tension
with medical orthodoxy that for so long had served as the botanics'
inner strength.[63] More damaging, the regulars "already possessed
an impressive plant materia medica, and numbered within their
ranks the most zealous and productive investigators." An aspiring
student of botanic medicine, commented one historian, "could get a
better botanic education at a Regular college and certain allopathic
medical schools."[64]

According to historian Alex Berman, botanical medical literature had existed on two separate levels. On one level, the literature
appealed to the lay consumer and the needs and desires of uneducated practitioners. The second level attracted educated readers
and provided the basis for "more ambitious students and practitioners." By 1839, the articles published in Thomsonian journals
had moved perceptibly from home-remedy advice and reports
of cures to articles that focused increasing attention on disease
processes. With this change to a more intellectualized therapeutics,
botanic medicine lost much of its grass-roots strength. Ironically,
those "who supported the Thomsonians began to mistrust their
own medical-school graduates for many of the reasons they dis-
trusted the allopaths."[65] As Berman has accurately observed, the

reform wing of the Thomsonians represented "the transformation of a movement which had for its base a mass of uneducated, fanatical patent right–holders into a botanic cult seeking survival in scientific respectability." Clearly, this was a direction opposite to what Thomson represented and had taught.[66]

In October 1840, Thomson held the first annual meeting of the United States Thomsonian Society. Attendance proved disappointing, with only the state society of Delaware announcing its adherence to the founder's system. Thomson railed against the mongrel practices that had emerged among the independents, their use of secret nostrums, and their willingness to use dangerous medicines, such as mandrake, iris, wild indigo, and bitterroot.[67] But, for all practical purposes, the heyday of orthodox Thomsonianism had passed. Old-guard Thomsonians never reconciled themselves to revisions in the system, and although they protested against being identified with those who undervalued education, they remained hostile toward the educational qualifications, the salaries, and the ritualistic symbols of orthodox medicine. In character, they chose to replenish their numbers from the ranks of their own people—hardworking citizens who had a healthy suspicion of authority and who kept alive the memory of their democratic origins.

For every advocate of old-guard Thomsonianism, there were two critics. According to L. Reuben, M.D., writing in 1849, reform medicine had an obligation to go beyond the system of Thomson. The founder had himself become "an impediment in the way of its immediate and perfect success." Thomson labored honestly in the vineyards of botanic medicine, but he remained "blinded" by "egotism," which prevented his system's full development. In truth, Reuben wrote, men were beginning to realize "that perfection cannot be expected from the labors of one man, and therefore, that modifications, enlargement, and improvement are possible, and even requisite, in the new system."[68] Yet another critic put it this way:

> Every enlightened friend to the Botanic practice must deplore the presumption of ignorant men, who imagine that by purchasing a Thomsonian book, and reading over a mass of heterogeneous nonsense, the sum total of Botanic medical science is obtained. The man who gives up his agricultural or mechanical pursuit, to acquire a livelihood as a botanic practitioner, may be

vain enough to think he has been transformed into a worker of miracles; but common sense should admonish the afflicted to guard against the general herd of Thomsonians, as much as against the prodigal practice of calomel and the lancet. To be a judicious and successful practitioner of the Botanic School, we contend that a radical knowledge of the vegetable kingdom is essentially necessary to give a claim to public confidence in the reformed practice of medicine. The miraculous power of transforming farmers and mechanics into doctors in a moment, is doubted in the present day.[69]

In the early days following the schism, Curtis called his followers *independent Thomsonians*. Soon afterwards, they began using the term *botanico-medicals*. At the Baltimore convention in 1851, Curtis recommended the name *physio-medical;* the convention, however, voted to adopt the name *medical reform*. But even this name faced dissension and, over the years, such labels as *physiopathic, physio-medical,* and *medical reformers* were used interchangeably. In time, Curtis' group became known as *physiopathists* in the eastern states and *physio-medicals* in the Midwest and South. Of all the appellations, *physio-medical* retained the greatest support and carried into the early twentieth century.[70]

In 1852, these various reformers held a national convention in Baltimore and organized themselves into the Reformed Medical Association of the United States, with Alva Curtis as president. In addition to the national society, Pennsylvania, Delaware, New Jersey, Maryland, and Virginia formed a Middle States Reformed Medical Society, and soon afterwards a Southern Reform Medical Association formed, composed of Virginia, Alabama, Mississippi, Arkansas, Tennessee, and Kentucky. Two years later, the Middle States Reformed Medical Society formed an alliance with the Eclectic Medical College of Pennsylvania and produced a statement of common principles, a situation that not all greeted with enthusiasm because it was unclear which would be the dominant party. Nevertheless, among physio-medicals in the middle states, the alliance was well received since they believed that the joining of the two new-school factions represented a watershed in the evolution of medical science. Despite gnawing concerns raised by Alva Curtis and other skeptics that the eclectics would soon usurp their power, the warnings went unheeded. Thus it was that the stronger eclectic movement took over both the Middle States Reformed Medical

Society and the Southern Reform Medical Association and resulted in a bitterness among the physio-medicals who then closed ranks around Alva Curtis and his followers in the Midwest. In the minds of these diehards, eclecticism had become the devil incarnate, more threatening and deceitful than even allopathy.[71]

Because so many uneducated and even illiterate men practiced medicine under the banner of Thomsonianism, societies that formed in the interest of botanic medicine began dropping the name and adopting other appellations. The Thomsonian Medical Society of the State of New York, for example, changed its name to the New York State Physiopathic Medical Society in 1849. Similar name changes occurred in the West and South. In large part, the name changes represented an effort to expand botanic judgment and opinions beyond strict Thomsonian practice. Many liberal Thomsonians adopted a system of practice that, as noted earlier, fell more appropriately under the eclectic rubric. Reflecting this new influence, the New York State Physiopathic Medical Society changed its name in 1858 to the New York State Association of Reformed Physicians, with noted eclectics Grover Coe, B. J. Stow, William W. Hadley, Henry S. Firth, and H. E. Firth as members.[72] This ecumenical spirit was short-lived as dissension soon erupted between the eclectic and physiopathic membership. In June 1863 in Albany, a committee met to form a new society, the Eclectic Medical Society of the State of New York.[73]

After the 1851 convention in Baltimore, the reformers did not meet again until 1883, when they convened in Indianapolis, Indiana, to again form a national association. This convention resulted in the creation of the American Association of Physio-medical Physicians and Surgeons. The last meeting of the association occurred in 1907, after which, remarked Berman, "The fate of the organization, if it still existed, is completely obscured through lack of a date."[74]

A Changing of the Guard

Historians remain divided in their assessments of the Thomsonians. Joseph Kett, author of a volume about the formation of the medical profession in America, attributed their decline to the waning of Jacksonianism, as well as to the decline of domestic practice itself.[75] For historian Daniel J. Wallace, however, Thomsonianism "was a viable medical sect only as long as it remained a grass-roots, popular movement. When certain leaders of the sect tried to improve it, they succeeded in diluting its force, and when they tried to professionalize illiterate frontiersmen, the movement fell apart."[76] William G. Rothstein reinforced this opinion by analyzing the sect's change "from a social movement of laymen to a movement dominated by professional healers." Seeking to pass beyond the limitations of a grass-roots, self-help movement, the reform Thomsonians set up infirmaries and state societies, all of which brought them more in line with traditional medical practice and militated against the need for restrictive licensing laws.[77] Generally speaking, Thomsonianism required persecution for there to be a catalyst keeping supporters in step; when a more liberal environment existed for any length of time, the reasons for maintaining their organization died away. Alexander Wilder pointed to political conditions that also intervened, in particular the sectional animosities of North and South and the events that precipitated the Civil War. These issues tended to "distract popular attention from medical questions," with the result that those medical schools with an especially narrow or characteristic philosophy tended to lose ground. Even in the South, where botanic medicine had gained a strong foothold, the events of secession and Civil War obscured sectarian philosophy and practice.[78]

To the exponents of regular medicine, for whom a correct reading of the materia medica or a book on therapeutics was of vital concern, Thomsonians represented the ultimate heresy. That one could, without study, without learning, interpret the signs of illness and disease and effectively intervene with sufficient insight and direction to be an agent of health seemed to conflict with the essential qualifications of medicine. That every family purchasing the right to Thomson's patent was qualified to practice medicine seemed a complete repudiation of the role of education in medicine and the destruction of all rationality in medical practice. Understandably, regulars viewed the Thomsonians as a threat to their own position, to medicine itself, and to education. Regular medicine was being bypassed by an extemporized form of practice that circumvented medical colleges and the traditional requirements of medical training.

As physicians began turning to the term *vital power* as a way of expressing *vis medicatrix naturae*, both botanics and regulars made the transition with a bit of discomfort. Regulars faced harsh criticism for their bleeding and purging regimens, while botanics faced similar criticism with their purging, puking, and sweating measures. The new age brought with it a greater recognition of the body's vital power and the need for drugs that would strengthen and stimulate. Here again, the botanics (with the exception of the old-school Thomsonians) and the regulars found themselves operating within a relatively similar set of premises regarding the body and its diseases. While older modes of treatment did not die, there was a perceptible shift to drugs that created a tonic effect on the system. General bloodletting and heroic dosages fell equally into disuse, as did blisters, counterirritations, and the heavy reliance on mercury. Even the language of disease entities changed for the two schools. And, finally, medicine witnessed a sequence of medical discoveries that were principally European in origin and that, in their totality, spelled the beginning of the end to America's sectarian years.

There is a tendency to remember sectarian medicine almost entirely for its faults, even for faults for which it was less culpable than the community in which it lived. This odious image, which Samuel Thomson came to epitomize, has dominated not only our popular lore but also our historical thinking. It must not be imagined, however, that these early sectarians were given over to a narrow view of medicine. Sectarian medicine produced a remarkable literature, which was speculative, as well as controversial; it formed the basis of an alternative system of medicine, which spread enlightenment, as well as confusion; fostered science, as well as pseudoscience; and served as midwife to orthodoxy's eventual reform.

3

Reformed Medicine, 1825–1856

Although virtually unknown outside the United States, reform physicians independent of the Thomsonians emerged in the 1820s, emphasizing single remedies; they gave special attention to the plant materia medica and supported in theory the importance of education and a scientific approach to medicine. Their popularity came at an auspicious time in medicine, a time in which doctors inside and outside allopathy were questioning the practice of purging, puking, and bleeding patients. Just as homeopathy and hydropathy owed their initial impetus to allopathy's reliance on heroic doses of jalap and calomel, not to mention leeches and the lancet, so this new breed of American reform physicians built its reputation on the elimination of the mineral remedies and the promotion of a less harmful plant materia medica.

One of the early proponents of reform medicine was Constantine Samuel "Schmaltz" Rafinesque (1783–1840), a professor of botany and natural history at Transylvania University for several years, who devoted a lifetime to the study of North American flora and to a scientific practice based upon vegetable medications. After immigrating to America in 1812, he spent several years observing the Choctaw, Chickasaw, and Cherokee of the South, as well as tribes living north of the Ohio River. During that time, he acquired an appreciation for the native plants used in self-medication. His journeys through the Mississippi Valley engendered a lifelong study of medical flora and resulted in his *Medical Flora: Or, Manual of the Medical Botany of the United States of North America* (1828–30), which contained figures and descriptions of medicinal plants, with their names, localities, properties, and histories. He classified plants into aliments, simples, poisons, flowers, and weeds (alimentary, medical, poisonous, ornamental, and useless). These plants included agrimony, aletris, aralia, arbutus, arum, asclepias, cactus, caulophyllum, chelone, chenopodium, chionanthus, cimicifuga (or macrotys), collinsonia, cypripedium, equisetum, erigeron, eupatorium, galium, gaultheria, gentian, geranium, geum (avens), hamamelis, hepatica, hydrastis, leptandra (Culvers root), lobelia, lycopus, monarda, phytolacca, podophyllum, snakeroot, sanguinaria, scutellaria, trillium, viburnum, and xanthoxylum. Each of these plants eventually became part of the later eclectic pharmacopoeia.[1]

According to Rafinesque, botanic medicine consisted of the application of empirical knowledge of vegetable substances first learned from the American Indians and shared among country practitioners, herbalists, empirics, and botanics. He believed it imperative to spread this medical knowledge among those in the established medical schools and through journals, pharmacopoeias, dispensatories, and general medical works.[2] Francis R. Packard wrote that Rafinesque attempted to pen a medical botany that would meet the needs of both the American physician and the American pharmacist. "He was an erratic genius," observed Packard, "and he frequently made rash statements, but if one reads his book with an open mind, it gives a most favorable impression of his honesty of purpose, and even if his views as to the value of certain plants have since been proved exaggerated or wholly erroneous, they are usually in accord with the ideas prevalent in his time."[3]

On the basis of his observations and natural curiosity, Rafinesque divided medical practitioners into three classes or groups: the rationalists, the theorists, and the empirics. The rationalists were liberal thinkers, neither intolerant nor deceitful, and ready to learn new methods. They were comprised of the improvers, experimentalists, and eclectics. The improvers studied nature and the human constitution and wrote their observations with the intent of improving medical knowledge. The experimentalists were directed by experience, experimentation, observation, dissection, and fact.[4] The eclectics, for whom Rafinesque had the greatest admiration, selected and adopted in practice whatever they deemed beneficial and changed their prescriptions "according to emergencies, circumstances and acquired knowledge." This classification, wrote eclectic physician and historian Alexander Wilder, "was the first occurring of the name eclectic in American Medicine, and from it the latter use of the designation appears to have been derived."[5] In writing to Wooster Beach, the originator of so-called reform medical practice, Rafinesque remarked: "I belong, like yourself, to a reformed school of medicine, and agree with you much better than with the Thomsonian, homeopathic and botanical empirics. Your system is a good one, if not perfect; it is better at any rate than most of the fashionable systems, Galenian, Brunonian or mineral."[6]

As for the theorists, Rafinesque observed that they had divided and subdivided into many different sects and almost always warred among themselves and their rivals. Illiberal and intolerant, the theorists included such diverse groups as the Brunonianists, Galenists, Mesmerists, skeptics, and calomelists; they followed a particular theory and mode of practice and employed few vegetable remedies. Finally, there were the empirics, whom Rafinesque described as "commonly illiterate, ignorant, deceitful and reserved; following a secret or absurd mode of practice, or dealing in patent remedies." The empirics included the herbalists, Indian or root doctors, steam doctors, quacks, and nostrum sellers—who followed secret modes of practice and often dealt in patent medicines.[7]

Rafinesque, who once refused Benjamin Rush's offer to serve as his mentor, opposed all exclusive medical systems, and he hoped that medical botany would become a work of general utility for all groups of enlightened physicians. Of nearly six hundred medical plants in the United States, he chose 105 as the most active and efficient. He objected to chemical manipulation of medicinal principles, believing that such processes did not suit the constitution. He also objected to polypharmacy, maintaining that it was proper to combine medicinal agents only if they were compatible in nature. Although some medical substances increased in power through combination, most exerted a negative effect on each other and on the intended medical result.[8]

Another advocate of reform medicine was Dr. George Andrew

Viesselius of Amwell, New Jersey, who is regarded as having laid the foundations for this particular practice of medicine in the 1760s and 1770s. Motivated by the Townshend Acts of 1767 and by the colonial nonimportation agreement, Viesselius and other physicians substituted native medicinal plants for the more popular imported plant and mineral drugs. According to Benjamin Smith Barton, Americans employed the dried and powdered berries of spicewood as a substitute for allspice (used for fever), the root bark of the magnolia tree (*Magnolia grandiflora*) in combination with snakeroot as a substitute for cinchona (Peruvian bark) in the treatment of intermittent fevers, and Bowman's root and ipecac as emetics.[9] Crude in many aspects, the plant discoveries of Viesselius still added materially to the stock of medical science. When Viesselius died, a young German named Jacob Tidd, who had helped the doctor make his washes, salves, and plasters, continued the practice. Tidd benefited from additional information gleaned from a relative who had learned of herbal medicines during his incarceration by Indians. "The hallmark of the botanics," wrote Harris L. Coulter, "was confidence in the traditional medical lore of the Indians and in the folk-medicine of the common people generally." Viesselius and Tidd were clearly a very real part of this tradition.[10] Although Tidd developed a lucrative practice, limited initially to external remedies acquired from his mentor, he soon augmented his armamentarium; and over a period of forty years of practice in the use of native plants, Tidd became famous in the region as an herb doctor.[11]

Beach's Reformed Medical Practice

Among those who attempted to learn Jacob Tidd's methods was Wooster Beach (1794–1868) of Trumbull, Connecticut. Initially spurned by Tidd, who refused to share his secrets, Beach did eventually earn his trust, becoming a valued assistant and ultimately taking over the practice. Beach later moved to New York City where he allegedly graduated from the Medical Department of the University of New York (established for a brief time by David Hosack and a group of seceders from the College of Physicians and Surgeons and operated under the authority of Rutgers, in New Brunswick, New Jersey) and joined the New York County Medical Society. While a member in good standing in the society, he took exception to the practice of bloodletting and to the use of strong mineral remedies, urging instead that physicians turn to herbs and roots. As the healing art developed, explained Beach, those who had made a profession of medicine stripped it of its simplicity and substituted speculative theories for observation and experiment. Physic eventually "became an abstruse science . . . out of the reach of ordinary men." Physicians filled their books with mysteries, introduced into practice an abundance of compound medicines, and labored to replace common sense with finespun theories.[12]

When Beach attempted to discuss openly his ideas of "reformed practice," he faced the sullen hostility of the profession. Undaunted, he began instructing students at his home in 1825 and, in the spring of 1827, opened the United States Infirmary on Eldridge Street in New York City, where he provided clinical support for his students. In the clinic's first year, he and his students treated twenty-one hundred patients without resorting to surgery, depletion, or mineral practices. In 1829, Beach changed the name of his infirmary to the Reformed Medical Academy and, a year later, to the Reformed Medical College of the City of New York, which, unchartered by the state, was prohibited from granting medical degrees. In lieu of a medical diploma, the college provided a printed certificate, which not surprisingly resembled a medical diploma.[13]

During the Asiatic cholera epidemic of July 1832, Alderman John Palmer appointed Beach health physician for poor patients in New York's Tenth Ward. Unlike regulars (who treated with calomel), Beach and his assistants undertook a nondrastic regimen with, as they alleged, highly successful results, claiming only a 20 percent mortality rate while regulars were lamenting a much greater 50 percent mortality. Also in 1832, Beach started his *Reformed Medical Journal*. In it, he and his disciples expounded the principles of reformed medical practice. The motto for the journal reflected his deep and abiding faith in reform: "The science of medicine, like the doric column, should stand simple, pure and majestic, having fact for its basis, induction for its pillar, and truth alone for its capital."[14] Like Elias Smith of Thomsonian fame, Beach also enjoyed dabbling in religious polemical writing. In addition to his medical works, he published several broadsheets known as the *Telescope* (1825–28), the *Ishmaelite* (dates unknown), and the

Battle-Axe (1837–40), which popularized his views on religion and sociology.

Beach was assisted in his early endeavors at the college by Thomas Vaughan Morrow, Ichabod Gibson Jones, and John J. Steele, all graduates of regular schools. This initial group formed the nucleus of the Reformed Medical Society of the United States with officers from Pennsylvania, New York, Kentucky, Maine, and Connecticut. Known as the "Fathers of Eclecticism," they also included Thompson Richardson of Marietta, Pennsylvania; G. W. Downing of New York City; Amzi Sanborn of Parsonsfield, Maine; and S. A. Stanley of Farmington, Connecticut.[15]

Although allopaths claimed that Wooster Beach and Samuel Thomson were spun from the same heretical cloth, reform medical practice was as unlike Thomsonianism as it was allopathy. To be sure, Beach adhered to a botanic system of cure; however, he did not share Thomson's strong anti-intellectual and class biases. Beach was educated, having reputedly attended the lectures of Philip W. Post, David Hosack, and Valentine Mott at the University of New York. Moreover, Beach insisted on a more catholic view of botanic medicine than the restrictive dogma of Thomson, having been grounded in a liberal foundation emphasizing professionalism and education as its twin pillars of strength. Beach intended his system "to release the mind from the dogmas of creeds and systems, the philosophy of medical schools, as they were then taught, and to direct it to an unlimited field of inquiry."[16]

Throughout reform medicine's history, however, Beach and his followers recognized Thomson as one of the intellectual antecedents. "No monument too lofty could be built," wrote Frank Stewart, M.D., "and no inscription too pure or beautiful could be written, for the moral courage and physical daring manifested under so many disadvantages and persecutions, in [Thomson's] endeavors to coin a system to prevent the destruction of life and benefit his fellow man."[17] These accolades aside, the reformers condemned Thomson's steam and puke methods as little more than quackery; his remedies were good in their proper place, but "to think of curing all diseases by them, is the height of empiricism and quackery." Those who discovered the folly of Thomson's system or declared themselves independent of the Thomsonians and who enlarged the area of their therapeutical views, as well as the vocabulary of their materia medica, preferred the more liberal appellation *reformed medical practice*.[18]

With respect to homeopathy, the reformers identified it as a foreign adaptation to the diseases of the United States. While dedicated to changing outmoded practices, they considered homeopathy little better than other imported Old World theories and systems. Moreover, homeopaths admittedly used infinitesimal doses and gave credence to poisonous and deleterious medicines, such as mercury, arsenic, and antimony. Reformers had little confidence in the principles of homeopathy, especially dynamization (the belief that the smaller the dose the more potent, speedy, and efficient the results). The etherealized globules of homeopathic cure, observed G. Price Smith in the *Eclectic Medical Journal*, had little perceptible effect "upon the obtuse sensibility of a Yankee." Nevertheless, reformers admitted that some advantages did derive from homeopathy, principally the belief that success depended upon the conservative powers of the natural constitution of the patient. Rather than encumber patients with heavy dosages of depletive medicines, homeopaths had rightly appealed to the natural efforts of the system to overcome or throw off disease.[19]

Concerned with what he considered to be the fallacies of old-school systems of practice, Beach met with Indian doctors, root and herb doctors, and eminent botanic physicians and even traveled abroad where he visited hospitals, colleges, and infirmaries in England, France, and Germany. From these experiences and observations, he concluded that the old-school system of practice required extensive modification. In 1833, he published his three-volume *The American Practice of Medicine*, which became the earliest textbook of the reformed medical practice. He wisely sent complimentary copies to the crowned heads of Europe and found himself quickly honored with medals and decorations by many who acknowledged his ideas and the importance of his vegetable-based medicines. Those whom Beach claimed had recognized his contributions included Professor Christoph Wilhelm Hufeland, first physician to the king of Prussia; King William IV of England; the kings of Holland, Saxony, and Württemberg; the grand duke of Saxony; and Pope Gregory XVI. And at home, Beach received praise from Harvard Professors Asa Gray and Louis Agassiz. Beach repeatedly used the various editions of his book to advertise these honors and acknowledgments.[20]

Beach believed that there must be first principles in medicine, as well as in philosophy, principles that, though simple, "are invariable and incontestable and that, like the stars of the firmament in guiding the mariner, will conduct the physician with assured aim through the different stages of disease."[21] These first principles included the admonition against using mercury and other minerals; opposition to salivation and long-continued regimens of depletion; bloodletting in all forms; and unnecessary surgery. The surgeon's knife had become a source of immense mischief to patients. Too often, argued Beach, physicians resembled "butchers eager to shed the blood of a poor animal."[22]

In addition to providing information on the nature, property, and employment of a given agent derived from the vegetable kingdom, Beach discussed the seasons for collecting vegetable medicines and methods for preparing extracts, infusions, and decoctions. His more popular medicines included wine bitters, made from goldenseal, whitewood bark, Indian hemp, and cayenne pepper; diuretic drops, made from sweet spirits of niter, balsam of copaiba, oil of almonds, and spirits of turpentine; antiemetic drops, made from salt, capsicum, and vinegar; and his rheumatic coction, made from Virginia snakeroot, white-pine bark, burdock seeds, and prickly ash bark. Beach marketed his medicines in packages, vials, and bottles that featured a picture of himself and his written signature. Sold under the label Beach's Medicines, they included Anti-Bilious Family Physic (a substitute for mercury) for dyspepsia, indigestion, and costiveness; Alterative Powder for rheumatism and impurities of the blood; Neutralizing Mixture for diarrhea and summer complaints; Pile Electuary for hemorrhoids; Vegetable Emetic for problems of the liver; Restorative Wine Bitters for debility, incipient consumption, and "inward complaints" peculiar to women; Pulmonary Powder for consumption; Female Pills for chlorosis or greensickness; Black Salve and Healing Salve for ulcers, sore nipples, and burns; Compound Tincture for dyspepsia; and Brown Ointment for "the itch." Orders for both his books and his medicines were available through James M'Alister of Fulton Street, New York City, the publisher of Beach's book.[23]

Beach's *American Practice of Medicine* fell within the accepted genre of advice literature and domestic medicine in the early nineteenth century, combining commonsense observations, uplifting poetry, domestic practice, popular wisdom, and testimonials (to advance his plan for proper living). Like many authors of advice books, he devoted pages to the importance of temperance, exercise, pure air, and proper clothing; the benefits of bathing; and the evils of tight lacing. He also gave rules for preserving health and obtaining longevity. He provided helpful hints to invalids and discussed the influences of the passions on "upright" living. He offered views on the frequency of sexual intercourse and the evils of onanism and self-pollution (masturbation). "The emission of semen," he wrote, "enfeebles the body more than the loss of twenty times the same quantity of blood, and more than violent cathartics, emetics, etc." In concert with food faddist and marriage adviser Sylvester Graham, he encouraged self-restraint even among married persons. "Never indulge in the propensity while it can well be avoided," Beach wrote. Hundreds of thousands of married couples hurried to premature graves or were made wretched by venereal diseases induced by excesses. As for onanism and masturbation, he said, persons who practiced these unnatural acts exposed themselves to the ruin of their health and morals. They laid the foundation for "incurable complaints," bad health, insanity, and eventual death.[24]

Beach was not especially meticulous when it came to recognizing and acknowledging those from whom he had drawn his information and illustrations. He borrowed from Rafinesque, William P. C. Barton, Jacob Bigelow, and Elisha Smith without giving them proper attribution. As Alex Berman appropriately noted, "One is forced to conclude, after reviewing Beach's work on the plant materia medica, that his contribution was noteworthy mainly for its mediocrity and excessive borrowing."[25] This fault aside, Beach's *American Practice of Medicine* quickly became one of the most popular works of botanical literature in the nineteenth century. He later condensed his treatise into a single volume, *The Family Physician*, which went through fifty-six editions, garnering a number of additional foreign medals and testimonials. When, in 1843, he received a medal from Louis-Philippe of France, the seventh such medal from a European head of state, news of the award brought a stinging rebuke from American medical orthodoxy. "What has this gentleman accomplished in the domain of medical science, to be honored by the bounty of kings?" asked the editors of the *Boston Medical and Surgical Journal*. "Nothing. He is neither known to men of science in his own country, nor acknowledged by intelligent men in the city of his residence, to have claims . . . upon the world on the score of superior sagacity or medical attainments. He has simply constructed a book which he calls a new system of medicine, but which is neither novel in its details, nor distinguished in its originality of thought."[26]

Worthington Medical College

The Reformed Medical Academy (1829), subsequently the Reformed Medical College of the City of New York (1830), the first sectarian medical college in the United States, flourished until 1838, having gathered together a group of physicians under the name of the Reformed Medical Society of the United States. Failing in their efforts to obtain a charter in New York, Beach and his colleagues looked westward, hoping to find a more favorable environment. At a meeting of the society in May 1830, the membership adopted the following resolutions:

> *Resolved*, That this society deems it expedient to establish an additional school in some town on the Ohio River, or some of its navigable tributaries, in order that the people of the West may avail themselves of the advantages resulting from a scientific knowledge of Botanic Medicine.
> *Resolved*, That Dr. John J. Steele be sent, on or before the middle of August next, to explore the towns on the Ohio River, from the head of navigation to Louisville, in order to fix upon an eligible site for a Reformed Medical Institution, and in case of failure, to proceed further west or south.
> *Resolved*, That those who contribute towards erecting the edifice for said school, shall be repaid in full, in medicine and attendance by our Faculty; or in the instruction of such young men as they may choose to have instructed in the principles of the new system.[27]

Acting upon the conviction that an indigenous medical system would have a better chance of taking root in the western territories, Beach distributed circulars to elicit invitations that might enable him and his colleagues to relocate the college in a more suitable environment.

Nearly thirty years earlier, in 1803, Colonel James Kilbourne, acting on behalf of the Scioto Land Company, located the town of Worthington in Franklin County, Sharon Township, Ohio, and drew to it emigrants from Hartford County, Connecticut, and

Hampshire County, Massachusetts. With its village square and spired churches, Worthington had the look of a typical New England village. The plan for Worthington included setting aside land for both a church and a school. The school, known as the Worthington Academy, was incorporated February 20, 1808, and eleven years later was incorporated again as Worthington College. The Reverend Philander Chase was appointed president of the new college; but, having also been elected to the Episcopal bishopric of Ohio, he turned the position over to his son, the Reverend Philander Chase, Jr.[28] At the time that Worthington College was established, there were only twenty-four states in the Union, and only two, Missouri and Louisiana, were west of the Mississippi River. In effect, the West included everything beyond New York and Pennsylvania.

On the advice of Colonel Kilbourne, the board of trustees of the college, having received a copy of Beach's circular, invited him to operate under their charter. Preparations were quickly made to open the Reformed Medical College of Ohio, better known as the Medical Department of Worthington College or simply as Worthington Medical College. (The old Worthington College reopened under a new charter as Kenyon College.) The institution opened for instruction in the winter of 1830 with eight students and John J. Steele, a reformed allopath, as its president. The college gave ten months of lectures, divided into spring-summer, fall-winter terms. When Steele found himself in trouble after "indulging in habits incompatible with the moral sense of the community," he vacated the position, which was then filled by Thomas Vaughan Morrow, a native of Kentucky who had been educated at Transylvania University and had graduated from a regular medical college in New York City, as well as from Beach's Reformed Medical College. Morrow was more a reformer than was Steele. Steele, observers noted, had been a recent "seceder from the old school." Only twenty-five years old, Morrow proved a good choice for the school, bringing energy and talent to the position. Known as "Old Macrotys" because of his preference for cimicifuga (*Cimicifuga racemosa*), he ultimately earned yet another honorific: "Father of Eclecticism in the West."[29]

For twelve years, the Medical Department at Worthington remained the most prominent institution for the instruction of reformed medical practice. In 1836, the department began publishing a monthly journal of medical and chirurgical science, the

Western Medical Reformer, which in its brief three-year history provided rules for the preservation of health, discussed the deleterious effects of bloodletting and mercury, argued for the importance of exercise, gave directions for the preparation and medicinal uses of the vegetable materia medica, advocated elements of hydropathy, and encouraged the philosophy of reform medical practice.[30] According to Jonathan R. Paddock, M.D., a member of the faculty, the object of the *Western Medical Reformer* was to expose and refute "such calumnies and slanders on the Reformed System of Practice, as, judging from their source, we may deem worthy of attention." He was particularly incensed by the criticisms of Charles Caldwell, M.D. (1772–1853), of Kentucky, who attacked the principles and deceitfulness of botanical medicine and reformed medical practice.[31] Paddock found Caldwell's remarks complete defamation. "Whether sober, or drunk with envy, hatred, and malice," he wrote, "it is evident that the learned Doctor has labored hard to combine incompatibles." There was all the difference in the world between the "dealers in steam" and the "dealers in the reformed practice."[32]

In 1837, the Worthington Infirmary opened for clinical instruction, and by 1838 the Medical Department had grown to ten faculty: John J. Steele, Ichabod Gibson Jones, Thomas Vaughan Morrow, W. Starrett, J. I. Riddell, Jonathan R. Paddock, D. L. Terry, Truman E. Mason, Joseph B. Day, and Richard P. Catley.[33] By 1840, two hundred reform physicians were practicing in the United States, all having gone forth from the New York and Worthington schools.[34]

Fees for the Medical Department at Worthington compared favorably with those of other medical schools of the day. The five-month fall-winter term in 1839 listed the following fee schedule:[35]

Anatomy and Physiology, T. V. Morrow, M.D., $12.00
Chemistry and Medical Jurisprudence, G. W. Chevais, M.D., $12.00
Theory and Practice of Medicine, and Midwifery, J. B. Day, M.D., $10.00
Surgery, Disease of Women and Children, I. G. Jones, M.D., $10.00
Botany, Materia Medica, and Pharmacy, J. R. Paddock, M.D., $10.00
Fees for spring and summer course each professor's ticket, $5.00
Use of dissection room, $5.00, optional. Graduation fee $10.00

Although the Worthington Medical College openly declared itself in favor of the improved botanical system of practice, it went out of its way to distinguish itself from the Thomsonian system. "Since Samuel Thomson obtained letters patent to enable him to steam and pepper the sick legally," observed the editor of the *Western Medical Reformer*, "and to authorize others to do the same, his system (if indeed it can be called one), has been so industriously puffed by interested agents and sub-agents, almost without number, that there can scarcely an individual be found, who has not heard more or less of the Thomsonian steam practice." Unfortunately, few laymen saw much difference between reformed medical practice and Thomson's steam and puke system.[36]

When Alva Curtis reported the success of his Botanico-Medical School of Columbus, Ohio, faculty at Worthington Medical College criticized the endeavor as a fraudulent effort to legitimize the steam and puke system with pretenses at science.[37] Not to be outdone, the supporters of physio-medicalism accused the reformers of being most like adherents of "non-committalism" or "nothing-ism." Curtis called the physicians of reformed medicine "the poisoning, blistering, cupping, bleeding, mongrelizing Beachites or eclectics." In rebuttal, the reformers accused physio-medicals of committing themselves "to all the crudities of an egotistical and embryotic system, which . . . claims to be a perfect science."[38] In response to a series of questions posed by the students at Worthington, Morrow claimed that reformers had introduced the true scientific botanic system of medicine and surgical practice without any knowledge of the system known as Thomsonianism. Essentially, Morrow disavowed any connection with the Thomsonian system and claimed for Worthington the full title to reformed medicine.[39] He asserted that the two systems were separate and that the intellectual origins of the reformed system had actually antedated Thomsonianism by several years. Morrow also objected to Thomson's belief that the practice of medicine did not require knowledge of anatomy or physiology; physicians should be persons of liberal culture, of strong character, possessed of a sound understanding of science and patient investigating procedures.[40]

Morrow's comments notwithstanding, Thomson accused the school of having questionable traits and practices and of having plagiarized ideas and techniques from his own medical system. He fought both the establishment of the Reformed Medical College of the City of New York and the Worthington Medical College in Ohio. According to Thomson,

> Finding that I should succeed in my Botanic practice, certain individuals of them have set up what they call a reformed college, in New York, where they have adopted my practice as far as they could obtain a knowledge of it from those who had bought the right of me, and would forfeit their word and honor to give them instruction. After finding that the Botanic practice gained very fast at the West, they [Beach, Morrow, and Steele] have established a branch of their reformed college in Worthington, Ohio. I saw Dr. Steele, last winter, who is the President of that Institution, I was introduced to him by Mr. Sealy, a member of the Senate, and Dr. Steele was introduced to me as President of said college. I asked him if he was president of that reform which was stolen from Thomson, in New York. This seemed to strike him dumb on the subject. At the same place, a few evenings after, I was introduced to one of the practitioners under this reform, who studied and was educated at the college in New York, and was one of the instructors at Worthington. I asked him if he ever saw any of my books in the college of New York. He said he had accidentally seen one there. I replied, then you accidentally confess that my books were studied in that college. I then asked him whether they used the lobelia. He said they did. I then named the cayenne, rheumatic drops, bayberry and nerve powders. He confessed they used them all in manner and form, as I had laid down in my book.[41]

The early years at Worthington were difficult ones for its professors. The college suffered from small classes and defects in organization. Dissent also became a part of its lot when Ichabod Gibson Jones returned to private practice, and the trustees invited Dr. D. L. Terry to replace him. This choice turned out to be unfortunate because he soon became a staunch Thomsonian, sowing discontent among the faculty and students. In May 1836, Terry went over to the Thomsonians, using the pages of the *Botanical Record* as his weapon against the reformers.[42]

Worthington was too small a town to become much of a medical center, and with the establishment of the Ohio Medical College under the control of regulars and subsidized by the state, the college faced difficult years. As a result of the financial crash of 1837, the faculty at Worthington lost their infirmary and had to suspend publication of the school's *Western Medical Reformer* in

December 1838. The college maintained a modest student body of about twenty but was constantly embarrassed by the lack of operating funds.[43] The faculty also found it difficult to procure anatomical materials and faced a hostile public, which accused them of grave robbing, or "resurrection skulduggery." For their part, the faculty constructed ingenious closets to hide dissection materials when, on occasion, the local sheriff and posse surrounded the college and searched the grounds and buildings for disinterred bodies. But not all criticism came from outside. Dr. Richard P. Catley, the chair of anatomy, became a bitter enemy of the school; after moving to Delaware, Ohio, he stirred popular resentment by circulating stories concerning the faculty's manner of procuring dissecting materials. Every effort was made to prevent the violation of family plots, but resurrections did occur, much to the dismay of school officials and, more importantly, to the indignation of the local community. As a consequence, the Medical Department was no exception to the so-called resurrection wars that broke out between town and gown in the nineteenth century.[44]

Like most medical colleges that existed as more than storefront operations, Worthington required students to take a course in practical anatomy. Ironically, as historian Linden F. Edwards recounted, medical faculty faced a paradoxical situation. "On the one hand, the public demanded of practitioners of medicine and surgery a practical knowledge of the anatomic structure of the human body, while on the other hand, the forces of human prejudice, ignorance, superstition, and piety in the legislative halls united in a conspiracy to prevent medical students from acquiring such knowledge by failing to provide for the legal acquisition of cadavers."[45] This meant that students and faculty became coconspirators in the business of obtaining dissection materials, depending upon their own ingenuity and the services of body snatchers or resurrectionists to obtain cadavers.[46]

Most medical schools depended upon the potter's fields of various cemeteries to obtain cadavers. However, the discovery of disturbed church graves that were not those of suicides, executed criminals, or paupers buried in a potter's field brought local communities to a riot pitch, demanding respect for the sanctity of burial grounds and vengeance against neighboring medical schools. Instances of mob violence occurred in Philadelphia in 1765 against Dr. William Shippen, Jr., and in 1788 when mobs forced themselves into the home of Dr. Charles F. Wiesenthal in Baltimore after he dissected an executed murderer with the help of a medical apprentice. The Doctors' Riot in New York City in 1788, which started when a medical student supposedly waved the arm of a cadaver from a window, required the militia to fire upon rioters, killing five before the tumult ended. Other examples include a dissection riot in 1807, which resulted in the destruction of Dr. John B. Davidge's Anatomy Hall in the Medical Department of the University of Maryland; mob action in 1811 in Zanesville, Ohio, with the discovery of an empty grave and the body's use as dissection material for students studying under a preceptor; and a mob storming Yale Medical College in 1824 to protest the violation of a grave. Similar riots occurred in 1830 at the Berkshire Medical Institution in Pittsfield, Massachusetts, the Vermont Medical College at Woodstock, and the Castleton Medical College in Vermont. Resurrection riots also took place in 1844 at the Missouri Medical College in St. Louis, in 1848 against the Medical Department of Illinois College in Jacksonville, and in 1849, when a mob attacked the home of the anatomy professor of Franklin Medical College in St. Charles, Illinois.[47]

In 1839, after nearly a decade of operation, Worthington Medical College became the focus of a serious resurrection riot, which resulted in the legislature's eventual repeal of its charter in 1840. Previous stories of the college disinterring bodies from family plots had exposed the faculty to several civil suits. However, the climax occurred when a Mrs. Cramm of Marietta, Ohio, died at the state insane asylum in Columbus and relatives did not arrive in time to claim the body. The asylum officials had buried her in a potter's field, from which the corpse was subsequently removed to the dissecting tables of the Medical Department. When the relatives found the empty grave, they quickly deduced that the Worthington medical students and faculty had masterminded the resurrection. This, plus the discovery of two additional empty graves, incited a mob armed with pistols and shotguns to march on the college. With the townspeople threatening bloodshed, Morrow wisely yielded on the guarantee that the faculty would be permitted to exit the college with their personal belongings. After Morrow and his colleagues withdrew, the rioters entered the building and found the body of Mrs. Cramm on the dissecting table and the body of a dead man on the grounds behind the college. In response to the furor gener-

ated by the citizenry, the Ohio legislature rescinded its authoriza-
tion to the trustees of the college to confer medical degrees. This
revocation, along with its chronic financial embarrassment,
brought an end to the reform experiment in Worthington.[48]

The Eclectic Medical Institute of Cincinnati

Morrow and his faculty struggled to offer medical education
at the Worthington Medical College after the repeal of its charter
in March 1840, but the effort proved fruitless. Morrow closed
the department and, at the invitation of Professor Alexander H.
Baldridge of Cincinnati, moved to Cincinnati, where he organized
a faculty comprised of Baldridge, Benjamin L. Hill, Lorenzo E.
Jones, Hiram Cox, and James H. Oliver and announced a course
of lectures for the winter of 1842–43 in the Hay Scales House at
the corner of Sixth and Vine Streets. The school, thus established,
became known as the Reformed Medical School of Cincinnati
(1842–45).[49]

After abortive efforts in 1843 and 1844 to receive a charter
and faced with the meddling of the Ohio Medical College, which
lobbied against incorporation, Morrow and his faculty succeeded
on March 10, 1845, in obtaining a charter under the name Eclectic
Medical Institute of Cincinnati (affectionately called the E. M. Institute or "Old E. M. I." by its faculty and alumni). The name *eclectic*
was adopted at the suggestion of one of the school's trustees (the
term had been earlier used by Constantine Samuel Rafinesque and
also by the Eclectic Botanic Medical Association of Pennsylvania
in 1840). The new college opened its doors in December 1845. In
a significant act of symbolism, the faculty elected Wooster Beach
chair of clinical medicine and surgery, thus drawing attention to
the fact that the E. M. Institute was the direct successor of the
Reformed Medical School of Cincinnati, which, in turn, had succeeded the Medical Department of Worthington Medical College,
the western branch of Beach's original Reformed Medical College
of the City of New York.

Unlike many medical schools of the day, the E. M. Institute
offered good physical facilities for medical instruction, an open
policy on the admission of female students, and a course of instruction similar to those of the better allopathic schools. In addition,
students had the use of Newton's Clinical Institute (named after
Robert S. Newton, who held the chair of surgery at the E. M.

Institute) on payment of a five-dollar fee. Before the clinic became available, E. M. students were without instruction in clinical medicine, having been refused access to Commercial Hospital in Cincinnati. Here, both Newton and Zoheth Freeman lectured on clinical medicine and surgery, performed operations, and treated patients. The clinic eventually was transferred to the lecture room of the E. M. Institute.

Between 1848 and 1855, the institute matriculated 2,145 students and graduated 593, exceeding the aggregate attendance of the five other medical schools of Cincinnati and outnumbering the classes of most medical colleges in the country (with the exception of the older schools of Philadelphia and New York). In an age when the size of the matriculating class was more important than quality, the college ranked high among the more popularly recognized medical schools in the country. The 1853 class numbered 233 students from twenty-one different states, including transfers from allopathic schools in Virginia; Charleston, South Carolina; Louisville, Kentucky; and St. Louis, as well as students from Philadelphia, the Ohio Medical College, and Worcester Medical School, Massachusetts. The sixteen-week session included seven lectures each day and extra courses of ten to fifteen lectures each, delivered at the request of the class by different members of the faculty. The faculty consisted of William Sherwood (special surgical and pathological anatomy), Joseph R. Buchanan (physiology and institutes of medicine), George Washington Lafayette Bickley (materia medica, therapeutics, and medical botany), Robert S. Newton (medical practice and pathology), John King (obstetrics and diseases of women and children), Zoheth Freeman (surgery), and John Wesley Hoyt (chemistry, pharmacy, and medical jurisprudence).[50]

Claiming that the mortality rate for those treated by eclectic practitioners averaged less than 2 percent (compared with 5 percent or more for the regulars), supporters confidently held that their reform system did not arise from discarding old and well-established truths but derived instead from "a close adherence to clinical experience . . . and the fruit of extensive observations upon the diseases of the United States in all climates, from Canada to Mexico."[51] In the cholera epidemic of 1849, the eclectics in Cincinnati reported a more successful cure rate than did the regulars: they claimed five deaths in 330, while regulars reported 116 deaths out of 432 cases.[52] The combination of new remedies derived from indigenous plants and cautious empiricism constituted the basis of eclectic medicine's claims of more successful cures.

A Matter of Definition

In the early days, the graduates of the New York and Worthington schools were designated as *botanic, reformed, American,* and even *Beachite.* By the mid 1840s, however, the title *eclectic* became their official designation. The name appears to have originated with Morrow, who employed the term in the *Western Medical Reformer* (when reissued at the E. M. Institute) as early as 1846. Nevertheless, the origin of the term remains somewhat muddied, with some suggesting that it derived from Rafinesque and others believing that it came from Calvin Newton, M.D., and even from a letter written by Dr. Benjamin Waterhouse of the Harvard Medical School to Samuel Thomson. Thomas Cooke, M.D., a botanic physician from Philadelphia, founded the *Botanic Medical Reformer and Home Physician,* a periodical intended to unite botanic physicians under one roof. Cooke adopted the term *eclectic* to designate his school of thinking and, in 1841, formed the Eclectic Botanic Medical Association of Pennsylvania, which lasted thirty years.[53] Beach had his own interpretation, recalling a discussion with Thomsonian physician Isaac J. Sperry of Connecticut. Sperry had disdainfully identified Beach as an eclectic, to which he supposedly responded: "You have given me the word which I have wanted; I am an Eclectic!"[54]

In their attempts to substantiate the intellectual origins of eclecticism, reform physicians were fond of turning to the medical ancients, beginning with Athenaeus of Attaleia and continuing with his pupil Claudius Agathinus of Sparta, the teacher of the Syrian Archigenes of Apamea. These men believed in the existence of an immaterial, active spirit, or pneuma, whose condition was considered the source of health and disease. Counted among the pneumatic or spiritualistic physicians, Athenaeus established a school of medicine built upon a rational and philosophical basis that he called *episythetic,* meaning accumulative or collective, drawing from all systems that which best served the needs of the sick.[55]

Others to whom the American eclectics attributed their intellectual origins included the alchemist and physician Paracelsus, who "disturbed the calm belief in Galenic medicine" by opposing the humoral theory of disease, teaching instead that diseases were specific entities curable by specific remedies; and the Belgian anatomist Andreas Vesalius (1514–64), one of the first to dissect the human body and the author of *De humani corporis fabrica libri septem* (1543). They also looked to Daniel Sennert (1572–1637), a professor at the University of Wittenberg in Germany, who attempted to draw from the conflicting doctrines of medicine a consistent set of principles, beginning with Hippocrates and extending through Paracelsus and his successors in medical theory and practice; English physician and anatomist William Harvey (1578–1657), with his discovery of the circulation of the blood; Dutch naturalist Antoni van Leeuwenhoek, who made simple microscopes through which he studied microorganisms, restoring observation to a leading position in the science of medicine; Edward Jenner (1749–1823), who announced his discovery of vaccination in 1798; and German physician and professor of pathology and therapeutics at the University of Berlin Christoph Wilhelm Hufeland (1762–1836), who started his *Journal of Practical Medicine* in 1795 to fight medical systems. Following in these mens footsteps came such individuals as Carl R. A. Wünderlich (1815–77), whose treatise on animal heat helped to found clinical thermometry; Czech clinician of the New Vienna School Joseph Skoda (1805–81); and Austrian physician Karl von Rokitansky (1804–78), whose work led to modern pathological anatomy. According to the American eclectics, each of these individuals helped to lay the foundations of the eclectics' therapeutic system.[56]

In addition to these men, the American eclectics also pointed to the period from 1830 to 1848, known as the Era of French Eclecticism. During those years, the Paris clinical school eschewed theories and dogmas, countenanced skepticism and political liberalism, and cultivated a variety of new methods and principles. E. H. Ackerknecht identified Auguste Chomel, Pierre Louis, Gabriel Andral, Pierre Rayer, Jean-Baptiste Bouillaud, Pierre-Aldolphe Piorry, Léon Rostan, and Armand Trousseau as among the more significant eclectics working at the Pitié, Salpêtrière, Charité, and Hotêl Dieu.[57] Alexander Wilder, apologist, defender, and official historian of reform medicine, explained that each of these individuals represented threads connecting the American eclectics with the past.[58]

In large part, French medical eclecticism derived from the

philosopher Victor Cousin (1792–1867). Cousin's *Fragments Philo-sophiques* (1826) formulated eclecticism as a philosophical method. Believing that all truth had probably been discovered, it was only necessary to pick and choose from that which already existed. But for biographer Jules Simon, the selection of ideas and methods that Cousin provided in his so-called eclecticism was not philosophy. Instead, it was "a sort of echo repeating all sounds."

> Once infatuated with eclecticism, a man is not only disinclined to think for himself, but he enters the schools of teachers utterly opposed to one another, in a settled spirit of docility and conciliation which induces him to accept a little from each and to unite opposites. This extreme aptness to conciliate has for its first effect to destroy the conciliator; he becomes a nobody because he belongs to everybody. He generalizes to excess, he overlooks distinctions, and without distinctions there are no ideas. . . . An eclectic is not a philosopher . . . nor is he an intelligence, for he admits all opinions; nor a will, since he belongs to anyone who will take him.[59]

In their early years, the American eclectics gave eloquent praise to the French clinical school and its glorification of observation and experiment. However, their premature focus on herbal medicines, their outward distrust of foreign influences, and their democratic approach to education caused them eventually to concentrate on a more nativistic blend of practical medicine.

With the establishment of the E. M. Institute, Morrow and his colleagues used the term *eclectic* to describe those persons who accepted the views of medical reform (i.e., that the practice of medicine should be free and untrammeled by a standard of faith or medical creed). Morrow intended for the school to become a catalyst for permanent reform of the healing art in "the most enlarged and liberal spirit of medical eclecticism." His purpose, as explained in the institute's official organ, the *Eclectic Medical Journal* (successor to the *Western Medical Reformer*), was to "draw from any and every source all such medicine and modes of treating disease as are found to be valuable, and at the same time, not necessarily attended by bad consequences."[60]

Democratic and empirical in their approach to medicine, the eclectics reflected the pretensions of the young republic. In a series of articles in the *Eclectic Medical Journal* highlighting the history of the institute, Bickley characterized eclecticism as that system of medical philosophy which rejects all theories not founded on well ascertained facts; which recognizes experiment as the basis of progressive medicine; which carefully scrutinizes all systems, and adopts such, and such only, as stand the tests of experience; and which rejects no theory, no opinion, without first submitting it to the ratiocination of inductive science.[61] Similarly, Harvey W. Felter's official history of the E. M. Institute begins in the same manner: "The history of the Eclectic Medical Institute is the history of the contest for freedom in medical thought and teaching. It is the history of the struggle of a few determined men . . . to build a great institution of learning; it is a history of success in the face of adversities and trials within and without the fold. It is, in brief, the history of the God-mother of American medicine."[62]

The E. M. Institute encouraged its graduates to draw from any and every source all medicines and modes of treating disease found to be of value. "We condemn nothing merely because it is used by others, nor do we adopt anything merely by the recommendation of others. We estimate the thing itself, regardless of the source from whence it emanated." The founders of reform medicine did, however, reject poisonous minerals in the belief that alternatives from the vegetable kingdom were safer and more efficacious in the cure of disease.[63]

Eclectic practitioners viewed the canon of medical literature as partly verifiable by experience but mostly as unacceptable and unreliable. The inconclusiveness of medicine meant that eclectics had to enlarge their experience, train their judgment, and then decide for themselves. They needed to learn to be guided in their decisions by the accumulated wisdom of medical predecessors but not to be bound by past wisdom because it was impossible to lay down absolute rules for all cases. Instead, the proponents of reformed medicine placed their faith in the common sense and decent instincts of fellow practitioners. The most reliable sign of medical progress lay in the realization that a few select men were able to practice without the conviction that they were obeying unalterable rules. These risk takers achieved what the great mass of practitioners failed to accomplish. The task of the modern eclectic was to teach mainstream medical practitioners to live as this small minority had lived and to understand that in the disbelief of past authorities lay the opportunity for physicians to practice independent, rational medicine.

The eclectics were strong believers in the proposition that the physician was the helper of or assistant to nature, thus they discarded most of the antiphlogistic and depletive practices of allopaths. Eclectic medicine encouraged practices that maintained the vitality of the patient and shunned those that celebrated the system of Sangradoism, which according to critics had felled more victims than had the sword. The reformers also avoided using remedies that produced results worse than the diseases they were intended to cure. They condemned outright the mercury and arsenic preparations, which changed the animal economy and deposited deleterious elements in the tissues. Reformers regarded it as their highest duty to assist the natural efforts of the system by administering remedies that acted in harmony with natural functions.[64]

Alexander Wilder (1823–1908), secretary of the National Eclectic Medical Association, viewed the American school of reform medical practice as having begun, like all world faiths, in an environment of persecution from orthodoxy. "This was not because of any malpractice or ill success," he observed, "but because of their fidelity and the certainty of a more successful rivalship." Even though the United States had moved out from under domination by England, its people had not yet found full expression in an indigenous set of principles. "The reign of the sceptre, the belt and the crosier" had departed, but elements of "worn-out despotisms" remained entrenched in certain dogmas, policies, and systems, including medical systems. Enlightened medical men, among them Benjamin Rush, objected to conferring "exclusive privileges upon certain bodies of physicians, and imposing disabilities upon others their equals." Extending to medicine the same doctrine as found in the Declaration of Independence—to which Rush was a signatory—he urged his colleagues to free themselves from the tyranny of schools of medical thought.[65]

Wilder applauded Rush's stand and urged America to take the lead in political, religious, and medical independence. The nation's doctors should emancipate medicine from the totalitarianism of exclusive systems and their privileged bodies of practitioners. "When any dogma, policy or system has been weighed in the balance by the most eminent of its adherents, and has been by them found wanting," wrote Wilder, "we are abundantly warranted in turning from it to seek a more excellent way." So it was, "in the exercise of a natural right, and in obedience to the call of duty," that the new American eclectic practice was born. Wilder's comment, which sounded much like Thomas Paine's *Common Sense* (1776) and the introduction to the Declaration of Independence, was not unlike what the early founders of reformed medicine stated and the embodiment of the kind of revolutionaries to whom they likened themselves.[66] As another eclectic remarked: "It is the republican element descended into the domain of science and philosophy; for eclecticism is Republicanism, par excellence, and stands out in striking antithesis to the servile, exclusive and pedantic dogmatism which so extensively characterizes the exanimate and fossilized systems of the past."[67]

Wilder was just one of many who viewed American reform medical practice as an important epoch in the history of medicine, the birth of a new art of healing that, like the colonies in their separation from England, symbolized the end of the reign of privilege and the beginning a new age "baptized in the fire and spirit of liberty."[68] Trusting in an American practice that relied on remedies supplied from the indigenous plant life of the Western Hemisphere, he advocated medicine grounded in vegetable remedies— yellow dock, sarsaparilla, wintergreen, birchbark, elecampane, comfrey, sassafras, plantain, whitewood, dandelion, snakeroot, hardhack, horseradish, and peppermint. As Wilder put it, the eclectic school "is essentially American. It was born on American soil; it was baptized by American blood; it has been championed by Americans during its whole existence. It has its colonies, but is American in its conception, American in its practices, and I hope to heaven that it will always be American in its nature."[69]

The intent of the words—*American system, American school of medicine, American reformed school, eclectic, reformed medicine,* and *reformed medical practice*—signified movement away from the dominant party in medicine. Had the art and science of medicine, as taught and practiced by the allopaths, been in keeping with their knowledge of the collateral sciences of medicine, wrote H. E. Firth, M.D., in 1878, "they would have been a useful power in the world, and a blessing to humanity, for their organization was complete. But the 'fallacy of the Faculty' was too apparent, and subsequent history has demonstrated that their whole philosophy of treating disease was incorrect." As practiced, allopathic medicine reduced the strength of the patient through bleeding, drastic purging, and puking in order to cure disease. Such drugs as tartar emetic, calomel, and other corrosive mineral poisons disorganized the blood, disintegrated the tissues, and paralyzed the brain and nervous system; similarly, allopaths tortured patients with blisters, setons, cupping, leeches, and actual cautery. The whole philosophy of allopathy, argued Firth, opposed "the efforts of nature and the best interests of the afflicted."[70]

Firth likened the beginnings of reform medicine to the technology and inventiveness of the nineteenth century: "Eclecticism, like railroads, steam and the electric telegraph, was but the natural outgrowth of an advanced civilization, and the legitimate result of republican institutions. Eclecticism was germinated, conceived and developed as the normal product of science, and was nourished amid those surroundings which have for their support fixed laws and principles." It was a philosophy that allied itself to no single body of belief, no particular system of practice, no listing of prescriptive principles. Instead, it claimed full freedom for choosing that which proved most useful in the interest of suffering humanity. Essentially, eclecticism represented "the antipode of prejudice and bigotry."[71]

Others who reflected on the origins of eclecticism were equally interested in establishing its measure of worth within the context of American culture. Trusting that reformation would take place in medicine to the same extent that reformation occurred in religion, G. W. Churchill, M.D., in an address before the Bay State Medical Reform Association in 1849, called for a reform spirit that would emancipate medicine from "rules and servile fear" and create a free exchange of sentiments on all subjects of inquiry. "A catholic Eclectic spirit," he argued, "can result in nothing short of an eradication of the errors and abuses we deplore, and the advance of science, skill and success in the use of means and modes of cure."[72]

To William Paine, M.D., professor of the principles and practice of medicine and pathology in the Eclectic Medical College of Pennsylvania, in Philadelphia, reform medicine differed from allopathic and sectarian practice in its determined effort to ascertain more precisely the natural causes and events of disease and the workings of medicines and in its continued research into the vegetable, mineral, and animal kingdoms for the resources to remove disease. To achieve these objectives, eclectics advocated a "spirit of liberality and progression," which dispensed with "creeds and cliques" in the profession. It became the duty of every physician to investigate each system of medicine, regardless of its origins, and to make all potential resources available for the relief of the sick. Like other reformers, Paine objected to the use of mercury, lead, zinc, arsenic, and any other mineral "incompatible with the organic tissues." Far better to leave the disease to the unaided efforts of nature "than attempt to remove it with medicine, unless its indications are demonstrated by observation and science." Indeed, like other eclectics, Paine discouraged the practice of constant drugging as intemperate and harmful. He urged the adoption of physiological and hygienic methods of curing and preventing disease, including regulation of the diet, temperature, and air purity; and he advocated bathing, friction, proper clothing, and mental and physical training.[73]

Not unlike other apologists for eclecticism, Paine believed that reform medicine advanced to the rank of an exact science by finding a middle ground between the extremes of ultraconservatism and fanatical reform. As conservatives, eclectics respected the labors and discoveries of their predecessors by adhering to those doctrines that long usage and extensive experience and science had demonstrated to be true. As reformers, however, eclectics boasted that they had extended their research into every direction that promised to expand the existing stock of medical knowledge, "paying no homage to the aristocracy and learned pedantry of the profession."[74] Paine also urged eclectics to inform the public on the true merits of the different systems and warned against trusting their health to those persons ignorant of their more enlightened principles and practice of medicine. In this manner, the spirit of true eclecticism became one of liberality and progression, based on scientific principles and inductive experience, devoted to the investigation of "all the therapeutic resources of every school," selecting from each "that which science and experience has proved beneficial in the treatment of disease."[75]

Others saw eclecticism as not so much a system as a "spirit, the inchoate condition of the incoming era of thought." It was neither an accident nor a discovery of any one individual but the "spontaneous and necessary out-birth of the reflective energies of the progressive element in human society." It did for the religions, sciences, and philosophies of the modern age what Socrates did for Greek philosophy. By starting with the principle of toleration and the belief that every system originated from the spontaneous intuition of man and contained some element of truth, eclecticism became "the arbitrator among the diverse systems." Though still in its infancy, eclecticism had "throttled the vast serpentine coils of the confused systems of modern times" through an ardent spirit of inquiry and an attempt to arrange the various elements of science and pull from its many errors the basis of reason. Believing that error proceeded from reflection and not from spontaneity, eclectics advanced their medicine as an action-oriented reform movement, based not on doctrine but on "the profoundest condition of thought itself." By introducing Socratic inquiry into the pretensions of past systems, reformed practitioners could interrogate claims "concealed in the mists of venerable darkness" and arrive at last at the enfranchisement of thought.[76]

Finally, there were those who objected to the identification of eclecticism with *any* of the more fashionable "-pathies," preferring instead to call it "PANTO-pathic." It was a system in which "its votaries have the largest liberty to choose, and which denies the right of any society or college to dictate a medical creed, or a limited routine of practice to the profession." As a philosophic position, eclecticism represented "a protest of American common sense and experience against the traditional dogmas, the antiquated theories, and the aristocratic rules which have cramped and degraded the medical profession."[77] In this regard, physician P. John from Millville, Pennsylvania, viewed eclectic medicine as "randoming," by which he meant the art of conjecturing or the science of guessing.[78]

The sectarian tide swept westward, mainly in the hands of the Thomsonians, eclectics, and homeopaths. The strongest intellectual tendencies were evinced by the homeopaths, who carried with them elements of romanticism, idealism, and middle- and upper-class affiliations. At the other extreme were the Thomsonians who were fiercely doctrinaire, appealing to the victims of regular medicine, and promising a much cheaper and understandable medical system. As noted earlier, they fell victim to authoritarianism and, unable to accept the professionalization of botanic medicine, remained aloof from change and slowly disappeared. Out of that schism within the Thomsonians, the physio-medicals developed a less doctrinaire version, which lasted into the early twentieth century. The eclectics, on the other hand, forged a place amid the ambiguities of medicine, asserting an openness to all of medicine's intellectual inheritance—provided, of course, that it worked.

One can only be impressed with the accomplishments of sectarian medicine since few regulars were left unaffected by its development. The sweeping gains made by the Thomsonians, eclectics, homeopaths, hydropaths, and others were evidence of the impulse to transform older medical structures. The early wave of reform medicine made converts in western New York and in the Midwest. Yet by mid-century, sectarianism had rebounded; it had moved back into the urban centers of the East as it consolidated its influence in such large cities as Boston, New York, and Baltimore, and in smaller towns in the new South and West. By this time, too, sectarians had founded their own journals, medical colleges, and educational societies.

Although immigrants took to the new sects, most preferred the security of the older medical systems. In large part, medical sectarianism remained a genuinely American phenomenon, which drew from Yankee stock and became a fellow traveler with the ideas of abolition, temperance, nativism, pacificism, and others. As such, it represented no aesthetic contemplation of a perfected universe but rather a patriotic assertion and vindication of democratic self-respect.

4

Buchanan's Feuds and Fads

In a certain sense, eclectic medicine was less a school of thought than a temperament, disposition, or attitude. It stood squarely at the center of American intellectual thinking at mid-century. At once romantic and nationalistic, chafing at the confinement of orthodox medical thinking, it represented the right hopes, the shared vision, and the curiosity that invigorated much of America. Proponents of reform medicine were filled with a moral imperative to seek the authority of their own convictions rather than the settled thinking of Old World medicine. Indeed, they reflected much of America's ambiguity in the nineteenth century, in that, at any one time, the prophet, idealist, evolutionist, optimist, and reformer labels seemed to apply without clarification or consistency.

Yet throughout its early and middle years, reform medicine was both enriched and embarrassed by colorful advocates who directed their passion and energy toward medical reform. In no mood for compromise, these medical iconoclasts drew strength in anticipation of controversy and interparty clashes. Few were peacemakers; instead, they showed contempt for other people's opinions and trumpeted the principles of their protestant inheritance. Although much of their scholarship was original, it was often coarse and dilettantish, filled with leaping non sequiturs that gave it buoyancy but little else. As tireless writers, their brilliance and literary flourish often overshadowed reason and good judgment. High-spirited, they admitted no regrets or misgivings. In a time when science had not yet come of age and few settled standards in medicine existed, they threw so many ideas into circulation and wrote so sincerely that few could ignore their words. Much of their work was ephemeral and much of it bound by regional and local needs; nonetheless, they remained in the mainstream of American thought and culture. What they insisted was universal, a final synthesis of medicine, turned out to be most often a regional (and sometimes national) reflection of American preoccupations.

For a homogeneous people, who lived close to the soil, who were cautious and doubtful of their place in world affairs, and who were intensely religious but unexpressed in arts and letters, these reformers represented the flowering of imagination that asserted their right to a role in the life of the mind. One of the best descriptions of this band of reformers came from John M. Scudder, himself an eclectic, who edited the *Eclectic Medical Journal* through much of its tumultuous history. "They were," he wrote, "very warlike, pugnacious as snapping turtles, but they had abundant cause for it; they were Ishmaelites, and every man's hand was against them, and they were inclined to turn their hands against other people."[1] Almost any of the early medical reformers could have fit Scudder's description; one individual, however—Joseph R. Buchanan (1814–99)—stands out among the eclectics.

A Dean's Dialectic

In 1842, Joseph R. Buchanan, who was described by contemporaries as a medical philosopher, investigator, speculative reasoner, scientist, and general scholar but who had "obtained no eminence as a practitioner of medicine," was briefly affiliated with the American Medical Institute (Independent Thomsonian) in Cincinnati, occupying its chair of institutes of medicine and diagnosis. There, he began teaching a neurological system, which he claimed had grown out of efforts in Europe and America to place the philosophy of man on a scientific basis.[2] The school's journal, the *True Thomsonian*, published several of his early papers. However, the institute failed to attract sufficient students; and Buchanan, ever anxious for a position from which to espouse his theories, made friends with the pioneers of the American reformed medical practice.

In March 1846, Buchanan joined the faculty of the E. M. Institute and, for a period of ten years, dominated its affairs and its journal, first as chair of physiology, then as professor of the institutes of medicine and medical jurisprudence, and finally, from 1850 to 1856, as dean of the faculty. A lecturer on phrenology and anthropology, Buchanan was a persuasive oral and written communicator, controlling discussions at faculty meetings, inciting cabals, and advocating his own idiosyncratic views of the world and of medicine. Although possessed of little medical knowledge, he claimed to have recognized the errors of medical orthodoxy and, as opportunity warranted, zealously defended the cause of reform medical practice. His favorite remedies included the extract of bullock's blood; gruel and beef tea; tapioca and cod-liver oil; bran loaf; various alkaline, conium and starch, creosote, iodine, sulfur, iron, oak-bark, and saltwater baths; and the preparations of pepsin, American hellebore, black snakeroot, quinine and belladonna, veratrine ointment, belladonna and monkshood (aconite), and podophyllum.

Buchanan's father, a highly literate man of unstable disposition, had dabbled in philosophy, education, medicine, and journalism. The son of this jack-of-all-trades seemed no less a prodigy, learning geometry and astronomy at six and studying Sir William Blackstone's *Commentaries on the Laws of England* at twelve. Following the death of his father, young Buchanan supported himself as a printer and then as a schoolteacher. He matriculated at the Medical Department of the University of Louisville after showing an interest in phrenology and cerebral physiology. A precocious medical student, he announced his discovery of two new sciences: one, which he labeled *psychometry*, demonstrated the influence of clairvoyance on the cerebral tissues of certain individuals; the other, *sarcognomy*, sought to determine the true relationship between mind and body. After graduation in 1842, Buchanan lectured throughout the North and South and later established a monthly periodical, *Journal of Man* (1849), which applied the principles of physiognomy, craniology, and psychometry in the analysis of individuals living and dead.[3]

The faculty at the E. M. Institute considered Buchanan "the ornamental element" of the school and set him to work as their official mouthpiece in representing the cause of eclecticism.[4] And, in point of fact, he was second to none in his role as spokesman for the school, its faculty, and its reform philosophy. One of his staunch admirers even put Buchanan to verse.

> But much, Daguerre, as has thy genius done
> In Educating this Latona's son,
> In thus educing, in the god of light,
> The power to paint so, at a single sight,
> BUCHANAN has transcended thee, as far
> As the sun's face outshines the polar star.[5]

To Buchanan, eclectic medicine had four important objectives to accomplish: *first*, the renovation and reform of the medical profession; *second*, the enlightenment of the public on reform medical practice; *third*, the accumulation of statistics demonstrating the superiority of the eclectics' practices; and *fourth*, the attainment of legal equality and increased professional standing of alternative medicine. To achieve the first objective, Buchanan urged reform physicians to send at least one student annually to a "liberal medical school" to ensure the "complete triumph of our principles, and the ultimate redemption of America from the curse of a destructive system of medication." He also encouraged reform medical schools to accept youths between fourteen and sixteen years of age rather than wait until they were twenty-five or older. By making this change, young men could begin their medical careers full of enthusiasm and energy much earlier and, over time, this youthful army would ensure the dominance of reform medicine. To realize his second objective, Buchanan recommended the publication of tracts to explain to the general public the facts of eclectic medicine. "With truth and justice on our side . . . we need nothing but a fair and full exhibition of arguments to impress and convince every candid mind." A few thousand copies in the hands of each eclectic physician would successfully propagate the cause and would rapidly change the current of public sentiment.[6] In his effort to collect statistics with which to demonstrate the superiority of eclectic practice, his third objective, Buchanan appealed to the practitioners of reform medicine to maintain accurate records of their cases. To assist in this process, he suggested a format that, if used, could be sent to the *Eclectic Medical Journal* and reported in its annual summaries. Lastly, Buchanan urged eclectic reformers to petition state legislatures with demands for equality with allopaths. In Cincinnati, he pushed for equal privileges with the Medical College of Ohio in the Commercial Hospital. He also insisted that the college's medical library be accessible to all physicians and their students, regardless of their beliefs.[7]

During his tenure at the institute, Buchanan reiterated several themes, which resonated among eclectic practitioners from New York to the South and to the West. The American republic, he observed, derived its greatness from those who fled Europe to escape the persecution of outworn systems and creeds. As medical protestants, eclectic reformers abhorred medical hierarchy and praised individual freedom. Recognizing but one medical profession, consisting of the accumulations of all ages, experiences, and observations, eclectics had made an ecumenical stand, candidly acknowledging all that was contributed to the healing art and neither despising nor rejecting anything that was the product of honest investigation. Until medicine outgrew its party affiliations and extinguished the need for medical sectarianism, every reform physician was obligated to understand the full range of medical sciences and communicate his observations to others.[8]

Like other eclectics, Buchanan looked to progressive reformers in the past and present who had triumphed over the hunkerism of conservative medical thinking. In former times, the friends of progress had battled for the doctrine of the circulation of the blood, the multiplicity of functions in the brain, the practice of inoculation and vaccination, the use of cold water and quinine in fever, the treatment of scurvy with acids and vegetables, the treatment of insanity by anodyne tonic and restorative measures, and the use of ether and chloroform as anesthetics. In his own day, Buchanan viewed medicine as struggling for improvements that, while not entirely established, were in hopeful transition, including the treatment of consumption with nutrient, tonic, and invigorating regimens; the treatment of cholera by alteratives and simple stimulants; the preservation of the vital powers in place of the lancet and other debilitating modes of treatment; the truth of the general principles of phrenology; the existence of extraordinary phenomena that were not yet fully understood but were observed in mesmeric experiments; and the improvement of the materia medica by more careful attention to botany and by the progressive disuse of older agents, such as mercury, arsenic, lead, antimony, and copper.[9]

In his lectures at the institute, the dean fondly placed reform medicine in the context of world history. The first quarter of the nineteenth century witnessed the development of the new science of phrenology, founded by Franz Joseph Gall and Johann Christoph Spurzheim. This science, an intellectual newcomer, "more pregnant with the germs of great thought, and great reforms, than any other form of human knowledge," promised to change significantly the understanding of the brain and its functions. The second quarter of the century became an American movement for the regeneration of the medical profession by means of a denial of the "absolute authority of its leaders to impose a creed upon its members." This initiative grew out of the influence of a "common sense" and a "common conscience" among American practitioners who achieved, with the assistance of their medical colleges and journals, the repeal of laws restricting the practice of medicine. Leaders, such as Wooster Beach, Thomas Vaughan Morrow, and Ichabod Gibson Jones, had accomplished in medicine what Daniel Boone, Meriwether Lewis, and William Clark had achieved in opening the West.[10] The third quarter of the nineteenth century, said Buchanan, found the eclectics vindicated and at the head of the reform movement, confirming their rights to freedom of thought and moving science to newer triumphs in clinical medicine. "The great feature of this second era of medical reform," he observed, "is the breaking down of the last fortification of Medical Hunkerism, leaving it entirely at the mercy of the people." No longer would medicine's quixotic voices impede the progressive spirit of the new generation. Warning against what he believed to be false systems and ancient wrongs, Buchanan advocated a truly democratic medicine, free from "despotic greed" and the "penalty of professional excommunication." Eclecticism represented the "giant intellect of Young America," which had banished past creeds and precepts for a pioneering spirit and its celebration of the self-reliant individual, unfettered by the dictates of the American Medical Association.[11]

Buchanan accused the allopathic schools of demanding full adherence to their doctrines. In St. Louis, for example, the medical faculty had placed physicians under their control for *life*, giving the faculty the power to expel graduates from the profession or to withdraw diplomas if they in later years deviated from orthodoxy. This insistence on medical hunkerism ran counter to the spirit of the age by attempting to compel the young men of the country "to wear the collar of professional servitude, while it hurls anathemas against honorable and independent cultivators of science."[12]

In "Song of the Reformers," written by Buchanan and sung to the tune of "The Star-Spangled Banner," the students and faculty at the E. M. Institute closed ranks to celebrate their origins and their mission.

Song of the Reformers

Come rouse up, Reformers! the night has gone by!
   Through the blue vault of Heaven the sunlight is beaming,
The clouds have departed, and beneath a clear sky,
   Our flag far and wide is now gallantly streaming.
We march as an army—united and true.
     Then rouse up, Reformers! the night has gone by,
     And our flag, far and wide, is now floating on high.

We battle against the dread armies of Death!
   And to God alone look for the biddings of duty;
Our oracles are not a frail mortal's breath—
   We kneel before Nature and worship her beauty.
And we march to a victory, bloodless and blessed!
'Tis to conquer Disease and relieve the distresed.
     Then rouse up, Reformers! the night has gone by,
     And our flag, far and wide, is now floating on high.

We've broken our fetters—they are trampled in dust,
   We've crushed every barrier in our career;
And conquer we will—and conquer we must!
   For the might of Jehovah shall go with us here.
Then on! like the Templar Knights, valiant of old,
Yet gentle and graceful, and winning as bold.
     Cry onward! Reformers! the night has gone by,
     And our flag, far and wide, is now floating on high.

Away with your systems of falsehood and wrong,
   That only were made for the dullard and craven;
When we battle for truth we are mighty and strong,
   And we dare to be free as the wild winds of Heaven!
Our watchword's Progression! our day is before us;
And the Sun of Reform has but dawned on its glories!
     Cry onward! Reformers! the night has gone by,
     And our flag, far and wide, is now floating on high![13]

Dissension

Buchanan, ever an enthusiastic believer, fluent speaker, and willing fighter, not only exposed the errors of old-school medicine but waged a noble war against its physic. An admirer of Samuel Hahnemann and his homeopathic theories on dynamization and drug potencies, Buchanan decided that the E. M. Institute could benefit from a broader medical program that would include these ideas. Partly in an attempt to counteract Dr. Hans Birch Gram's efforts to set up a homeopathic college in Cleveland, Ohio, Buchanan and Benjamin L. Hill (1813–71) urged their colleagues to establish a chair of homeopathy.[14] One consequence of Buchanan's effective lobbying was that Morrow issued a circular in 1849 inviting homeopathic physicians to nominate a professor for the institute. Several weeks later, a convention of homeopathic physicians representing the northern part of the state recommended Dr. Storm Rosa (1791–1864) of Painesville for the professorship. As a further demonstration of openness, the *Eclectic Medical Journal* offered its columns to Dr. David Sheppard to present the opinions, theories, and therapeutic practices of homeopathy.

These actions, however liberal (or strategic) their intent, resulted in a heated debate among the institute's faculty, with Professors Alexander H. Baldridge and James H. Oliver resigning and Wooster Beach forced into retirement. As reported by Buchanan, the faculty discovered the "utter incompetency" of Beach, accusing him of providing a "silly and undignified professional course and literary plagiarism," which only reflected his "age and mental weakness." Baldridge, on the other hand, was accused of giving "dull, tedious, illiterate and uninstructive" lectures. Fired from his lectureship, Baldridge proceeded to establish the American Reform Medical Institute in Louisville in 1849, anticipating that, with the internecine problems continuing at the E. M. Institute, the new college might eventually become the center of reform medicine in the southwestern states. Unfortunately for Baldridge, the college and his expectations died for lack of students.[15]

Horatio P. Gatchell, M.D., a noted homeopath, filled the vacancy created by Baldridge's departure. With Gatchell in special, general, and pathological anatomy and with Storm Rosa in principles and practice of homeopathy, delivering the first homeopathic lectures in the West, the institute came to the first critical crossroads in its history. Essentially, the faculty found itself in the peculiar position of advocating the best of all systems yet giving special recognition to homeopathy as first among equals. In the end, the experiment proved an embarrassment, with both homeopaths and eclectics demanding a clarification of the institute's future direction. Buchanan belatedly realized the problems and contradictions of the undertaking and, in his presentation of the views of the faculty before the institute's trustees, argued that, "although the eclectic principles are sufficiently comprehensive·to harmonize with all forms of truth, and although the two systems coincide in rejecting blood-letting, mercurial poisoning and other abuses, the eclectic and homeopathic parties cannot harmoniously cooperate until the latter shall have changed its character." Specifically, "a party governed by one idea alone, and rejecting everything else, will not harmonize with eclectic reformers, who hold fast to the results of experience, and present reform in a conservative instead of destructive manner."[16]

At the close of the 1849–50 session, the faculty voted to abolish the chairs, forcing Rosa to move to Cleveland, where he accepted an appointment in obstetrics at the newly formed Western College of Homeopathy. Gatchell accepted the chair of anatomy at the same school but later moved to Chicago, Illinois, where he served as professor of physiology at the Hahnemann Medical College. Nevertheless, before the coalition ended, six students graduated from the E. M. Institute with both eclectic and homeopathic diplomas.[17]

When Morrow died in July 1850, confusion enveloped the school. Dr. Ichabod Gibson Jones became dean of the college but failed to fill Morrow's shoes; in addition, the faculty seemed unable to rise above personal animosities, ambitions, and jealousies to carry forward the educational mission of the institute. With the business side of the college becoming a "mass of confusion," the trustees invited Professor Robert S. Newton (1818–81) of the Memphis Medical Institute in Tennessee to take charge of the school. Newton's medical education had begun as a regular under Daniel Drake, Samuel D. Gross, Lansford P. Yandell, and Charles Caldwell at the Medical Department of the University of Louisville, where he had matriculated in 1839 and had graduated in 1841; in 1845, however, he had broken with allopathy. He then united with the advocates of reformed medical practice. From 1851 until 1862, Newton taught surgery at the E. M. Institute, and during part of that time, he and Buchanan were coeditors of the the *Eclectic Medical Journal.*

In addition to offering Newton the management of the institute, the trustees and faculty invited William Byrd Powell (1799–1866), Zoheth Freeman (1826–98), and J. Milton Sanders to abandon their teaching positions at Memphis Medical Institute and accept chairs in the school. Freeman and Sanders agreed to the offer but, Powell refused to associate with what he considered to be Buchanan's idiosyncratic views. Powell had devoted a lifetime to physiological studies and especially the brain and the theory of temperaments. A student of Caldwell and a graduate of the Transylvania University Medical Department in 1823, he held that the human temperament could be read from the cranium alone, without need of hair, eyes, flesh, or even the remainder of the skeleton. Eventually, he accepted the chair of cerebral physiology at the E. M. Institute—but only after Buchanan's expulsion.[18]

Free-School Movement

Buchanan had originally expressed a desire to purchase the E. M. Institute; however, lacking sufficient capital, he settled for succeeding Jones as dean of the faculty and using his new administrative title to leverage support for some of his more progressive educational ideas. The first of his educational reforms was implemented in 1852 when he inaugurated a scheme of free, no-cost education. The plan was immediately divisive. Freeman and Sanders left in disgust, and the financial integrity of the college was nearly wrecked.[19]

Buchanan's argument was deceptively simple: it postulated the belief that society had started from a platform of individual self-interest. In this early environment, education became a matter of "mercenary speculation," which deprived the poorer classes of its benefits. Eventually, however, every great nation took an interest in its citizens, looking to improve their intelligence, thereby creating well-disciplined minds, generous sentiments, and strong moral character. Instead of taxing the diffusion of knowledge, enlightened governments endeavored to encourage the welfare of the community by increasing knowledge of the corporate society.[20] Buchanan then argued that medical schools had become perfect models of practical efficiency, imparting a greater amount of knowledge than possible from any other institution or plan of education. Medical schools were "among the most remarkable labor saving apparatus of this age of steam" and the cheapest route for young men entering the profession. Among the many schools, the eclectics stood for a more accessible system, presenting themselves as the prophets of democratic medicine, that is, open to men and women "not supplied with the gifts of fortune" nor "disposed to bow beneath the yoke of medical orthodoxy."[21]

Over and over again, Buchanan accused the allopaths of having become aristocratic and elitist, no longer providing access to impoverished young men of talent and determination. Along with its elitism, Buchanan charged allopathic schools with deliberately making themselves inaccessible to these students by increasing the number of required courses and lectures. Such was the nature of the restrictive learning advocated by those who had been educated abroad or who admired European educational systems. In countering this aristocratic bias, Buchanan urged that medical education become as free as primary education, promising that the change would end quarrelsome rivalries among schools and elevate the entire tone of medical discourse. The diploma would be awarded on merit alone, not simply upon those who could afford to purchase it. Free medical education, he argued, would end the "host of half-educated practitioners" who swarmed over the countryside. Buchanan looked to France and Germany, where students enrolled in courses free of tuition; those who aspired to the degree paid only for the diploma itself and examinations.[22]

Beguiled by the dean's eloquence (and intimidated by his threats), the faculty voluntarily renounced the usual fees and renamed the school: it became the Central Free Medical College of America. "We have decided to lay aside our professor's fees as an encumbrance to our reform," stated Buchanan, "and we have done it with alacrity, as an army upon the march would resolve to burn all its baggage, however valuable, if necessary to its rapid progress."[23] Just as America had the honor of striking the first effective blow for political freedom, so Cincinnati would now strike a blow for professional freedom. As a catalyst, Buchanan warned the faculty that the city of Cleveland had already expressed similar free-school intentions and, unless they took the initiative, Cleveland would no doubt become the model for education in the West. But if successful, Cincinnati could eventually establish a free national university and stake its claim to leadership in the West. The faculty were reluctant to ignore Buchanan's challenge given the fierce competition among urban centers in the early nineteenth century.[24]

Buchanan's free-school movement actually had less to do with a philosophy of education, or even competition with Cleveland, than with a desire for increased remuneration via a radically different marketing plan, which would leave the institute in undisputed control of eclectic medical education in the United States. Before inaugurating his plan, annual enrollment averaged one hundred students, producing an income of sixty-four hundred dollars, including tuition and diploma fees. The dean then divided revenues between stock dividends and salaries for professors. Under the free-school movement (which competing colleges interpreted as little more than a hostile takeover), the faculty anticipated enrollments of five hundred students in the fall and eight hundred in the winter and spring sessions. At twenty dollars each (fifteen for a matriculation fee and five for a clinical ticket), they expected to generate sixteen thousand dollars, plus the diploma fee; with more than two hundred diplomas conferred at twenty dollars each, the institute would collect another four thousand dollars, for a total income of twenty thousand instead of sixty-four hundred. One critic called the free-school movement little more than "a blind to entrap students, to sustain private pay lectures, to increase the sale of books, etc., and not to elevate or dignify the profession."[25]

The plans may have been promising, but reality proved otherwise as greater enrollment failed to materialize. Rather than having provided a harvest of new students and increased revenues, the plan resulted in a decline in income, an exodus of faculty, and a serious problem with financial instability. One member of the faculty felt that the scheme proved suicidal for, while it did not increase the size of the classes as expected, it did lower the dignity of the school, cut the salaries of the faculty, and increase the hostility from competing medical colleges. "It drove other colleges to the adoption of a reduced fee bill, and caused many honorable young gentlemen to shun the western schools" for fear of being identified as "charity students."[26] To the editor of the *Worcester Journal of Medicine*, the Cincinnati experiment simply attracted indigent students looking for a quick profession and an even quicker income, a situation that created unfortunate instances of "indolence and rowdyism" that detracted from the reputation of reform practice.[27]

After four years of disappointment, the institute quietly reversed its policy and asserted the claim for "all competent teachers [to receive] a salary sufficient to support them in good style, and to furnish them with all the incidental requirements of so responsible a position."[28] The 1855–56 session marked the end of the free-education scheme (and of the name Central Free Medical College of America) when the announcement noted a five-dollar matriculation fee, twenty dollars for tuition, twenty-five for graduation, and five for the anatomy ticket. In addition, the faculty were permitted to take on private students.[29]

Internecine feuds continued to plague the school. One particularly vicious controversy erupted around Lorenzo E. Jones, M.D., who publicly criticized the teaching abilities of several colleagues and accused Buchanan of deception by offering a private course of lectures at the Mechanic's Institute, Cincinnati, while enforcing the free-tuition scheme at his own school. In his defense, Buchanan considered the private lectures distinct from his regular college course and insisted that students attending the lectures did so on an entirely voluntary basis. When Jones took exception to the dean's explanation and wrote a scurrilous pamphlet objecting to the course, Buchanan responded in the pages of the *Eclectic Medical Journal* by accusing Jones of being "intensely selfish, avaricious and penurious, destitute of all liberal progressive and generous impulses."[30] In addition, Buchanan brought Jones before the board of trustees, who forced Jones to make the following pledge: "That no member of the Faculty shall bring before the class any subject of Faculty action, and no member of the Faculty shall address the members of the class, either publicly or privately, in a manner disparaging or unfriendly to his colleagues."[31]

So vicious had the Jones affair become that the announcement of the spring 1853 session contained a caution: "Do not permit young men to be deluded by the thousand falsehoods set afloat in flying rumors by a traitor and condemned slanderer."[32] Following continued animosity between the two men, the trustees asked Jones to resign and, when he refused, expelled him. In recalling the first time he met Jones, faculty member George Washington Lafayette Bickley commented: "I was satisfied, merely from the appearance of the man, that, if there was any truth in the philosophy of Gall,

Spurzheim, Combe, and Buchanan, he must be a very selfish man," a man who "would strive to make the rest of the Faculty submit to him in matters pertaining to the Institute."[33] Only later did Bickley discover that Buchanan had deceived the faculty regarding the charges against Jones. "Not one of us dreamed of the injustice we were doing Prof. Jones," wrote a contrite Bickley, "because we believed the statements of Prof. Buchanan, and acting upon that belief, we were united in our opinion that he ought to be expelled."[34]

Following his expulsion, Jones founded the American Medical College of Ohio. Many of the disaffected, who had originally been friends of Morrow in the institute, moved to the new school; they included T. J. Wright, Alexander H. Baldridge, Stephen H. Potter, E. H. Stockwell, W. B. Witt, J. L. Galloway, and F. D. Hill. The school soon closed for lack of students.[35]

The Crucible: Phrenology and Mesmerism

With the departure of Jones and his allies from the faculty, Buchanan had free rein to teach his favorite subjects: phrenology, neurology, psychometry, and spiritualism. His ideas on clairvoyance and spiritual communications, then better known as "the night side of nature," became leading articles in the 1849 and 1850 issues of his *Journal of Man*. During his tenure as dean, he wrote extensively on the "rappings" of the Fox sisters, the significance of scientist-mystic Emanuel Swedenborg, and the Stratford knockings, as well as on "heavenly talks" with the deceased, galvanic and electrical communication with spirits and demons, and mesmeric cures.[36]

Buchanan claimed, above all else, to be a devotee of the science of phrenology, which had begun with the anatomical research of Franz Joseph Gall (1758–1828), a German doctor who suggested a plausible account of the relationship between mind and brain. Gall assumed that specific functional significance existed in different parts of the brain. Along with his assistant, Dr. Johann Christoph Spurzheim (1776–1832), Gall built this science on three broad principles: first, that the brain was the organ of the mind; second, that the brain consisted of a number of separate organs, each related to a distinct mental faculty; and third, that the size and shape of each organ represented the measure of its power.[37] Gall's system recognized twenty-seven organs in the brain; Spurzheim revised the nomenclature and suggested thirty-five (later thirty-seven) organs, which quickly superseded those of Gall in the popular culture. The system of phrenology as taught in England and the United States became substantially the system of Spurzheim.[38]

George Combe (1788–1858) became Spurzheim's leading disciple in England and the exponent of phrenology at Edinburgh. Others included Dr. Andrew Combe (1797–1847), Sir G. S. Mackenzie, Hewett C. Watson (1804–81), and the Reverend David Welsh (1793–1845). George Combe, in *The Constitution of Man* (1828), the bible of phrenological advocates in the nineteenth century, accepted Victorian science and social science and worked them into a knowledge scheme based on familiar ideas that were grounded in physiognomy and the temperaments. According to historian David de Guistino, phrenology was "an easy philosophy, expressed in ordinary language. It was a guide to reform and to knowledge; it was a new basis of morality. It was logical and slightly mysterious, precise but flexible, awesome in judgment and yet humanely hopeful. It meant amusement and improvement, common sense and social liberation."[39]

Combe's interest in the science of phrenology waned following publication of *The Constitution of Man*; he then concentrated most of his energies on its social, political, and religious implications. Thereafter, phrenology became more social and less scientific in its direction.[40] Steven Shapin called British phrenology "a social reformist movement of the greatest significance," with Combe and his circle of friends advocating penal reform, better treatment of the insane, education of women, modification of capital punishment, and improved education for the working classes; they also recommended a reconsideration of British colonial policy. Phrenology became an instrument of individual awareness and of change based on the principles of "a social optimism which maintained that the manipulation of environmental factors could improve the human constitution."[41]

While the European users of phrenology tended toward a more conservative interpretation, focusing on the hereditary rather than the environmental nature of the brain and its functions, American phrenologists followed their English cousins in seeing it as a mechanism for ameliorative change. It represented an eminently useful science for personal, social, and political ends. Nevertheless, the methodology of phrenology was profoundly superficial, claiming the correlation between a person's moral and intellectual faculties, the size of the cerebral organs, and the observable external surface of the skull. The ability to "read" an individual's mental character derived from a desire to build an intellectual bridge between the mind and the body, between the physical landscape of the person and his or her sociological and psychological manifestations.

Spurzheim traveled to the United States in August 1832 as a missionary of the new science and was lionized by the popular press and the intellectual community. He gave lectures at Harvard, including in his audiences the medical faculty; and, although he died in November 1832, adoption of his ideas led to the formation of numerous phrenological societies. When George Combe visited the United States in 1838, he was welcomed into a community whose leading minds had already been influenced by Spurzheim and had become willing believers in the new science. Public debates—on such issues as "is phrenology true?—usually resulted in favorable responses both from the public and from the professionals. In addition, national personages like Horace Greeley, Henry Ward Beecher, Charles Caldwell, and Walt Whitman lent respectability to its claims. On the business side, the firm of Fowler and Wells Co., based in New York, "turned phrenology into a national industry," establishing parlors in New York, Boston, and Philadelphia. Their publications, lecture tours, and paraphernalia became common discussion points among aspiring intellectuals across the United States. Phrenology became the popular psychology of the day, appealing to the religious and the secular minded alike. The proponents of phrenology, glib and triumphant in the early decades of the nineteenth century, concluded that the division of the brain into different organs had the endorsement of the leading men of science. Most importantly, they concluded that phrenology was a science of practical utility that harmonized nature with natural and revealed religion. The skull became the window of the soul; and in a short time, phrenology was transformed into an American cult of huge proportions.[42]

William H. Cook, editor of the *American Medical and Surgical Journal*, said that phrenology stood before the world not only as a science but "in all the majesty of unerring Truth." Its practical advantages existed in law and government, religion and education; it also provided physicians with a window into the study of physic.

Indeed, medical faculty had the responsibility of introducing phrenology into medical schools as a part of the regular studies. In view of this commitment, Cook dedicated a continuing portion of his journal to the science of phrenology.[43]

Along with phrenology, both Americans and Europeans had an interest in the peregrinations of Franz Mesmer (1734–1815), a graduate in medicine from the University of Vienna, who introduced the phenomenon of "mesmerism" or "animal magnetism" into popular and scientific thought. Mesmer, although blessed with a respectable educational background, felt constrained by the limitations of orthodox medicine and, seeking alternatives to existing knowledge and practices, turned to the phenomena of planetary influence and to what he called the invisible "universal fluid," which enveloped the world and through which it was possible for one individual to communicate with another. Mesmer's theory of animal magnetism combined the idea of an invisible universal fluid with that of personal charisma. As a man of sentiment more than of science, wishing to make a sweeping synthesis of religious, medical, political, and social theory, Mesmer revolted against the strict rationalism of the eighteenth century. It was the "nature" of Jean-Jacques Rousseau, not that of Locke or Newton, that Mesmer and his followers worshiped. All bodies—from people to planets—were influenced by the forces of the universal fluid, and the social virtue of empathy that existed between human bodies became analogous to the forces of magnetic attraction between celestial bodies. Although what he created was insubstantial and at times even grotesque in its eccentricities, animal magnetism provided a counterforce to conventional therapy and, in retrospect, became the eventual spawning ground for hypnotism and psychoanalysis. The theory of animal magnetism represented an effort to reduce such terminology as *suggestion* and *personality* to quantifiable physical forces within the context of eighteenth-century rationalism. Animal magnetism was a subtle, invisible, and omnipresent force, but Mesmer gave it a "scientific" explanation, an explanation that reinforced the harmony among the universe, mind, body, and social adaptation.[44]

The medical faculty of the University of Paris repudiated Mesmer's claims, yet his doctrines won numerous adherents, including British physician and physiologist John Elliotson (1791–1868) and British surgeon James Braid (1795–1860). Braid, with a medical degree from the University of Edinburgh, distinguished the phenomenon of neurohypnotism, or hypnosis, from the more quackish claims of Mesmer and his followers. In his book, *Neurypnology* (1843), he attempted to prove that hypnosis could be induced without the accompanying mysticism and universal fluid postulated by Mesmer. The president of the Phrenological Society, John Elliotson, who had trained both at Edinburgh and at Cambridge University and had graduated in medicine, became aware of the medical possibilities of mesmerism from Richard Chenevix, a second-generation disciple of Mesmer. Chenevix, through his articles in the *London Medical and Physiological Journal* in 1829, encouraged further inquiry into potential medical use of the phenomenon at St. Thomas's Hospital.[45]

Phrenology and animal magnetism became almost symbiotic in their relationship after 1838. Elliotson, for example, insisted on the close relationship between the two and began using the term *phreno-magnetism*, suggesting that a patient in a mesmeric trance evidenced behavior that corresponded directly to the phrenological stimulation applied to the cranium by the mesmeric operator. In 1843, he founded the *Zoist*, a journal dedicated to the study and application of cerebral physiology and mesmerism.[46]

Buchanan's Synthesis: Sarcognomy

Gall's name stood preeminent in phrenology, but Joseph R. Buchanan claimed that his own neurological system extended the theories of Gall by perfecting the doctrine of cerebral subdivision and establishing the newer faculties of organology, modality, antagonism, cooperation, unity, and duality. The Gallian system failed to explain the laws of sympathy between mind and body, while Buchanan's neurological system demonstrated that every portion of the brain sympathized with and was connected to a corresponding portion of the body. The connection between the brain and the corporeal organs made it possible, he believed, to construct a psychological map of the body corresponding to that of the brain. Buchanan identified this newfound knowledge as *sarcognomy*. Just as physiognomy interpreted the character of the face, so sarcognomy interpreted the character of the body, revealing its laws, connections, and sympathies to the physician.[47] Sarcognomy corrected the errors of phrenology and animal magnetism by bringing "the chaos of benevolent empiricism under the jurisdiction of science."[48]

Buchanan coined the word *sarcognomy* in 1842 while he was

affiliated with the American Medical Institute in Cincinnati. Derived from *sarx* or *sarcos* (flesh) and *gnoma* (opinion), the term meant "a knowledge of the flesh, or recognition of its character and relations." From a practical standpoint, the new science implied a knowledge of the physiological and psychological powers that belonged to the body in health and in disease, and it implied the understanding of the correlation of soul, brain, and body in that relationship. The "soul of life" operated through the brain to the body. When an emotion or a passion of the soul (e.g., love or anger) worked through the brain, it expressed itself in the body by voice, action, and circulation of the blood. Similarly, the conditions of the body in health and disease acted upon the brain and soul. Thus, alcohol, fever, and some traumatic physical forces would modify the conditions of the body and its relation to the brain and soul. No physiological process or condition existed in the body that did not result in a corresponding action in the brain. The exercise of every psychic faculty (emotion, impulse, etc.) produced a characteristic effect on the body, while the exercise of any portion of the body produced a characteristic effect within the brain and mind, the locality of which could be specified on the brain. In this regard, diseases had mental as well as physical symptomatologies; in other words, the entire surface of the brain corresponded to the entire surface of the body.[49]

As a vitalist, Buchanan lamented the materialism of the reigning medical philosophies of his day, particularly the theories of French scientist and philosopher René Descartes (1596–1650) and the modern skeptic Thomas Huxley (1825–95). The Cartesian attitude of "limiting the mind to the conception of physical facts" had transformed humans and animals into "mere machines, operating without consciousness or thought, as a clock or any other physical apparatus." Buchanan also rejected Huxley's beliefs as gross scientific materialism which destroyed both religion and pneumatology (the area in which science entered the sphere of wisdom and love). Objecting strenuously to the proposition that life was only a condition of matter, Buchanan, as stated earlier, postulated the pneuma as the essence of vitality. In this regard, he allied himself with the philosophical views of English physiologist and microscopist Lionel S. Beale (1828–1906), who held, Buchanan said, that life was entirely distinct from the operation of physical forces.[50]

Buchanan considered himself a philosophical evolutionist in keeping with the tenets of Herbert Spencer, Henry Drummond, and Ralph Waldo Emerson. "Spirit perpetually struggles with matter to which it is bound," he wrote. "This was a struggle which, in the progress of evolution, would eventually result in the mastery of spirit over the conditions of the material world. At the present stage in man's development, however, we can only look to a higher stage of life which remains encumbered by matter."[51]

Buchanan spoke of the invisible and "limitless ocean" of unembodied life, the "over-soul" of the universe, which sustained and developed life, and the "divine nature," which consisted of will, wisdom, and love. These linguistic tools became the anchors of his romantic idealism, within which was discerned truth in insight and intuition and within which the external world became little more than an expression of mind. Like Emerson of Concord, Massachusetts, Buchanan subscribed to the over-soul as the appropriate metaphor connecting the individual to the universe, to nature, and to the all-encompassing existence of spirit. Emerson published the essays "The Over-Soul" in 1841 and "Nature" in 1844. From his position as editor of the *Journal of Man*, Buchanan took notice of Emerson's lectures in Cincinnati, describing him as "the most remarkable specimen, now living, of highly cultivated and intense Ideality."[52]

Buchanan also identified himself with the vitalistic doctrines of Jan Baptista van Helmont (1579–1644), George Ernst Stahl (1660–1734), John Hunter (1728–93), William Harvey, Georges Cuvier (1769–1832), and Marie-François Xavier Bichat. The philosophical basis of sarcognomy, he argued, was to be found in "the very intimate sympathy and parallelism of soul, brain and body, which enables us, through any one of the three, to affect the other two in a corresponding manner." Acting on this principle, he maintained that the treatment of disease was to support the vital force of the body, using animal magnetism, massage, electrotherapeutics, hygiene, and drugs. While he did not subscribe to the metaphysical medicine of Christian Science regarding the unreality of disease, he did approve of many of its methods.[53]

Nervauric Treatment

What others practiced as animal magnetism, Buchanan preferred to call *nervauric treatment* to circumvent hostility from the medical profession toward the original name. The "unyielding spirit of materialism," which dominated all scientific and medical circles, had effectively denigrated the cures of animal magnetism. The regulars had "shamefully neglected and discouraged therapeutic magnetism, because it could be practiced by persons without a medical education, whom they regarded as ignoble rivals." Ignoring animal magnetism, the profession confined its attention to the simple technique for producing hypnotism, carefully avoiding the claims of clairvoyants. For the medical profession to profess its support of hypnotism without recognizing the vital influence of animal magnetism represented to Buchanan a further sign of orthodox medicine's conspiracy to disregard or otherwise defame the influence of the mind as a healing factor.[54]

Buchanan held that every human being exuded a vital emanation of what he called *nervaura*, or animal magnetism. The nervaura continually and unconsciously influenced all with whom the individual came in contact. "We see this in the diffusion of smallpox and virulent fevers, in the contagious influences that rule public assemblies, and in the assimilation of those who associate together." It was especially evident in the power and "healing presence" of the physician who, under certain circumstances, could cure without medicine and even without contact with the patient. It was also realized "whenever the hands [were] placed upon the patient, whether there be any purpose or not." The influence of the hand was sufficient apart from will; but when the determined influence of the will combined with the hand, an astonishing influence came over the individual.[55]

The specific areas on the surface of the brain and body could be reached and stimulated (or tranquilized) by nervauric methods, as well as by electricity, heat, cold, and other medical applications. Each individual, however, differed from another in response to the healing arts. Highly impressionable persons (distinguished by the breadth and height of the front of the head and by large pupils) responded readily to nervauric treatment, and for them Buchanan recommended placing hands on the body to heal them. While a select few could be treated "by the soul power alone"—without any physical contact—for most, contact with the skin was essential for the most complete healing effect. Using percussion, friction, and "dispersive passes," the healer produced local and physiological effects on the body that became psychic "in proportion as the brain sympathizes with the spot."[56]

Buchanan recommended six methods of treatment. The first, manual treatment, included touch and gentle percussion for stimulation, dispersive passes with the hand, and moderate friction for stimulation. His second and third methods involved the use of galvanic and faradic currents applied to the spine or affected organ. His fourth method included various mechanical treatments, such as dry cupping, hot or cold water, and ice. The fifth consisted of stimulant and tonic plasters applied to the spine. California laurel, for example, restored spinal energy, especially in paralytic conditions. Buchanan's sixth and final method was counterirritation on the spine, which he recommended when obstinate or chronic difficulties resisted other therapeutic measures. For this technique, the healer applied mustard plasters, cantharides, ammonia, and concentrated acetic acid, as well as moxa and hot metallic buttons, which were heated to the temperature of boiling water and applied to the spine to remove pain. Another effective counterirritant from the eclectic dispensatory was the compound tar plaster.[57]

Professor Isaac Miller Comings of Manchester, Massachusetts, writing in the *Eclectic Medical Journal* in 1853, advocated the application of electrical medication under the rubric of psychology, mesmerism, and mental alchemy. Although many doubted the truths of electrical medication, considering it both visionary and impractical, Comings found it in perfect harmony with the reformed notions of medical practice and urged its use as a "powerful auxiliary to the medical practitioner." Among his recommendations was the need for "sensitive persons" to sleep with their heads pointing north to harmonize with the magnetic currents constantly passing around the earth. Comings also claimed to have successfully relieved severe back pain in a woman through "several [mesmeric] passes over the seat of the pain." For this problem, as well as for females, children, somnambulists, and individuals laboring under various nervous diseases, Comings advocated his reformed medicine.[58] Similarly, Powell and Newton gave particular deference to the ideas of George Combe and his *Constitution of Man*; to the works of Gall, Spurzheim, Andrew Combe, and other writers; to the psychological influence of the mother on the fetus; and to the importance of the moral faculties.[59]

The eclectics, as exponents of new ideas, found themselves enamored with the possibilities of phrenology and mesmerism. Admittedly, Buchanan's presence on the faculty had much to do with this influence. During his ten years at the E. M. Institute, both the school and its journal reflected his special interest in phrenology, the study of human temperaments, the importance of mesmerism in therapeutics, and his own crafted theory of cerebral physiology. For many medical-school faculties—regular and sectarian alike—the claims made by the advocates of phrenology and mesmerism could not be ignored, nor could their implications for medicine. Eclectics, as reformers, found them especially appealing for within the elaborate scheme of these two new "sciences" were the elements of a romantic and revolutionary sentiment. Clearly, as John H. Warner has explained, the E. M. Institute may have used some of the same physiology textbooks that regular schools used, but the content of physiological instruction was notably different. Buchanan's interest in the functions of the brain and in its mental powers affected the focus of physiological teaching at the E. M. Institute, the texts of the faculty during the early decades of the institute's existence, and the choice and tenor of articles in the early issues of the *Eclectic Medical Journal*.[60]

Psychometry

Buchanan identified the final piece of his system as psychometry, first discussed in his essays in the *Journal of Man* in 1849 and later incorporated into his *Outlines of Lectures on the Neurological System of Anthropology* (1854). By the term *psychometry*, derived from the Greek terms *psyche* (soul) and *metron* (measure), Buchanan meant "soul-measuring," or the measurement of an individual's psychic or soul capacity, which he considered analogous to thermometry, barometry, electrometry, and similar precise measurement systems. Buchanan believed that the soul-measuring abilities of an accomplished psychometrist could move into the darkened "underworld of the intellect" and illuminate the meaning of rare, anomalous, mysterious, and inexplicable facts of life. As a science and as a philosophy, psychometry could utilize psychic abilities in the investigation of character, disease, physiology, biography, history, paleontology, anthropology, medicine, geology, astronomy, theology, supernatural life, and destiny.[61]

Buchanan claimed to have discovered this new science in the autumn of 1842, shortly after graduating from the Medical Department of the University of Louisville. Working for a brief time in New York City with Charles Inman (the younger brother of artist Henry Inman), Buchanan found that the young man could discern the entire character of an individual merely by placing his hands upon different portions of the head.[62] But Buchanan did not stop there. On the basis of his work with Inman, he postulated that people could identify and even taste materials that were only touched. This phenomenon was significant for Buchanan because he then concluded that medicinal substances could affect patients without being consumed. So important was this discovery that he made it a part of the medical instruction at the E. M. Institute, distributing among his students various drugs concealed in paper wrappings, telling them to hold the wrappers in their hands while listening to his lecture. According to Buchanan, sensitive students soon discerned the nature of the medicines and were visibly affected by the vigorous emetic, cathartic, or stimulant effects they mentally imparted to their systems.[63]

In 1849, the members of Buchanan's medical class signed a document attesting to the witness of this event: "We, the undersigned members of the medical class of the Eclectic Medical Institute of Cincinnati . . . formed the experiment of holding in our hands, for a short time (generally from five to twenty minutes), various medicines, enveloped in paper." Although the drug properties contained in these papers were unknown to the class, they were convinced that "distinct effects were produced upon us strictly similar to those which would be produced by the action of the same medicines administered in the ordinary method." Forty-two out of 130 students testified to these effects, as did several fellow professors: Benjamin L. Hill, William Sherwood, Daniel Vaughan, Horatio P. Gatchell, and John King.[64]

Buchanan concluded from these experiments that "no consumption of medicine [was] absolutely necessary to produce medical effects." In this regard, he allied himself with the homeopaths who, using their infinitesimal doses and the principle of dynamization, claimed no diminution in drug potency as it underwent attenuation. Buchanan, however, went one step further. "The same vial of medicine may be used successfully for the medication of a thousand or of ten thousand patients," he observed, "and if well sealed it will have lost no portion of the medical substance, so far as we can discover."[65]

Disappointments

Throughout his stormy career, Buchanan complained bitterly that the medical and scientific communities had not given his ideas a fair hearing. Of major disappointment was the decision by the *Phrenological Journal* of Edinburgh to refuse publication of his investigations of the brain. Equally devastating to his pride, the Academy of Arts and Sciences in Boston refused to review his claims and test his results. In 1851, Buchanan attempted to give a paper on cerebral embryology before the American Association for the Advancement of Science meeting in Cincinnati. In his paper, entitled "On the Facts of Cerebral Embryology, and Comparative Anatomy—The Inferences Deducible Therefrom, and Their Bearing on the Science of Ethnology," he intended to shed light on the characteristics of the races as illustrated by comparative anatomy. Louis Agassiz, president of the association, accepted the paper on the basis of its title (the paper itself was not presented for review) and scheduled it for delivery on the last day of the session. However, the association omitted the paper from its published proceedings. Upon learning of Agassiz's decision, Buchanan criticized the association for not fulfilling its educational purpose. "Our so-called American Association for the Advancement of Science," he complained, "is not an association for the advancement of all sciences, but merely an association for the accumulation of physical knowledge in preference to more valuable sciences, thus serving to lay a foundation for more comprehensive science and philosophy."[66]

A similar application to the American Medical Association, formed in 1847, and its presiding officer, Samuel D. Gross, M.D., met with another disappointing response. The discoveries could not be brought under the notice of the association or subjected to investigation because, Gross said, Buchanan was not a member of the dominant medical party.[67] "I thought it useless to seek any further decision by any authoritative scientific tribunal," Buchanan wrote in disgust, and thus "[I] united with other unconquerable liberals in the medical profession to establish a liberal system of medical education and break the unreformable intellectual despotism which had held and still holds the great mass of the medical profession."[68] Years later, in 1877, Buchanan requested that an investigating committee of the Kentucky State Medical Society be assigned to examine the claims of psychometry and its relationship to the actions of medicines. A committee did form, but it did "nothing whatever in performance of [its] duty," and Buchanan left for New York City convinced once again "that it was utterly useless to lay any psychic facts before the dogmatic profession, or to invite them to investigate anything beyond their narrow routine of thought and action."[69]

Faced with these disappointments, Buchanan instead began to claim that he had demonstrated his theories before public audiences in New York and Boston and referred vaguely to investigative committees at Indiana University, Boston, and New York, which had allegedly supported his findings. He relied as well on testimonials of former students, medical professors, and colleagues at the E. M. Institute. In addition, Buchanan noted, his experiments were repeated by Professor J. K. Mitchell of the Jefferson Medical College of Philadelphia. Unfortunately, Mitchell did not have the "moral courage" to continue with the experiments. "I soon found," remarked Buchanan, "that the well-disciplined army of the followers of the European system were determined not to investigate a demonstrable, but revolutionary science, and that I was as obnoxious as Harvey ever was."[70]

Exodus

However creative his theories on neurology and sarcognomy, Joseph R. Buchanan's poor management, his bombast, his intimidation of colleagues, his free-tuition debacle, and his thirst for control brought the E. M. Institute to the brink of financial ruin. The style of his leadership as dean and his truculent disposition also exposed the school to a number of other problems, including the frustration of having continuously to confront the prejudices of regulars and the tensions of maintaining the rhetoric and substance of reform medicine. While these issues simmered for years, the elements changed abruptly following the failure of the free-school movement and the beginnings of a quarrel between Robert S. Newton and Charles H. Cleaveland over the efficacy of certain medicines known as eclectic concentrations. Cleaveland took particular exception to the medicines manufactured by B. Keith and Co.; while Newton, who owned and managed the *Eclectic Medical Journal* and also *Newton's Express*, lauded Keith's medicines. When supporters of Cleaveland (Buchanan and William Sherwood) offered to buy out Newton's interest in the journal, Newton refused, whereupon a substantial number of E. M. faculty denounced the journal and established the *College Journal of Medical Sciences* with Ichabod Gibson Jones as editor. Newton then entered into an agreement with B. Keith and Co. to publish a revised *American*

Eclectic Dispensatory that would bring the concentrated medicines into favor among eclectic physicians. The feud quickly escalated into a major battle between the Newton forces on one side and the Buchanan and Cleaveland forces on the other, with control of the *Eclectic Medical Journal* and author credit for the *American Eclectic Dispensatory* as the eventual prizes. Faculty members—who before had been so intimidated that only the brave and the foolish seemed willing to take a stand—openly challenged Buchanan and his allies. Further complicating the situation, Buchanan and his clique repudiated the National Eclectic Medical Association, which was supported by Newton and Zoheth Freeman.[71]

As treasurer for the board of trustees, Newton felt that matters at the institute had gotten precariously close to being out of control and that the financial affairs of the corporation were being "unwisely and fraudulently managed." In particular, he accused Buchanan of having collected tuition fees for both the winter and spring sessions and of having appropriated most of the money for his personal use.[72] In response to Newton's demand for the tuition money, Buchanan brazenly claimed that he had loaned the money to a friend. Newton reported the details to the faculty on March 24, 1856, and then told Buchanan to pay the balance of the money or he would place the matter before the board of trustees. Newton notified students not to pay any more money to the dean in an effort to prevent further erosion of the school's finances.[73]

In answer to Newton's threat, Buchanan, William Sherwood, Charles H. Cleaveland, John King, and John Wesley Hoyt met on April 5 and issued seven thousand dollars' worth of new stock without giving notice to the trustees, stockholders, or treasurer. They intended with the stock sale to change stockholder constituency, giving the majority to Buchanan and his friends. With this accomplished, the group met again on April 7 and voted in a new, bogus board of trustees. Sherwood, as representative of the new board, changed the locks on the doors of the institute and placed the school under the protection of the Cincinnati police.[74]

On the same day that Buchanan and his colleagues voted in the bogus board, the legal stockholders met at Newton's office and unanimously passed a resolution accusing Buchanan, Sherwood, King, Cleaveland, and Hoyt of fraudulently issuing the new stock as a means of "preventing the legitimate stockholders . . . from electing such a Board of Trustees as will protect their interest, and prevent the affairs of the Institute from being continued under the control of said faculty." The stockholders then elected a new board of trustees, which included W. B. Pierce, J. P. Mayer, A. Death, J. C. C. Holenshade, W. F. Hurlburt, H. Leonard, J. P. Cunningham, C. S. G. Wright, H. M. Ritter, J. G. Henshall, Dr. Robert S. Newton, Dr. Lorenzo E. Jones, Dr. Zoheth Freeman, Dr. Alexander H. Baldridge, and Dr. O. E. Newton. In its final motion on that day, the board appointed a committee consisting of Robert S. Newton, Lorenzo E. Jones, and J. P. Mayer to consider legal action against Buchanan and his colleagues for their involvement in the stock scheme.[75]

At a subsequent meeting of the board on April 29, the trustees passed a resolution accusing the five faculty members of violating the institute's act of incorporation by issuing illegal stock. They also removed the men from their chairs as professors, expelled them from the school, ordered Newton to take possession of the grounds, and notified students to cease paying fees to the former dean. When Cleaveland attempted a lockout of the school, Newton countered by obtaining a set of keys from the janitor's wife. Cleaveland then responded by changing the locks. Finding an open door, Newton and his band armed themselves with weapons and took possession of the building. The siege lasted nearly twenty-four hours, with Cleaveland and his forces circling the institute, armed with knives, pistols, and clubs. Undaunted, Newton dragged a six-pound cannon to the school's entrance, and the Cleavelandites wisely decided to allow the courts to resolve the issue.[76]

The five former faculty members, following their expulsion, published a resolution declaring the incompetence of Newton to fill the professorship vacated by Buchanan. As an added sign of their contempt, they urged graduates of the school not to place the word *eclectic* on their signs or business cards; rather, they recommended that they use the word *physician* since it embodied the full meaning of the medical practitioner. Furthermore, the exiled faculty issued diplomas in the name of the E. M. Institute to seventeen students who had sided with their cause.[77]

On October 25, 1856, the judge of the District Court of Cincinnati decided that the legitimate stockholders had selected Newton's office as the proper place for holding the election and that they had legally voted to reconstitute its board of trustees. The decision also declared illegal the seven thousand dollars in stock issued by

Buchanan and his colleagues, called it a fraud upon the charter, and pronounced it void.[78]

With Newton's group judged the lawful controllers of the institute and its stock, Buchanan filed in Hamilton County, Ohio, to create the Eclectic College of Medicine. The new college, with Buchanan as dean, opened in October 1856 and was composed of the faculty who had left the school and the students who had followed them. The schism proved an embarrassment for both faculties, as well as for reform medicine. In 1859, the faculties (minus Buchanan) after negotiations reunited, as did their journals, under the title *Eclectic Medical and College Journal*. Part of the reason for this merger stemmed from the events leading to the Civil War and the resulting lack of students from the southern states. For the faculty of both schools, it became evident that two rival eclectic institutions could not compete within the same region.[79]

The Final Years

Following Buchanan's expulsion from the institute, his former colleagues took a renewed interest in his writings, seeking to establish that his doctrines were actually antagonistic to reform medical practice. Calling him "J. R. Buchanan the Great," the faculty portrayed the former dean as a "frothy specimen of a medical man" who had imbibed too heavily of the subtle and ethereal whims of metaphysics and spiritualism. As Buchanan knew little of true eclectic philosophy, he turned the kindness of colleagues into efforts to aggrandize his own position. Buchanan had demonstrated his true character after he had received his professorship by having charged the school's founder with ignorance and incompetency and having conspired to have him expelled. Later, when Thomas Vaughan Morrow became seriously ill, Buchanan had even "pompously volunteered his services as the medical attendant" and, "together with his consummate arrogance and self-importance," had directed a form of treatment that eventually resulted in the founder's death in 1850.[80] According to former colleagues, Buchanan tyrannized the faculty, forcing many to resign, and expelling others in an effort to move the school toward homeopathy. Newton accused the former dean and editor of having engineered the appointment of homeopaths into their ranks and also accused him of conspiring to remove *eclectic* from the institute's name in order to place it on an allopathic basis.[81]

In 1863, Buchanan campaigned unsuccessfully for U.S. Congress as a Peace party candidate. Changing careers, he moved to Syracuse, New York, where, for a brief time, he manufactured salt. He moved once again, this time to New York City in 1867, where he joined the faculty of the Eclectic Medical College as professor of physiology. He remained on the faculty until 1881, whereupon he established the College of Therapeutics in Boston to demonstrate the use of electric and manual treatment as "a grand agency for the prevention of disease and development of health."[82]

During the 1880s, Buchanan continued to support the legal rights of eclectic and homeopathic medicine. He addressed the Rhode Island House of Representatives in 1887 on the subject of restrictive medical legislation; and in 1889, he spoke before the Judicial Committee of the Massachusetts House of Representatives about the "collegiate bigotry" of the American Medical Association. He also condemned regulars for their "knife quackery" in the treatment of cancer and appealed to state legislators to recognize the achievements of those who, "without collegiate permission," successfully cured cancer with alternative techniques.[83]

Buchanan later moved to California. There, he attempted to reestablish his College of Therapeutics in San Francisco, but when his health began to fail, he moved to San Jose where he prepared his last work, *Primitive Christianity*, which represented the culmination of his sixty years' labor. As he stated in the book's preface, a lifetime of investigations had led him "up from anatomy, physiology and therapeutics to the brain, the soul, and the eternal life of man."[84] Science, in its perfected state, harmonized with religion; the relationship between mortality and immortality merged ultimately in the psychometric powers of the new-age scientist. Using psychometric skills, Buchanan wrote *Primitive Christianity* based on "messages" received from the "high world." Messages, he said, came to him from George Washington in 1855; from St. John, while he was sitting on the platform of the Ladies Aid Society in Boston; and from Moses in 1891. He also "spoke freely" with the spirits of Abraham Lincoln, Lucretia Mott, Horace Mann, Robert Dale Owen, Samuel Hahnemann, John Wycliffe, Justin Martyr, St. James the Apostle, and the Greek biographer Plutarch.[85] Buchanan's ability to cross from the visible to the spiritual world followed a pattern set earlier by Swedish philosopher Emanuel Swedenborg (1688–1772) whose "communications" with angels and his doctrine of "influx" (one man's influence over another) led, not surprisingly, to numerous therapeutic systems based on mind cure.[86]

Buchanan continued his old association with the E. M. Institute, writing to John Uri Lloyd on occasion and informing him of his latest research. To the end, he urged the importance of magnetic healing, electrotherapeutics, psychometry, and sarcognomy. He viewed eclectic and homeopathic medicine as offering a "healthy beginning" for reform practice. However, they had failed to carry reform practice into the higher levels of healing. "If I could tumble down the old and pull out the good new timber for a true temple of science, how eagerly would I begin. But it is too near sunset unless I can conquer the table of mortality which nearly conquered me in 1897." But disappointments with state governments, which refused to recognize alternative medicine, and the unwillingness of the scientific world to test his breakthroughs in psychometry had made him bitter. All he saw was a "ram shackle corrupt Republic, fit to match our rum shackle [sic] materia medica."[87]

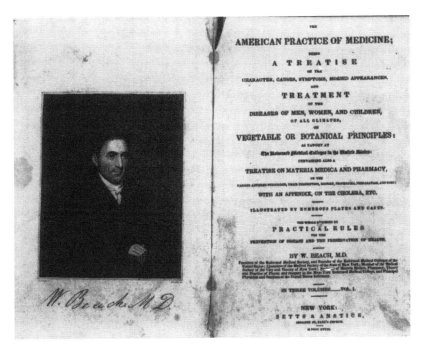

Wooster Beach, *The American Practice of Medicine* (3 vols. New York: Betts and Antice, 1833). Courtesy of the Southern Illinois University School of Medicine Library, Springfield.

NEW-YORK

REFORMED MEDICAL COLLEGE,

ELDRIDGE-STREET.

CIRCULAR.

THE happy effects of the botanical system of practice, more especially of late, employed in the cure of diseases, are such as entitle it to a high rank among modern improvements. The opinion long entertained in its favour by many of the judicious, a thorough experience has now demonstrated to be well founded; and with the number and variety of its salutary achievements, its reputation is increasing.

It must be evident to every discerning mind, that the present prevailing practice of medicine, which rejects this botanical aid, is at variance with our nature and our happiness.

MERCURY, the LANCET, and the KNIFE, are chiefly relied upon by physicians and surgeons of the present day, for the removal of almost all the diseases incident to the human body, notwithstanding the effects of those deleterious agents are evidently fatal to multitudes. Deeply impressed with these facts, and with a view of reforming the science and practice of medicine, an individual in this city, in the year 1827, procured a lot of ground, and erected a handsome and convenient edifice for an Institution, denominated the United States Infirmary, expressly for employing a reformed system of practice in the treatment of diseases: the remedial sources being chiefly derived from the productions of our own country. The course of treatment adopted by this Institution, was principally the result of nearly forty years' experience of a distinguished medical reformer; which course, we are happy to state, has been crowned with success, and proved to a demonstration that, without mercury, that boasted champion of the materia medica, or other poisonous drugs, diseases generally may be cured by those more safe and salutary means which the God of nature has so liberally scattered around us.

Animated by the past success, and with the hope of benefiting future generations, an irrepressible desire has been felt, that measures commensurate with the importance of the object should be taken to promulgate this valuable system of practice, and thereby improve and reform the noble and important science of medicine.

After reflecting for years on the most prudent and successful method of effecting so desirable an object, it has been deemed expedient to establish a Medical School, with competent teachers, where students may receive board and education, until they are fully qualified to practice in the various branches of the healing art, upon the reformed system. We are now happy to announce, that a building for such an Institution has been erected, and opened for the reception of students, who can commence at any period.

The building is large and commodious, situated in Eldridge-street, between Grand and Broome streets, adjoining the present United States Infirmary. It is in a healthy and retired part of the city, and has been completed at a great expense.

2 M

Advertisement for the New York Reformed Medical College, from Wooster Beach, *The American Practice of Medicine* (3 vols. New York: Betts and Anstice, 1833), I, 1–2. Courtesy of the Southern Illinois University School of Medicine Library, Springfield.

AMERICAN
MEDICAL AND SURGICAL
JOURNAL.

EDITED BY

S. H. POTTER, M. D.

VOL. I.   DECEMBER, 1851.   NO. 12.

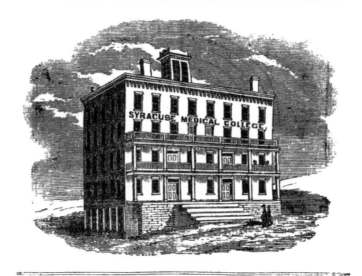

PUBLISHED BY

DRS. POTTER & RUSSELL,

SYRACUSE, N. Y.

TERMS—ONE DOLLAR PER ANNUM.

Printed at the Office of the Syracuse Daily Star.

Syracuse Medical College, from the *American Medical and Surgical Journal*, I (1851). Courtesy of the Lloyd Library and Museum, Cincinnati.

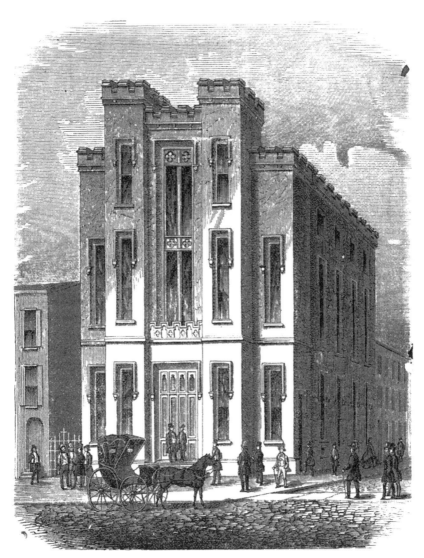

THE

PHILADELPHIA UNIVERSITY OF MEDICINE AND SURGERY

Ninth Street, below Locust, South of the Continental Hotel.

The Philadelphia University of Medicine and Surgery, from William Paine, "Announcement," *Philadelphia University Journal of Medicine and Surgery*, XIII (1869–70). Courtesy of the Lloyd Library and Museum, Cincinnati.

CHARTERED 1874.

SESSION OF 1883-4

ST. LOUIS
ECLECTIC MEDICAL COLLEGE,
Session of 1883-4.

FACULTY.

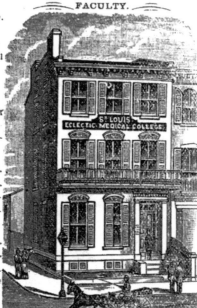

G. H. FIELD, M.D.
608 N. 13th Street.
Professor of Sur
gery and Surgical
Pathology.

* * *

* * *

Street. Profesor of
Obstetrics Gyne
cology and Disea-
ses of Children.

T. Butterfiel , M. D.
Ellersville. S. L. Mo.
Professor of Phys-
iology and practi-
cal Microscopy.

J. MUELLER M.D.
9th. Washington Ave.
Professor of Anat.
omy, Descriptive
and Surgical.

* * *

* * Street.
Professor of Prin
ciples & Practice
of Medicine.

L. C. WASHBURN,
M. D. 701 N. 14th.
Street. Professor of
Materia Medica &
Therapeutics

P. A. MEDLIN, M.D
9th. Washington Ave.
Professor of Chem-
istry, Pharmacy &
Toxicology.

* * * *

Lecturer on Medi-
cal Jurisprudence.

Prof. J. MUELLER
M.D. Demonstrator

Special Lectures by different members of the Faculty, on

Throat and Lungs, Genital. Vaginal and Urinary Organs. Eye and Ear,
Chronic Diseases, Anatomical Landmarks, Etc.
Regularly During the Session.

Regular Session opens the second Monday in October, and continues twenty weeks.
Good clinical and practical advantages.

FEES—Matriculation, $5.00 Demonstrator, $5.00: Practical Chemistry $5.00;
Prof. Tickets, $50.00. Graduting, Fee, Twenty-five Dollars; Scholarship, $125.00.

Good opportunities, and cheap material for studying Practical Anatomy.

College Building located at Northwest corner of Fourteenth street and Lucas Avenue.

L. C. WASHBURN, M. D., PRESIDENT,

GEO. H. FIELD, M.D., DEAN,

Office 608 North 13th. Street, ST. LOUIS, MO.

The St. Louis Eclectic Medical College, from "Announcement," *St. Louis Eclectic Medical Journal*, X (1883). Courtesy of the Lloyd Library and Museum, Cincinnati.

Lincoln Medical College,
Lincoln, Nebraska, 1904.
Courtesy of the Lloyd Library
and Museum, Cincinnati.

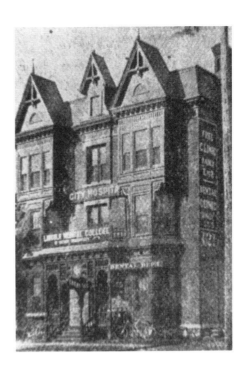

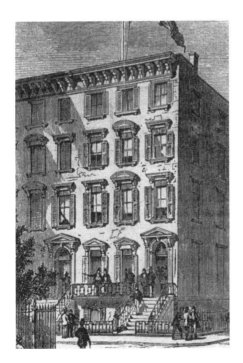

Eclectic Medical College of the
City of New York, 1880.
Courtesy of the Lloyd Library
and Museum, Cincinnati.

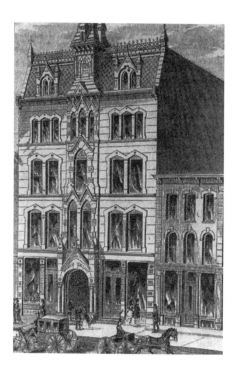

Bennett College of Eclectic
Medicine and Surgery,
Chicago, 1878. Courtesy of the
Lloyd Library and Museum,
Cincinnati.

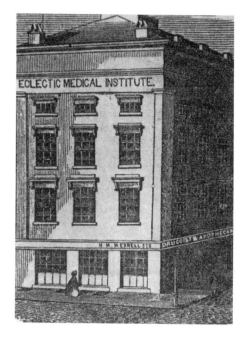

Eclectic Medical Institute,
Court and Plum Streets,
Cincinnati, erected in 1845.
Note the drug manufacturer
W. H. Merrell and Co. offices
on the first floor. Courtesy of
the Lloyd Library and
Museum, Cincinnati.

Joseph R. Buchanan (ca. 1855). Courtesy of the Lloyd Library and Museum, Cincinnati.

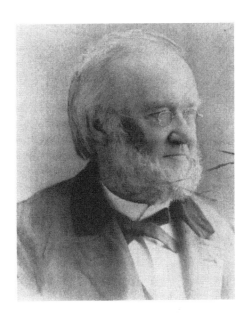

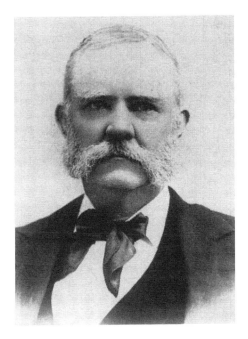

John M. Scudder (1860). Courtesy of the Lloyd Library and Museum, Cincinnati.

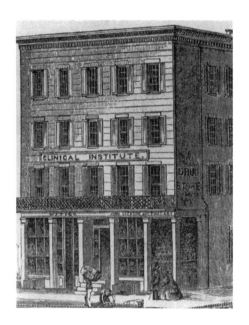

Newton Clinical Institute, Cincinnati, 1859. Used by students and faculty of the Eclectic Medical Institute. Note the John Dickson Apothecary offices on the first floor. Courtesy of the Lloyd Library and Museum, Cincinnati.

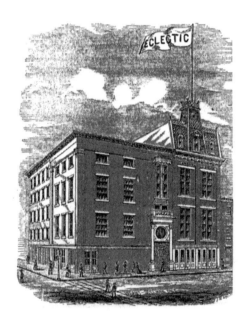

Eclectic Medical Institute, Court and Plum Streets, Cincinnati (1883). Courtesy of the Lloyd Library and Museum, Cincinnati.

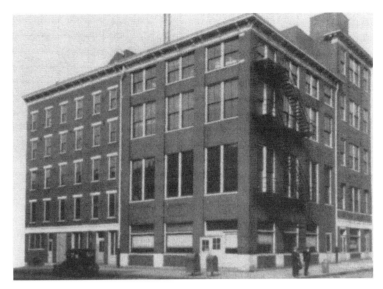

Lloyd Brothers Laboratory (formerly the home of the Eclectic Medical Institute), Court and Plum Streets, Cincinnati (ca. 1930). The older college building on the corner, erected in 1845, was rebuilt to accommodate the business department of Lloyd Brothers Laboratory. The five-story building to the left, formerly the dormitory of the Eclectic Medical College, was reconstructed and connected to the other buildings. The two upper stories were devoted to the laboratory offices, a working library, a research laboratory room, and the museum of plant materials. Courtesy of the Lloyd Library and Museum, Cincinnati.

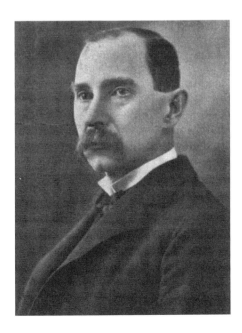

John Uri Lloyd (1895). Courtesy of the Lloyd Library and Museum, Cincinnati.

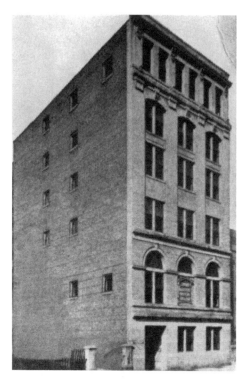

Eclectic Medical College, 630 West Sixth Street, Cincinnati (1931). Courtesy of the Lloyd Library and Museum, Cincinnati.

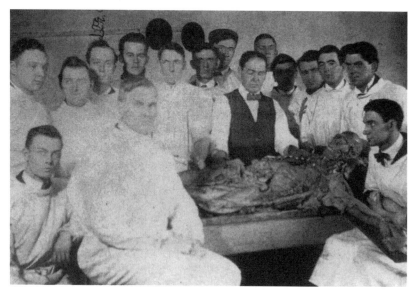

Students with cadaver (ca. 1890). Eclectic Medical Institute, Cincinnati. Courtesy of the Lloyd Library and Museum, Cincinnati.

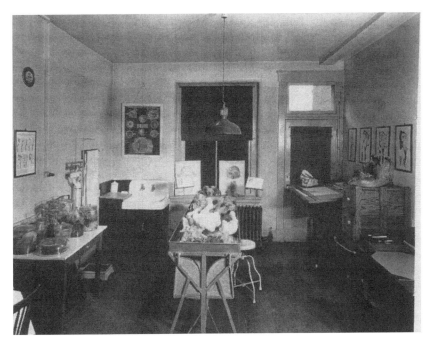

Preparation room in the Department of Anatomy, Eclectic Medical College, Cincinnati (1933). Note the dissecting table, which keeps the body in position; the numerous charts on the wall; the jars containing special prosecting specimens; the files for student notebooks; and the special drawing board. Courtesy of the Lloyd Library and Museum, Cincinnati.

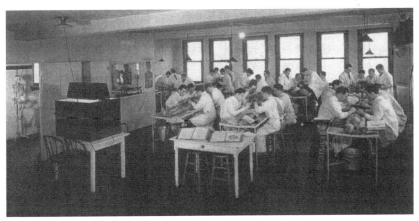

Anatomy lab, Eclectic Medical College, Cincinnati (1933). Courtesy of the Lloyd Library and Museum, Cincinnati.

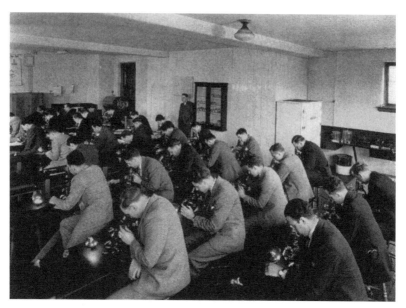

Histology and embryology laboratory at the Eclectic Medical College, Cincinnati (1933). Note the sterilizer, incubator, large refrigerator, and microtones. Each student had access to a microscope. Courtesy of the Lloyd Library and Museum, Cincinnati.

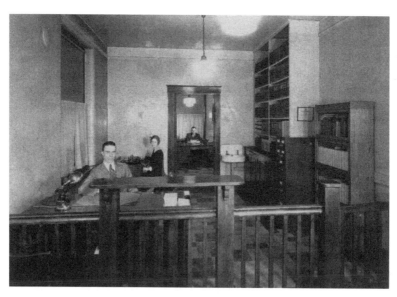

The administrative offices, situated on the second floor of the Eclectic Medical College, Cincinnati (1933), contained all student files, including grades and attendance records; minutes of regular and special meetings of the board of trustees and faculty; and textbooks and supplies for students. Courtesy of the Lloyd Library and Museum, Cincinnati.

5
Consolidation, 1856–1875

As noted earlier, eclecticism was more than just an alternative approach to regular medical practice. It also offered itself to the American people as the common man's access to medical education—a topic hotly debated in the early years of the American Medical Association. In contrast with those who looked to Europe for models of medical education, the eclectic medical schools of the nineteenth century ensured a place for those who sought a more nativistic option. Medical students of means took their training abroad in the teaching wards of Paris, Germany, Italy, and England, but those without resources could still take preceptorships, graduate from eclectic medical colleges, and move into respectable practices in almost any part of the country. In rural areas and small towns, their presence was especially welcome and offered a modicum of medical care for a population that, to this day, is often underserved. The educational and professional stature of the eclectic clearly did not undergo the same evolution in status experienced by the regular practitioner, and few ever obtained a reputation that went beyond the local region. Nevertheless, for those communities they served, the eclectics provided much-needed care, and the relationship they had with their patients remained one of their more noteworthy strengths. According to historian Joseph Kett, for every ten regulars in the United States in 1860, there was roughly one sectarian. This was a smaller proportion than what the Thomsonians had held decades earlier; moreover, it was a ratio that would continue to shrink with the change in popular attitude and the movement toward academic medicine and an identifiable profession. Until that time, however, the eclectics and other sectarians saw themselves as providing a functional alternative for American society.

The Scudder Years

By 1857, matriculants at the E. M. Institute numbered 2,555, an average yearly number of almost 213 students. By the outbreak of the Civil War, the college had established a place in American medical education, having graduated more than 850 students. Applying almost any standard, the college was no better or worse than most medical schools at mid-century. Its faculty, facilities, curriculum, and time devoted to clinical instruction and anatomy could be equated to those of mainstream allopathy. Nevertheless, complications created by Buchanan's poor management, plus the financial depression of 1857, forced the school to reduce its fees to sixty dollars per session. Then, too, the issues of slavery and secession undermined the effects of reform medicine by focusing the nation's attention on the impending national crisis. The school, never financially strong, saw its fiscal integrity further eroded with the loss of students during the war, the refusal of the Union army to accept eclectics as assistant surgeons and surgeons, and the continued internecine feuding among the faculty. Six months into the war, the *Eclectic Medical Journal*, the official organ of the college, suspended operations.[1]

The college, formed as a joint-stock company, stabilized only when John M. Scudder took control in 1862. Under Scudder's careful management, the college rebounded from the damage caused by its petty quarrels and financial distress. A sharp businessman, Scudder moved quickly to secure the financial underpinning of the institute, including the revival of the journal, which he edited from 1862 to 1894. Scudder, himself a graduate of the institute in 1856 and valedictorian of his class, had been selected by the faculty to be professor of general, special, and pathological anatomy. From 1858 to 1860, he filled the chair of obstetrics and diseases of women and children and then transferred to the chair of pathology and principles and practice of medicine, a position he held until 1887.[2] In addition to his strong administrative abilities, Scudder became a spokesman for eclectic practice through his contributions to the *Family Journal of Health* (1860) and the *Eclectic* (1870–71), both of which were general family magazines. He introduced in 1869 the concept of specific medication, which transformed the eclectic school from one of openness to all therapeutic measures to one of distinctive practices of direct medications based on specific diagnoses. Under his leadership, the E. M. Institute became the flagship of eclectic medical schools, its faculty having contributed the majority of textbooks for the reform system of medical practice.[3]

The institute under Scudder's stewardship remained free of divisions, and the faculty devoted themselves to teaching and writing textbooks and to explaining the eclectic philosophy. In effect, the school became "respectable" in the context of other nineteenth-century medical schools, having disassociated itself from the vagaries of Buchanan's cerebral physiology. To set an example for his colleagues, Scudder authored the popular *A Practical Treatise on the Diseases of Women* (1857); *Eclectic Practice of Medicine* (1864); *The Principles of Medicine* (1867); *The Eclectic Practice in Diseases of Children* (1869); *Specific Medication and Specific Medicines* (1870); *On the Reproductive Organs, and the Venereal* (1874); *Specific Diagnosis* (1874); *The Eclectic Practice of Medicine for Families* (1876); and with Lorenzo E. Jones, *American Eclectic Materia Medica and Therapeutics* (1858). By 1888, he and the E. M. faculty had written eighteen textbooks.

Two early publications by institute faculty included Benjamin L. Hill's *Lectures on the American Eclectic System of Surgery* (1850) and Ichabod Gibson Jones' and Thomas Vaughan Morrow's two-volume *The American Eclectic Practice of Medicine* (1854). This latter work embodied the general principles and practice of medicine, adapted to the wants of the American West's physicians, students, and professors, and set out to correct and remove erroneous impressions of the eclectic system. Jones and Morrow had been associates at the Worthington Medical College and had been partners in practice for many years. As proselytizers of reform medicine, they opened their book with an instructive overview of eclectic practice, demonstrating to the interested reader how it had grown from obscure beginnings and against blind superstition and exclusivity.[4]

Similarly, William Byrd Powell and Robert S. Newton, authors of *The Eclectic Practice of Medicine* (1858), used the early chapters to explain the principles of reform practice more fully. In the book's preface, the authors described how they had been educated in

> strictly orthodox Allopathy—that they believe[d] themselves to have abandoned no fact and no truly-founded [sic] principle which they acquired, and that, inasmuch as they were not bound, by an oath of allegiance, to the false doctrines and mischievous practice that were taught to them . . . they felt, and still feel, that they have not forfeited their right to private judgment, nor their privilege to abandon errors, when discovered, no matter whence obtained.

This revealing comment went far in explaining both the philosophy of the eclectics and the rationale for maintaining their separateness. The authors saw their obligation not in advancing "authority" for every opinion presented but rather in investigating every practice or system and then, "by the standards of reason and experience," adopting those practices that "we deem to be the best."[5]

Another popular eclectic writer was John King (1813–93), who graduated from Beach's school in 1838 and set up practice in New Bedford, Massachusetts. With the move of reform medicine westward to Worthington Medical College in Ohio, King decided in 1845 to locate in the growing West, moving first to Sharpsburg, Kentucky, where he practiced medicine and wrote articles for the *Western Medical Reformer*. He later called for the first National Convention of Reform Medical Practitioners in Cincinnati in 1848. In 1849, he moved to Memphis, where he filled the chair of materia medica at the Memphis Medical Institute until resigning in 1851; he then became a professor of obstetrics and diseases of women and children at the E. M. Institute.

During his years in Cincinnati, he became a vocal abolitionist and affiliated with the Republican party. King threw himself into the 1856 controversy between Newton and Buchanan, taking sides with the latter. With the expulsion of the Cleavelandites, he and other exiles established the Cincinnati College of Eclectic Medicine and Surgery. King returned to the E. M. Institute after a reconcilation in 1859 and for forty years provided exemplary instruction. In 1870, he published the eighth edition of *The American Dispensatory*, which became the standard authority on vegetable remedies and contained an account of the medicinal plants indigenous to the United States; listed the pharmaceutical compounds entitled to the rank of "official," which were in general use among reform physicians; and offered a full account of objectionable medicines. In 1878, he became president of the National Eclectic Medical Association. His publications included *American Eclectic Obstetrics* (1855), *Women—Their Diseases and Their Treatment* (1858), *The Microscopist's Companion* (1859), *The American Family Physician* (1860), *The American Dispensatory* (1864), and *The Causes, Symptoms, Diagnosis, Pathology and Treatment of Chronic Diseases* (1867). Not limited to medical writings, King, who opposed all forms of class legislation, wrote *The Coming Freeman* (1886), which he dedicated to the Knights of Labor and in which he proposed a new representative form of government that would ensure the rights of rich and poor alike.[6]

Under the direction of Newton, of Buchanan, and later of Scudder (and even later, of his son, John King Scudder), the *Eclectic Medical Journal* became the sheet anchor of reform medical practice and defended its principles against eastern elitists (who found it hard to imagine a scientific journal, let alone a respectable medical college, in the West).[7] Articles in the first years of the journal reflected the need to define eclecticism and to argue the superiority of reformed medicine against existing systems and -pathies; later issues focused on a wider array of topics, many drawn from other journals, which proposed new treatments and clinical practices. Except for editorial comments and articles on the materia medica, little differentiated this journal from those of regular medicine. Scudder railed against the practice of bleeding, the use of opiates (especially for children), the too-frequent purging of infants and children, and the use of mercury. Each issue provided information about other eclectic schools, their enrollments, and their contributions to reform medicine. In particular, the journal apprised readers of beginning sessions, lectures, and commencements at local medical colleges; the journal also noted the establishment of new colleges and whether they maintained healthy enrollments. In the January 1853 issue, for example, the journal discussed attendance at the eclectic colleges at Syracuse and Philadelphia, as well as the success of the botanical medical schools at Macon, Georgia, and at

Memphis. The journal also took offense when the Ohio Medical College faculty tried to rescind the diploma of any graduate accused of departing from the proscribed teachings.[8]

During the final decades of the nineteenth century, the *Eclectic Medical Journal* turned to such topics as electrotherapeutics (galvanic, franklinitic, and faradic), reviews of new allopathic and homeopathic textbooks, and its continuing interest in plant pharmacy. Not unlike allopathic editors, the Scudders took frequent pokes at Mary Baker Eddy and her Christian Science Church and at various medical quacks who treated cancer. Also, as did many contemporary publications, the journal contained notes and republished articles from other journals, including the *American Medical Review*, the *Medical News*, the *Western Druggist*, the *Gaillards's Medical Journal*, various state and European journals, and such journals as the *American Journal of Medical Sciences*, the *Medical Record*, the *British Medical Journal* and even the *Journal of the American Medical Association*.

Other Eclectic Schools

Botanic medicine, representing an expansion of domestic medicine, eventually sired nearly two-thirds of the more than one hundred irregular medical colleges that emerged in the nineteenth century. Following the opening of the Reformed Medical School of Cincinnati in 1840 and its incorporation as the Eclectic Medical Institute in 1845, other eclectic schools also began organizing in New York, California, Georgia, Indiana, Maine, and Iowa, and in Boston, Chicago, and St. Louis. H. E. Firth, who maintained meticulous records of eclecticism, was less than enamored of New York's reform medical colleges. "The west," he admitted, "seems to be the 'garden spot' of eclecticism so far as medical colleges are concerned."[9] Firth recognized the E. M. Institute as the most successful of all reform schools and the center from which emanated most of the medical texts on reform practice and surgery. New York State, on the other hand, had three types of reformers: the radical Thomsonians, the physiopaths (the physio-medicals), and the eclectics. The eclectics viewed the radical Thomsonians with much the same hostility as they did the allopaths. While the physiopaths were closer in philosophy to the eclectics and were often united with them, attempts to merge their medical colleges proved difficult and the parties concerned too fractious, even for the most liberal among them. Other reasons for reform medicine's failure in New York included the tendency toward poor financial management, the nomadic existence of its schools, and the "inharmony among the professors and the medical men who conducted the enterprises."[10]

The Eclectic Medical Institute of New York, created in 1847 by Stephen H. Potter and Orin Davis as the Medical School of Fredonia, New York, moved to Rochester, New York, in 1848, merging with the Randolph Eclectic Medical Institute; in 1849, it moved to Syracuse, becoming the Central Medical College of New York. The faculty of the college, many of whom were affiliated with the E. M. Institute, included Zoheth Freeman in anatomy and surgery; Lorenzo E. Jones in theory and practice, materia medica, and botany; Orin Davis in obstetrics; Benjamin L. Hill in physiology, clinical surgery, and medical jurisprudence; and William W. Hadley in chemistry and pharmacy. According to Hadley, dean of the faculty, the prerequisites for graduation included three years of study in the office of an established and respectable practitioner of medicine; attendance at two full courses of medical lectures, the last of which had to be in the college; and a satisfactory thesis, written about a subject connected with medicine or surgery. He encouraged ministers of the gospel, as well as students who had prepaid for their attendance at the E. M. Institute in Cincinnati, to attend the lectures. Students attending the college would be credited for the course work if they subsequently went to Cincinnati. Not having procured an act of incorporation, the college existed solely as a private enterprise espousing eclectic medical philosophy. In 1850, it moved back to Rochester and closed in 1852.[11]

The Metropolitan Medical College of the City of New York, so constituted that both eclectics and physiopaths served as trustees and faculty, incorporated in 1853 and continued until the repeal of its charter in 1862, whereupon many of its students transferred to other eclectic colleges.[12]

Another school, the Eclectic Medical College of the City of New York, opened in 1865 under the leadership of the Honorable William F. Havemeyer, one of the city's former mayors. Among the school's professors were Robert S. Newton, Paul W. Allen, William W. Hadley, and Edwin Freeman. Until it closed in 1913, it offered hospital advantages unsurpassed by most medical schools, having clinical observation and training available to its students at New York Hospital, Bellevue Hospital, Emigrant Hospital, St. Vincent's Hospital, Jews' Hospital, St. Luke's Hospital, Women's Hospital, Blackwell's Island Hospital, and at the Eye and Ear Infirmary and the Colored Home, as well as at various dispensaries. Its own dispensary, located at 135 East Twenty-sixth Street, between Second and Third Avenues, opened every day but Sunday for persons in need of medical attention. In an effort to reduce the cost of operation, the trustees and faculty invited the cooperation of drug companies and dealers to furnish free supplies and medicines for its work.[13] The *New York Eclectic Medical Review*, begun in 1866, was the official organ of the college and became the "unflinching advocate" of reform medical practice.[14] Horace Greeley, always a gadfly for reform efforts, spoke at the school's 1866–67 class commencement. Representing himself as a champion of voluntarism, Greeley heralded the college as a protest against medical abuses and a "palpable expression of a desire for free thought." Greeley predicted that medical etiquette would ultimately prevail, at which time homeopaths, eclectics, and allopaths would consult together in a "spirit of Christian conciliation" rather than continue their stance of persecution and intolerance of one another.[15]

Dr. Lanaier Bankston's Southern Botanico-Medical College (1839) at Forsyth, Georgia, led a particularly nomadic existence. It began as a school devoted to physio-medicalism and to the ideas originally put forth by Alva Curtis, but it soon became a battleground for the Curtisites and eclectics. In 1845, the college moved to the state capital at Macon, where it changed its name to the Reformed Medical College of Georgia, reflecting the dominant influence of eclectic thinking within the faculty. Among its patrons were U.S. House of Representatives member Alexander Stephens (later, vice president of the Confederacy), Governor Joseph Brown, and Brigadier General Robert A. Toombs. It suspended activities in 1861 but started again in 1867 and subsequently changed its name to the American College of Medicine and Surgery in 1874. In 1881, the college moved to Atlanta, where it merged with the Georgia Eclectic Medical College (1867) and continued until its closing in 1916.[16]

Calvin Newton (1800–1853), a Baptist preacher and theologian, studied medicine at the Berkshire Medical Institution and began practicing medicine in 1845. A fellow of the Massachusetts

Medical Society, he rebelled against the therapeutics of allopathy and became a collaborator with Samuel Thomson in advocating a botanic materia medica. He found much in the accomplishments of Thomson and Curtis, but he was no slavish admirer, considering each to be superficial and each as having too many shortcomings. He believed in the unification of all botanic physicians and organized the Worcester Medical School (physiopathic) in 1846; however, because of opposition from the Massachusetts Medical Society, Newton failed to obtain a charter for the college. Undaunted, he came to an understanding with Isaac Miller Comings (1812–89) of the Southern Botanico-Medical College in Macon. Worcester would become a "branch" of Comings' college, and thus students would be granted degrees under the auspices of the Georgia charter. Accordingly, the school changed its name to the Worcester Botanico-Medical College and began granting degrees in 1847. A year later, after signing a more lucrative agreement with an institution in Petersburg, Virginia, and obtaining the authority to grant degrees under the aegis of the Virginia charter, the college again changed its name, becoming the New England Botanico-Medical College.[17]

Calvin Newton disavowed any further association with the "uncompromising stiffness of Samuel Thomson" in an address to the college at the close of its fourth course of lectures in June 1849. Instead, he expressed the importance for the graduates of adopting "a suitable eclecticism" in order to position themselves in the field of true science, reason, and common sense. The objective of the college was to train candidates for medicine by pointing out the errors of past medical systems, presenting the results of original investigations and discoveries, and inviting students to adopt "the truest eclecticism." This meant becoming "fearless of the charge of innovation" and liberated from "servile allegiance to any theory, however plausible," in the pursuit of truth.[18]

After it secured its own charter in 1851 and returned to its original name, the Worcester Medical School saw attendance increase; and in 1852, Newton gained an affiliation with the Syracuse Medical College. Following Calvin Newton's death in 1853, surgeon Walter Burnham (1808–83) assumed duties as the school's new president, serving also as president of the National Eclectic Medical Association. The school evinced a genuine spirit of fraternity with eclectics and homeopaths, and over the next several years, a number of its faculty became teachers in eclectic medical colleges. Burnham, however, lacked Newton's energy and reform spirit, and the college soon fell into financial difficulties. To make matters worse, he repudiated eclectic theory in 1863. In a last-gasp effort, the trustees moved the school to Boston in 1856; however, it was dying and closed its doors in 1859.

The Eclectic Medical College of Pennsylvania, chartered in 1850 by Drs. Thomas Cooke, Joseph Sites, and Henry Hollemback, opened in Philadelphia and continued until 1880. Throughout its thirty-year history, the school suffered severe quality problems and was seldom in good standing among eclectics. The *American Medical and Surgical Journal,* was established under the patronage of the New York eclectic societies and the faculties of the Eclectic Medical College of Pennsylvania and Syracuse Medical College. Editor Stephen H. Potter, professor of principles and practice of surgery and obstetrics at Syracuse, and Thomas Cooke, professor of theory and practice of medicine at Philadelphia, represented the union of the two schools. Philadelphia reflected the eclectic interests of the East and South, Syracuse reputedly those of the North and West.[19]

The American College of Medicine, chartered in 1853 as a rival to the Eclectic Medical College of Pennsylvania, failed as a successful competitor and reorganized in 1858 to become two associate institutions, the Eclectic Medical College of Philadelphia and the American College of Medicine in Philadelphia. John Buchanan (no relation to Joseph R. Buchanan) operated the former as a diploma mill, while William Paine, a graduate of the Berkshire Medical Institution, managed the latter. After the Civil War, Paine sold the American College of Medicine to three Methodist ministers who changed its name to the Philadelphia University of Medicine and Surgery. Graduates of the university came chiefly from Pennsylvania, Maryland, Virginia, and North Carolina. As its first president, Paine published several textbooks and served as editor of the *Philadelphia University Journal of Medicine and Surgery.* The school styled itself as separate from the "fine-spun theories of homeopathy" and the "conglomerate garbage of modern eclecticism," yet it was decidedly in the camp of eclectic thinking, espousing botanic medicines and concentrations, opposing mineral drugs and bloodletting, and maintaining a close association with Joseph R. Buchanan and his nervauric theories.[20]

Requiring two full courses of lectures and three years' study, the Medical Department of the Philadelphia University of Medicine and Surgery offered the following curriculum. The first session, which ran from October until March, embraced physiology, materia medica, practice, obstetrics, anatomy, practical and demonstrative anatomy, military and plastic surgery, pathology, diseases of women and children, diseases of the eye and ear, clinical medicine and surgery, medical jurisprudence, and chemistry. The second session, during spring and summer, included surgical, microscopic, pathological, descriptive, and demonstrative anatomy; plastic, military, and operative surgery; analytic and organic chemistry; pharmacy; materia medica, including practical botany; obstetrics and diseases of women and children; comparative and human physiology; auscultation and percussion; practical instruction on the use of the microscope, laryngoscope, stethoscope, ophthalmoscope, auriscope (otoscope), and rhinoscope; practical instruction in the use of the speculum, catheter, and bougie; principles and practice of medicine and pathology; clinical medicine and surgery; general and special technology; and clinical instruction in the use of atomizers, nebulizers, hypodermic needles, and inhalators. The Medical Department claimed ample means of illustrating and teaching clinical medicine and surgery and diseases of women and children through the use of local hospitals and dispensaries. In addition, the department offered intern and resident physician appointments at Pennsylvania Hospital, Episcopal Hospital, St. Joseph's Hospital, Wills' Hospital for the Eye, City Lying-in Hospital, and Children's Hospital.[21] When Surgeon General Joseph K. Barnes refused to accept its graduates as assistant surgeons in the United States Army, Paine accused Barnes of "forgetting his position as a servant of the people" by becoming "a drummer for his favored medical colleges."[22]

During the 1870s, critics accused both the Eclectic Medical College of Philadelphia and the Philadelphia University of Medicine and Surgery of selling diplomas in the United States, Europe, and Latin America. John Buchanan eventually admitted to having sold sixty thousand diplomas over a forty-year period at prices ranging from ten to two hundred dollars. When the editor of the *Medical and Surgical Reporter* charged Paine with similar fraud, Paine responded that the diplomas in question had been obtained from parties separate from the university and that, besides, the traffic in medical deceptions applied to other schools as well.[23] However, the issue of bogus diplomas continued to dog him as inquiries and accusations connected the college to one A. J. Hale, who claimed to be the "medical agent" for the Philadelphia University of Medicine and Surgery. According to Paine's own investigation into the matter, A. J. Hale, who worked in close association with Buchanan, awarded diplomas upon "receipt of a certificate of [good] standing in the community and fifty dollars" and offered to print the diplomas in the names of Jefferson Medical College, the University of Pennsylvania, Boston University Homeopathic College, the Eclectic Medical College of Philadelphia, and the American University of Philadelphia. Notwithstanding his many denials, critics claimed that Paine had sold more than ninety thousand dollars worth of bogus diplomas. The Philadelphia University of Medicine and Surgery finally closed its doors in 1880.[24]

Another reform college in Pennsylvania was the Penn Medical College (later renamed Penn Medical University of Philadelphia), established in 1853 by Joseph S. Longshore. Founded on the twin principles of eclecticism and the chronothermal system of Samuel Dickson of London, the school instituted one of the earliest graded curricula; Longshore also established a "coordinate education" system in which men and women took the same courses but at different times. Unfortunately, the college sullied its reputation by selling diplomas and closed its doors in 1881. Yet another school, the American University of Philadelphia, organized in 1867 as a diploma mill controlled by John Buchanan, began as a branch of Buchanan's Eclectic Medical College of Philadelphia under the pretense of educating blacks. The school's name was deliberately chosen to deceive many in other parts of the country into believing that it was synonymous with the University of Pennsylvania or with the Philadelphia University of Medicine and Surgery. Authorities eventually arrested John Buchanan—but not before he had sold thousands of bogus diplomas.[25]

In Chicago, the pillar of reform medicine was Bennett College of Eclectic Medicine and Surgery, incorporated in 1868 and named after John Hughes Bennett (1812–75) of Edinburgh, whose medical sentiments were closely allied with those of the eclectics.[26] Although off to an auspicious start in a four-story marble structure on Washington Street, the college burned to the ground in the Chicago fire of 1871. Its trustees then purchased lots on Clark and

State Streets; there, they erected a new school. The college's official organ, the *Chicago Medical Times*, the second-oldest eclectic journal in existence, boasted the largest circulation of any medical journal in the state. Its editors were John Forman, dean of the faculty and professor of anatomy and clinical medicine, and Robert A. Gunn, professor of surgery. The journal later merged into the *American Journal of Clinical Medicine* (subsequently renamed *Clinical Medicine and Surgery* in 1894), which in 1906, became again the *American Journal of Clinical Medicine*.

Other reform medical schools included the American Medical College of St. Louis, founded in 1870, which had access to City Hospital. Following a faculty schism, a rump group split off and formed the St. Louis Medical College. The two schools existed as rivals in the St. Louis area until the National Eclectic Medical Association ruled in 1878 in favor of the American Medical College of St. Louis.[27]

Fierce competition proved ruinous for many of these sectarian schools, causing them to strike out at sister institutions with the same vigor and animosity they directed toward allopathy. Attempting to elevate their own colleges at the expense of rivals, they made claims and cast aspersions that went far beyond their usual attacks against allopathic schools. John Buchanan, for example, felt that, of the nine existing eclectic colleges in 1874, only the Eclectic Medical College of Pennsylvania and the American College of Medicine and Surgery in Macon taught the true principles of reform practice. He called the rest "mongrel, chaotic, and brainless," little more than "a burlesque on medical teaching."[28] More specifically, he called the American Medical College of St. Louis "a port slaughter house, possessing no legal status"; the Bennett College of Eclectic Medicine and Surgery as having "no more force than the charter of a tobacconist"; and the E. M. Institute as "simply a common school."[29]

Some of the more notable journals to derive from these assorted schools included the *American Medical Journal* of St. Louis, edited by two professors, E. Younkin and M. M. Hamlin, and published between the years 1890 and 1900. In its pages, the American Medical College of St. Louis faculty authored articles ranging in topic from the materia medica to brain surgery. The *Chicago Medical Times*, later edited by Professors Finley Ellingwood and A. L. Clark of the Bennett College of Eclectic Medicine and Surgery, embraced seventeen volumes from 1890 to 1906, after which it was "betrayed into the hands of the enemy and ceased to exist as [an] Eclectic institution." *Ellingwood's Therapeutics* originated with Finley Ellingwood's withdrawal from the editorial staff of the *Chicago Medical Times*; and the *Eclectic Review* of New York, edited by George W. Boskowitz, was the official forum for the Eclectic Medical College of the City of New York. The *Eclectic Medical Gleaner* of Cincinnati, a bimonthly, was edited by Professor William E. Bloyer and Dr. William C. Cooper during its early years and later by Alexander Wilder and Harvey W. Felter. Publication of the *Eclectic Medical Gleaner* lasted twenty-two years. Other publications included the *Georgia Eclectic Medical Journal* of Atlanta, published between 1891 and 1903; the *New Jersey Eclectic Medical and Surgical Journal*, beginning in 1875; the *Eclectic Medical Journal* of St. Louis, which stressed the importance of specific medication; the *Transactions* of the National Eclectic Medical Association, which encompassed twenty-one volumes, ending with the 1908 Kansas City, Missouri, meeting (recording the work of the national organization and its twenty-one presidents); and the *Annual of Eclectic Medicine and Surgery*, which covered the years 1891 through 1898 and published the best literature from the state eclectic societies.[30]

Women Practitioners

Medical knowledge was often attributed to women, especially among the native Americans, the Negro slaves, and the Caucasian plantation society. Women served as nurses, midwives, and doctors to remote families and populations. They did most of the doctoring on the frontier and in rural areas, relying on a combination of home remedies, practical experience, superstition, and herb and root concoctions. A disproportion between the sexes contributed to the temper of the times, providing leverage for the growth of feminine prestige. While in the East fashion dictated lighter exercise, stuffy rooms, tight stays, and poor diet for the "gentler sex," the frontier and younger towns in the West divided responsibility more evenly between the sexes. Western custom allowed girls more freedom but compensated by increased duties and roles. To be sure, romantic sentimentality and double standards prevailed to some extent, but the inhibitions surrounding feminine social life seemed measurably more relaxed in the West than in the East.

When orthodox medical schools in Philadelphia and New York

denied admission to Elizabeth Blackwell (1821–1910), Joseph R. Buchanan, dean of the faculty at the E. M. Institute, and Stephen H. Potter of the Central Medical College of New York each offered her a place to study. Before she could matriculate at either, Geneva Medical College in rural western New York State, in the heart of the burned-over district, consented to receive her. The college, after presenting Blackwell in 1849 with the first regular medical degree conferred on a woman in the United States, refused to accept additional women applicants. In contrast, the eclectic colleges at Worcester, Syracuse, Rochester, and Cincinnati opened their doors to women, as did most homeopathic schools. Syracuse Medical College, as stated earlier, opened in 1851 with a class of eighty students and offered to register women "on the same terms, and enjoy[ing] equal advantages with those of the other sex." Four women took advantage of the opportunity.[31]

Most regulars objected to women in the medical profession except as midwives. The thought of a woman leaving her proper sphere within the home circle engendered hostility, repugnance, and noticeable jeering; those few who did enter practice were treated not unlike irregulars and quacks. Such manly pursuits, argued regulars, destroyed true femininity, taxed a woman beyond her natural intellectual capacity, and threatened to undermine morality. Hostility kept most women out of regular medical schools; and in the years before the Civil War, only sectarian medical colleges, notably eclectic colleges, welcomed women. These included the Boston Female Medical College, formed in 1848 by Samuel and George Gregory; the Female Medical College of Pennsylvania in 1850; and the Women's Medical College of the New York Infirmary for Women and Children in 1868, where Blackwell briefly held a chair in hygiene.

In 1852, the Boston Female Medical College took the name New England Female College and expanded its curriculum to parallel that of other medical schools. Nevertheless, few students finished the course of study. As of 1855, only six women had graduated from the school's program out of a population of more than one hundred students. In 1874, the institution merged with the Boston University School of Medicine, which espoused homeopathic theory and practice.

The National Eclectic Medical Association in 1855 endorsed coeducation; and by the start of the Civil War, nearly three hundred women had received medical degrees from its various schools.[32] "It was the eclectics who introduced woman into the medical profession, who admitted her first to membership and equal favor in medical societies, who in every way recognized whatever ability and talent she possessed," remarked Alexander Wilder, "and if she loves justice as well as she does compliments, she will remember who her first friends were." Ironically, orthodoxy's rigid stance against women physicians had two unintended effects. First, many women in their efforts to obtain a medical education were forced by prejudice to apply to sectarian schools, whereupon regulars criticized not only their choice to become physicians but also the sectarian schools they entered. Second, sectarians found it easier to win acceptance, or at least toleration, from regulars when they chose to exclude women from their ranks.[33]

The stigma of feminism was both a strength and a handicap to the sectarians, a mark of their insulation from the main currents of American medical thinking. And, even among eclectics, the issue was not firmly settled. George Washington Lafayette Bickley, M.D., took issue with those of his colleagues who offered to educate women along with men in the medical arts. "The proper sphere of woman is limited to the duties of companion, wife, and mother," he remarked, "and when the true character of these positions is well understood, it will be seen that her parts on the grand stage of life are quite extensive enough for all ordinary ambitions." A woman who went beyond her sphere "unsexed" herself and "at once [became a] dangerous citizen, who should then relinquish all claims upon the protection of man." A creature of impulse who followed the dictates of affection rather than of calm reason, and a creature who, like a child, was imitative, woman faced the consequences of abuse if educated outside her natural sphere. While the E. M. Institute had graduated "some very excellent ladies," Bickley believed, as a rule, "they will find that a general practice of the healing art is by no means adapted to the tastes of a refined lady." Bickley urged young women to seek instead satisfaction in nursing, while older and more experienced women could find useful careers as midwives. In considering the problems of coeducation, Bickley recommended the establishment of female colleges and suggested that women study midwifery and the diseases common to their sex. Women required only "a knowledge of the art of obstetrics, and a due acquaintance with physiology and hygiene, to enable them to become useful members of the community." In compensation for this, women were conceded to embody a far greater moral purity than men, and they could make this purity effective in the world through their influence within the home circle. But the realm of medicine, with its stark immediacy to death, disease, and social impurities, would only unsex the woman physician in a perverse and dehumanizing way.[34]

In the August 1857 issue of the *Eclectic Medical Journal*, the E. M. Institute renounced its support of coeducational medical colleges. "While we do not oppose the medical education of ladies, we would advise all such students to avail themselves of the ample opportunities now afforded them at medical schools established for their exclusive benefit. . . . [H]ereafter no female students will be admitted in the Eclectic Medical Institute of Cincinnati."[35] Two months later, the editor of the journal noted that courses at the institute would commence on October 12 and that, "females having evacuated our halls, the gentlemen who attend may expect a full and legitimate course of lectures, without the annoyances incident to the presence of 'hoops' in the lecture room."[36]

In rescinding its policy of female admittance, the institute reflected the prejudices of regular medicine, and—even among the few eclectic women practitioners—there seemed to be an acquiescence to woman's supportive role. "The true physician never need fear being pushed aside by a woman," wrote Dr. Mary B. Morey in the *Eclectic Medical Journal* in 1904. "She may be just as capable, stronger in judgment through intuition, quick to see and act, and yet save more lives through her conservatism, but she can never take the place of the old family physician. She must be satisfied with less."[37]

A break in this conservative mentality came with the admittance of women to the Boston University Homeopathic College in 1874, followed by the Cleveland Homeopathic Hospital College, the University of Michigan Homeopathic Medical College, the Hahnemann Medical College in Chicago, and the Homeopathic Medical Department of the State University of Iowa. In 1876, the American Medical Association (AMA) admitted its first woman member when Sarah Hackett Stevenson took her seat at the Philadelphia convention that year. The E. M. Institute in 1877–78 proposed a women's hospital, where women could pursue courses in obstetrics, diseases of women, and nursing; and the institute offered to provide separate entrances, waiting rooms, and dissecting rooms; but the effort failed to elicit support and quickly died. Not until 1884 did the Massachusetts Medical Society admit women, followed four years later by the Philadelphia County Medical Society. In 1893, Johns Hopkins University accepted an endowment from Mary E. Garrett on condition that women be admitted to medical training on equal terms with men. In 1899, Cornell University Medical College turned down merger with the Women's Medical College of the New York Infirmary for Women and Children and chose to admit women. This decision, followed by similar decisions by other university-affiliated medical schools, resulted in the closure of most of the remaining women's medical colleges, except for the one in Philadelphia. Despite this seemingly liberal trend, these ostensibly coeducational colleges in reality admitted only token numbers of women. For many women seeking a career in medicine, the choice was between sectarian medicine, which offered an uncertain future and a problematic foundation, and opportunities abroad, principally in Switzerland and France.[38]

Although the E. M. Institute reversed its position and endorsed women physicians, the faculty mandated a more circumscribed role for the woman practitioner. "There is no reason why the woman physician should not excel in pediatrics," explained Harvey W. Felter in an editorial in the college's journal in 1918, "nor is there any reason why she should not make the needed examinations of women for insurance and other organizations. The refined and tactful woman physician, with a liberal education and good, sound sense, should be able to hold her own in this work, and this is, in fact, what she is doing in many localities."[39]

Education and the American Medical Association

Regulars meeting in New York City in 1846 to consider a national medical association did so amid the turmoil of a nation increasingly embroiled in the issues of slavery, industrialization, manifest destiny, tariffs, and the nature of western expansion. The agenda, therefore, faced initial indifference. The majority of delegates came from New York, and two-thirds of the medical colleges in the country had no representation. The next year's meeting produced a greater turnout, with representatives from twenty-two states and the District of Columbia attending the convention in Philadelphia. This meeting in 1847 officially organized the AMA.[40]

No sooner had the AMA organized than it advised lengthening the period of instruction in medical schools from four months to six, with courses taught by at least seven professors; carefully monitoring student performance; and enforcing a yearlong preceptorship prior to beginning college study. Some of the strongest critics of these recommendations were Harvard's medical faculty, who were content with the four-month curriculum. Of course, Harvard's curriculum existed within a system of personal study under the close guidance of mentors, and this system worked reasonably well with self-motivated students and with private teachers, but elsewhere, without mentors, it had a distinct leveling effect on the broad mainstream of medical education.

In 1848, the Committee on Education of the newly formed AMA reported that, in all the "most enlightened nations of Europe," the standards of qualification essential to the attainment of the medical degree were "far higher than . . . in the United States."

> The preliminary education is broader and more thorough; the term of medical study is from one to two years longer; the curriculum includes a greater diversity of subjects, the series of lectures are more prolonged and the examinations more elaborate, searching, and practical. But beyond all this, there is one feature in the medical schools of Europe which stands in marked contrast with many of those in the United States. At Paris, at Strasbourg, at Montpellier, at Vienna, at St. Petersburg, at Berlin, at Edinburgh, at Dublin, at London, a great hospital forms a part of the scene, and furnishes an essential constituent of the material of instruction. In the United States alone is continued an absolute system of teaching demonstrative science by description, of teaching the manipulations of surgery, and the art of recognizing and healing diseases without exhibiting the practice of either, and of explaining the movements and changes of living bodies to those who are ignorant of the laws which govern inert matter.[41]

This statement, damning in its analysis of the American medical-education system, was equally critical of the laissez-faire nature of proprietary medical institutions, which, left to pecuniary self-interest and unaffiliated with universities, operated beyond the control of any national, state, or local governmental body.

Apart from the meager fare of medical education, certain changes did take place. In 1847, the University of Pennsylvania in Philadelphia and the College of Physicians and Surgeons of New York extended their terms of instruction to five and one-half months and five months, respectively; and Buffalo Medical College in upstate New York increased its term of lectures to five months, with a preliminary month devoted to dissection. Not to be out-classed, the medical faculties of the Geneva Medical College and the Rush Medical College in Illinois agreed to extend their terms provided that other institutions did the same.[42]

In 1853, the Committee on Medical Education of the AMA recommended the study of the classics and the natural sciences, as well as mathematics and metaphysics as good preliminary training for medical school. It also considered botany, zoology, and meteorology important stepping-stones. In other words, the committee endorsed a strong general-education program as an essential foundation for medical education.[43]

When the Penn Medical University of Philadelphia distributed a pamphlet in 1855 announcing its plan to extend the period of graded instruction from October through June, requiring four successive sessions instead of the more typical repetitive curriculum common to most medical colleges at the time, the editor of the *Eclectic Medical Journal* thought the plan well-intentioned but feared that the prolonged course of instruction would result in a decline in numbers of students. The plan, introduced by William Schmoele, required twenty-four courses of lectures. Under the existing system, the professor condensed, in four months, the most essential knowledge of his department and repeated it every session. With the proposed new calendar, the professor would extend his subject through a period of sixteen or eighteen months. Students would presumably not repeat the expanded program as had been the case in the former system. The faculty soon abandoned the experiment when competing schools failed to take it up. The school, chartered in 1853, eventually closed its doors in 1881.[44]

In 1867, the Committee on Medical Education of the AMA reported that "the curriculum of instruction . . . has undergone no thorough improvement except in a very few of the schools, during the last half century. It is, in fact, essentially the same now as it was at the death of Dr. Rush, in 1813."[45] The committee noted again the importance of English, sufficient Greek and Latin to understand the technicalities of medicine, a working knowledge of French and German, and competency in logic, mathematics, history, and geography. In 1871, the committee stressed the importance of English, literature, geography, elementary physics, history, algebra, geometry, and elementary chemistry, as well as Latin, geology, mineralogy, zoology, botany, and a familiarity with French and German.[46]

In looking at the whole of American medical education, critics uniformly believed the situation had deteriorated rather than improved. Although this was hardly the case among elite medical schools, advocates of reform were not averse to making such claims in order to encourage additional change. Samuel D. Gross's comment in 1876, that "not one [medical thesis] in fifty affords the slightest evidence of competency, proficiency, or ability in the candidate for graduation," served as grist for demands for a three-year curriculum, examinations for licensing, and tougher boards of examiners. While Gross's remarks were directed at mainstream medical education, including the Jefferson Medical College in Philadelphia where he taught, they ignored a growing reform consensus that had emerged among elite institutions several decades earlier and that had become the preoccupation among the new breed of German-trained physicians. However, when viewed in the context of all medical schools, Gross's remarks were probably well-founded.[47] As John Shaw Billings explained in 1886, "In America we have over eighty gates, a number of turnstiles and a good deal of ground in unenclosed common."[48]

Reform Medicine's Merger Efforts

Heartened by Thomas Cooke's statewide efforts to form the Eclectic Botanic Medical Association of Pennsylvania (1841), which lasted thirty years, Thomas Vaughan Morrow attempted to bring the various factions of botanic medicine together in a national organization. His intent was defensive in nature: he feared that, unless the reform sects presented a united front against regulars, they would become easy targets for adverse medical legislation. Morrow not only called for a national convention of reformed physicians but proposed the establishment of a national medical university at a central location, capable of accommodating between five hundred and one thousand students. This ambitious plan met with considerable hostility from those already associated with reform medical departments. Undaunted by rejection, Morrow hoped to establish a national association of botanic physicians based on the principles of justice and liberality. This, too, failed to elicit support. The creation of the AMA in 1847, however, jolted botanics out of their complacency.[49]

The first national gathering of eclectic physicians took place on May 25, 1848, at the E. M. Institute. The convention met for three days and resulted in the formation of the American Eclectic Medical Association, whose original members included Morrow, Wooster Beach, Joseph R. Buchanan, Lorenzo E. Jones, Ichabod Gibson Jones, John King, Orin Davis, Thomas Cooke, Benjamin L. Hill, and John H. Jordan. The association, which also included Alva Curtis's independent Thomsonians, urged the formation of state and local societies and the compilation of statistics to document the success of reform medical practice. Shortly afterwards, the name of the association changed to the National Eclectic Medical Association, with Morrow as president and John King and Lorenzo E. Jones as secretaries. Morrow vowed that the association would combat the conspiratorial designs on the part of the AMA to monopolize medicine and medical practice. "The great struggle of the day in the medical profession," he announced to the assembly, "is between the spirit of freedom on the one hand, which is seeking for truth in science, and the spirit of conservative despotism on the other, which aims to perpetuate its power and doctrines by organized combinations, and by discountenancing or suppressing every attempt at reform, whatever may be its merits or its source."[50]

Morrow made every effort during his presidency to unite the competing schools of reform physicians. In contrast, when Joseph R. Buchanan became president in 1850, he encouraged the dissolution of the national organization and suggested instead the establishment of regional conventions. His attitude reflected a growing belief in regional differences (and biases), competition among schools, and the incompatibility of their ideas.[51] Ironically, Buchanan's efforts to establish committees on theory and practice, obstetrics, surgery, physiology, materia medica, medical botany, chemistry, pharmacy, statistics, hydropathy, homeopathy, utility of neurology, the chronothermal system, and one that would study the comparative merits of the different systems of medicine did much to expand rather than limit the role of the organization. Moreover, his insistence that statistics ranked as one of the seven principal branches of medical science had the effect of strengthening national ties because, if for no other reason, it would make available comparative data on eclectic practices and successes. His support of statistics also reflected the early compatibility of eclectic thinking with the Paris clinical school of Pierre Louis.[52]

When the association met in New York in 1851, it adopted a platform that condemned any therapeutic regimen that impaired the vital powers through bloodletting, mercury, tartar emetic, or other depletive methods. The convention also voted to recognize the merger of physiopathic and eclectic physicians under the name *reform medical physicians*, and it renounced all other appellations. Numerous reform medical societies formed as a result, while the older physio-medical and eclectic societies proceeded to adopt the new name. However, the union of physiopaths and eclectics did not meet with uniform acceptance outside New York; indeed, considerable criticism came from both the South and the West. Buchanan vehemently opposed the merger, as did the editor of the *Southern Medical Reformer*, representing the interests of physiopaths. Not surprisingly, the organization of the reform medical physicians collapsed, and the efforts under way for establishing a national reform medical association failed as well.[53]

At a third meeting of the National Eclectic Medical Association at Rochester in May 1852, the membership elected Calvin Newton as president, adopted the designation *eclectic*, announced the association's intention to establish the eclectic theory of medicine on a scientific basis, and passed a resolution condemning the free-lecture system of the E. M. Institute as injurious to other reform colleges.[54] The association also adopted eight principles. These included the demand for freedom of thought and investigation; the cultivation of a liberal spirit in medical science, particularly in the development of the vegetable materia medica; the adoption of inductive (Baconian) reasoning in investigations; the emphasis on assisting nature in its recuperative efforts on the body; the selection of remedies based upon the nature of the disease and upon the character of the agents employed to treat the disease; the avoidance of all medicines or treatments intended to permanently depress the constitution; a preference for vegetable remedies but not to the extent of favoring an exclusive system of herbalism; and an opposition to harmful agents, such as mercury, arsenic, and antimony. The association approved a later addition to these principles in 1855 when it elected Dr. Wooster Beach president of the society. At that time, the membership adopted a new platform, which declared that, in the administration of healing agents, eclectics would use "only those [in] which the therapeutic action is physiological and not pathologic" and only if the disease was not a "vital action, but that condition of a part which disqualifies it for the performance of its function in a normal manner."[55]

Throughout the 1850s, eclectics and independent Thomsonians lamented the divisiveness of party spirit and the mutual jealousies that paralyzed their energies. In their animosity, however destructive, they underestimated the resolution of sectarian practitioners to maintain their separate identities; moreover, many sectarians feared the potential power of a national association—even their own. On the surface, the National Eclectic Medical Association prospered, providing occasion for much oratory about the glories of cooperation and the haunting specter of orthodoxy's sinister powers. In reality, the association existed because it had accepted the individuality of its many parts.

The Civil War had a deleterious effect on reform medicine, resulting in a demonstrable decline in interest in eclectic issues and practice. Also, repeal of state legislation, which had restricted the practice of irregular doctors, had the unintended effect of eliminating the perceived need for reformers to organize in defense of their interests.[56] Eclectics by 1866 had gained considerable confidence in their future and were gratified that their numbers were increasing at the expense of "grim, tyrannous Allopathy, with all its bluster, presumption, bigotry, intolerance, and incapacity." Notwithstanding the power that the regulars exerted in bolstering their own professional status, reformers confidently felt that they were taking the place of "the swarm of old fogy non-progressives of the tottering, and unscrupulous allopathic school."[57]

J. M. Toner's statistical sketch of the medical profession in the 1870s provided a profile of regular, homeopathic, hydropathic, and eclectic strengths in the states and territories. As expected, the eclectics showed their greatest strength in the Midwest (Illinois, Indiana, Iowa, and Ohio), where they averaged 13 percent of the practicing physicians; a cadre in the Northeast (New York, Massachusetts, and Connecticut); and smaller numbers scattered throughout the South and West. In most instances, their chief sectarian rivals were the homeopaths, except in the South, where the numbers of miscellaneous practitioners (many of them hold-overs from Thomsonianism) continued to vie even with the regulars. Overall, regulars amounted to 78 percent of practicing physicians, with homeopaths accounting for 5.9 percent, eclectics for 5.7 percent. Nearly 10 percent of medical practitioners were undefined, leaving one to believe that a considerable number of poorly educated irregular practitioners were practicing as a result of weak or nonexistent examining boards and licensing standards. Such states and territories as Arkansas, Georgia, Idaho, Illinois, Indiana, Massachusetts, Michigan, New York, Ohio, and Pennsylvania had great numbers of such irregulars. In Arkansas, unde-fined irregulars actually outnumbered regulars, homeopaths, eclectics, and hydropaths combined.[58]

In 1870, the Reformed Medical Association of the United States worked with other state organizations to revive the national associa-tion, which had become dormant after 1856. A convention there-fore met in Chicago that same year, reestablishing the National Eclectic Medical Association. Dr. John Wesley Johnson, a professor in the college at Worcester, was elected president; and Robert A. Gunn, professor of surgery at Bennett College of Eclectic Medicine and Surgery, Chicago, became secretary. Membership in the associ-ation included men *and* women graduates of reform medicine, and it adopted as its official organ the *Transactions* of the National Eclectic Medical Association.[59] The association met regularly in New York City, Indianapolis, Columbus, Boston, and Springfield, Illinois, and in the District of Columbia. Besides the national associ-ation, state societies operated in Maine, New Hampshire, Vermont, Massachusetts, Connecticut, New York, New Jersey, Pennsylvania, Ohio, Michigan, Indiana, Illinois, Wisconsin, Minnesota, Iowa, Missouri, Nebraska, Kansas, Oregon, and California. Outside the United States, eclectics found support in Canada and in England.

Beach introduced his reformed medical practice into England following a series of public lectures there in 1848, resulting in his publication of *The British and American Reformed Practice of Medicine: Embracing a Treatise on the Causes, Symptoms and Treatment of Diseases Generally, on Eclectic Principles: Including a Synopsis of Physiology and Midwifery* in 1859. Thomas Simmons, a Scottish surgeon, became a vocal advocate of Beach's ideas and assisted in spreading his

Medical Protestants

Table 5.1
Numbers of Physicians, 1873

States and Territories	Regular	Homeo-pathic	Hydro.	Eclectic	Misc.	Total
Alabama	853	5	—	—	—	858
Arizona	20	—	—	—	20	40
Arkansas	453	4	2	4	518	981
California	643	31	9	33	89	905
Colorado	40	2	—	5	6	53
Connecticut	430	46	2	47	56	581
Dakota	15	2	1	—	2	20
Delaware	113	14	1	7	3	138
Dist. of Columbia	174	887	—	5	14	200
Florida	139	—	—	—	—	139
Georgia	649	69	4	37	226	985
Idaho	19	—	—	1	1	21
Illinois	3,202	267	11	406	329	4,215
Indiana	2,463	115	3	358	221	3,161
Iowa	1,139	95	16	146	218	1,614
Kansas	443	7	—	6	164	620
Kentucky	1,996	41	2	60	99	2,198
Louisiana	560	18	—	2	21	601
Maine	527	45	1	29	54	656
Maryland	961	23	—	14	76	1,074
Massachusetts	1,120	190	3	136	432	1,881
Michigan	1,274	204	3	162	218	1,862
Minnesota	320	38	6	16	63	443

beliefs into English practice. A "zealous radical," Simmons identi-
fied with the causes of John Stuart Mill, Harriet Martineau, Eliza
Cook, William Cobbett, and others. He later moved to Canada
and then to Hartford, Connecticut.[60] In 1862, the British Medical
Reform Association organized with one hundred fifty members
under the leadership of James Skelton, Thomas Shotwell, William
Hitchman, Dennis Turnbull, J. H. Blunt, and J. F. Payne. The
Eclectic Medical Journal began publishing in 1864, followed by the
New Era of Eclecticism in 1869, which became the official journal
of the association. Along with the Americans, the British eclectics
denounced mineral remedies; but unlike their cousins, the British

Table 5.1 (continued)

States and Territories	Regular	Homeo-pathic	Hydro.	Eclectic	Misc.	Total
Mississippi	646	13	2	29	18	708
Missouri	2,140	67	3	124	149	2,483
Montana	22	2	—	—	11	35
Nebraska	117	8	—	18	50	193
Nevada	52	3	—	1	13	69
New Hampshire	371	32	3	43	38	487
New Jersey	750	102	4	30	67	953
New Mexico	21	—	1	1	1	24
New York	4,153	601	28	278	514	5,574
North Carolina	811	3	—	13	38	865
Ohio	3,032	263	16	378	364	4,053
Oregon	143	5	—	. 9	22	179
Pennsylvania	3,392	357	7	168	249	4,173
Rhode Island	134	33	—	23	67	257
South Carolina	583	1	1	—	1	586
Tennessee	1,434	24	2	64	81	1,528
Texas	1,186	21	2	22	49	1,280
Utah	9	1	—	7	1	18
Vermont	392	46	—	38	38	514
Virginia	1,195	4	—	6	18	1,223
Washington	26	1	—	7	7	41
West Virginia	401	16	—	69	95	581
Wisconsin	645	129	4	54	127	959
Wyoming	8	—	—	1	3	12
TOTAL	39,219	2,955	137	2,857	4,832	50,000

assailed the use of ether and chloroform in surgery as increasing the rate of mortality in operations and denounced vaccination as "an outrage upon the known laws of health and physiology." In effect, British eclecticism preferred a more conservative approach to medicine and a return to simpler therapeutic measures.[61]

Eclecticism also made inroads into upper Canada, the Canadian West, and Ontario due to the English-speaking fraternity of practicing physicians, their accessibility to American travelers and settlers, and the proximity of the latter province to Ohio, Pennsylvania, New York, and Michigan, which were hotbeds of sectarian activity. While some of these eclectics were simply converts from Thomsonianism and therefore without formal medical training, by the late 1850s and 1860s, trained Canadian practitioners began to graduate from colleges in Philadelphia, New York, and Cincinnati.[62]

6
Eclectic Materia Medica

Although eclectics did not always agree on why or how their medicines worked, they held certain things more or less basic, that is, agents that impaired the vital power should be discarded; one disease could be cured by producing another; and noxious drugs should be avoided.[1] In this category, calomel, tartar emetic, lead, tin, copper, and arsenic became the pariahs of reform medicine. These pillars of old-school therapeutics illustrated the harshness of allopathic medicine while ignoring the proven use of harmless, innocent, and well-tried substitutes. In addition to their stand against mineral drugs, eclectics opposed blistering, bleeding, and drastic purging. They also objected to the use of opium, except with extraordinary precautions, and refused to use greasy cerates and ointments as medical carriers.[2] Instead, they chose a liniment base consisting of a saturated solution of ammonium chloride to which they added medicinal preparations, such as the tincture of monkshood (aconite) and camphor.[3]

"We refuse to bleed," wrote one eclectic, "because we consider it unscientific, injurious to the constitution and often dangerous to life." Physicians had the responsibility of promoting recovery and of abstaining from those things that would worsen "debility, or break down that vital power upon which . . . recovery depends."

Reformers liked to point to the trials conducted by Joseph Dietl (1804–78) of Vienna on 380 pneumonia patients in the wards of the Hôpital de la Charité in the 1860s, which demonstrated the mortality rates from bleeding and from tartar emetic compared with the "unassisted resources of nature"—*vis medicatrix naturae*. In the experiment, 189 people were treated by diet and rest alone, with fourteen deaths, or 7.4 percent mortality; 106 were treated by large doses of tartar emetic, with twenty-two deaths, or 20.7 percent mortality; and eighty-five were treated by bleeding, with seventeen deaths, or 20.4 percent mortality. John Hughes Bennett and Joseph Skoda performed similar tests that confirmed Dietl's findings. "Wherever the blood-letting treatment has been subjected . . . to a careful scientific investigation," wrote one eclectic, "the result has proved that it has no power to control inflammation, but, on the contrary, by increasing the weaknesses and irritability of the constitution, it renders the inflammatory process more dangerous and destructive." Eclectics frequently referred to the clinical work of Gabriel Andral, Jules Gavarret, François Majendie (1783–1855), and Leon Simon, who opposed bloodletting as destructive of the vitality of consumptive constitutions.[4]

Reform practitioners supported preventive medicine and believed in sustaining the vital forces; and, although they did not practice general venesection, they did sometimes resort to localized bleeding in certain types of congestion. In most cases, however, they substituted gelsemine, veratrine, or hyoscyamine. They also rejected cupping and leeching, as well as mush jackets and poultices of any kind. They instead recommended the use of larded cloth dusted with emetic powder or parchment lightly spread with Libradol. And, as part of their attempt to utilize the truths of all medical systems, eclectics openly adopted hydropathic treatment in the 1850s.[5]

Even though they were enthusiastic users of electrical apparatuses, eclectics objected to electric belts and chairs, which had become the property of quacks and charlatans. Yet, because of the open-ended nature of reform medical practice, professors at the E. M. Institute, as well as their graduates, often strayed into idiosyncratic fields of therapeutic theory and practice. This meant promoting their own therapeutic theories, selling their own medicines, and feuding with colleagues regarding the efficacy of their special regimens. Institute faculty experimented extensively with the use of galvanic and magneto-voltaic batteries to relieve patients of the consequences of old-school treatment by removing mercury and other metals from the body. Essentially, they offered to electrolyze "obnoxious metals" from the system by using a sponge moistened with a solution of salt, which they attached to a positive pole and passed along the patient's spine. They then attached a negative pole to a copper plate and placed it in a footbath, where the patient rested his or her feet. If mercury, lead, arsenic, antimony, and other deleterious metals existed in the system, they were withdrawn by electrolysis to the copper plate.[6] "One electrolysis is generally sufficient," commented J. Milton Sanders, "but it sometimes requires two or three sittings in order to withdraw entirely from the body all the mercury that may be lingering there."[7]

The Medium System

Every system of medicine touted some feature that distinguished it from all others. For the allopaths, a remedy, to be efficacious, produced a morbid state in the body different from the one already existing, thus justifying their predilection for puking, purging, and depleting patients with calomel, tartar emetic, blistering agents, and bloodletting. In contradistinction to this theory, homeopaths claimed to cure disease by using drugs that in a healthy person produced symptoms similar to those of the disease (*similia similiabus curantur*). Samuel Hahnemann (1755–1843) and his disciples, refusing to administer doses in conventional amounts, chose remedies in small quantities, in infinitesimal amounts.

Eclectics introduced the "medium system" into the materia medica as an alternative to the allopathic and homeopathic systems of the period. The originator of the medium system, Johann Martin Honigberger, M.D. (1795–1869), a native of Kronstadt in Transylvania, practiced medicine for thirty-five years in the East (Turkey, Syria, Bukhara, and Hindustan) between 1815 and 1850. During those years, he managed several hospitals and dispensaries where he tested the effects of various reform theories. He devoted his energies in particular to investigating the materia medica and the competing claims of allopaths and homeopaths. Because of his accomplishments, eclectics declared that Honigberger had built a monument "that will tower as far above the heads of his compeers as the Pyramid of Cheops is loftier than the Sphinx."[8]

Honigberger divided medicines into three classes: those containing milder plants, earths, charcoals, salts, metals, and the weaker vegetable acids; those containing acrid plants, some of the crystallized vegetable acids, and the mild chemical preparations; and those containing all so-called poisons of the animal, vegetable, and mineral families. He administered remedies of the first class in doses of $1/25$ to $1/5$ grain; those of the second class from $1/50$ to $1/25$ grain; and those of the third class in doses of from $1/100$ to $1/50$ grain. He dispensed all medicines as tinctures or triturations made into powders or lozenges.[9] In addition, he urged physicians to prepare their own medicines (or at least to oversee their preparation), never trusting them to ordinary apothecaries. Following his advice, most eclectics chose to dispense their own medicines, a practice that encouraged them to prescribe the best remedies they could purchase from wholesale pharmacies, relying on the reputation of the manufacturer for purity and strength.[10] The practice also inspired the confidence of each patient, who knew that the physician was doubly interested in his or her case. By dispensing their own medicines, reform practitioners kept in close touch with patients, learning more thoroughly their conditions and the subtle aspects of the various drug therapies.[11] Reform medical colleges placed a special emphasis in their curricula on pharmacotherapeutics, a factor that reflected their origins, as well as their persistent opposition to allopathic medicines. Industrial pharmacists eventually recognized the financial possibilities of catering to the needs of these predominantly botanic physicians. Only when this occurred did eclectics relinquish their custom of preparing stock medicines, and even then, most persisted in dispensing their own medicines from their offices and during visits to the sick.[12]

In spite of the eclectics' dedication to the medium system and the purity and accuracy of their materia medica, the reluctance of reform medical schools and their pharmaceutical manufacturers to embark on a full scientific study of their medicines "doomed . . . much of eclectic pharmacy to scientific sterility and gross empiricism."[13] True, many physicians representing the scientific side of medicine applauded eclectics for their emphasis on a botanical and indigenous materia medica; nevertheless, they also criticized them for their lack of original research and their failure to be objective. And William Proctor (1817–74), professor of pharmacy at the Philadelphia College of Pharmacy and editor of the *American Journal of Pharmacy*, admonished eclectics for promoting vegetable medicines without understanding the exact chemical nature of each.[14]

Eclectic Calomel and the Concentrations

In 1831, William Hodgson, Jr., analyzed podophyllum rhizome and published his results in the *American Journal of Pharmacy*. Several years later, in 1846, John King, considered the analytical pharmacologist of eclectic medicine, described the resin of podophyllum and began prescribing it to patients.[15] Months later, John R. Lewis published a separate analysis of the rhizome, describing the resins and suggesting that six or seven grains acted as a drastic cathartic, accompanied by vomiting. While King and Lewis wrote independently of one another, King recommended the resin as a therapeutic agent, touting the virtues of the drug before his classes at the E. M. Institute and advocating it as a substitute for calomel.[16]

Besides his work on podophyllum, King experimented with the the resin of macrotys (*Cimicifuga racemosa*) and the oleoresins of iris, black cohosh, and Culvers root (leptandra).[17] Oleoresins (sometimes called *soft resinoids* or *gum resins*) were the medicinal principles of plants precipitated by water from their alcoholic solutions. They maintained the same degree of medicinal power and purity as resins but were semifluid in character and could not be manufactured in powdered form without decomposing. Thus, they were processed in the form of soft extracts or thick oils. Oleoresins included apocynin from dogbane, aletrin from star root (devil's bit), asclepidin from pleurisy root (butterfly weed), liatrin from button snakeroot, and oil of lobelia from the lobelia seed.[18]

King gave the name podophyll*um* to his discovery but eventually accepted the more popular term podophyll*in*. William S. Merrell, pharmaceutical manufacturer and proprietor of Union Drug Store in Cincinnati, prepared the drug in 1847 for commercial use and introduced the name *resinoid* in place of *resin* and also defended the *-in* suffix for the resinous principle on the authority of George B. Wood, professor at the Philadelphia College of Pharmacy and, as stated earlier, coeditor with Franklin Bache (1792–1864) of the *U.S. Dispensatory*.[19] When the *U.S. Pharmacopoeia* officially recognized Resina Podophylli in 1860, it did so with the name formulated by the editors of the *U.S. Dispensatory*, a fact frequently overlooked by the opponents of reform medicine who considered that *name* an exclusively eclectic term. Opponents included physician and pharmaceutical manufacturer Edward R. Squibb (1819–1900), who accused eclectics of ignoring the drug's true nature, having given it a name that was "vulgar and inelegant." Understandably, physicians and their patients confused podophyll*in* and similar resins with the termination -*ine* already established in alkaloidal chemistry and in such drugs as morphine and quinine manufactured by Squibb.[20] These criticisms aside, podophyllin (or podophyllum) quickly assumed a position of importance in the vegetable materia medica, becoming known to many as Eclectic Calomel.[21]

Eclectics credit William S. Merrell with having established the industrial side of reform pharmacy by having manufactured its earliest concentrated medicines. A native of Oneida County in western New York, Merrell graduated from Hamilton College in Clinton, New York, in 1823 and then moved west, opening a preparatory school in Cincinnati, where he taught chemistry and allied sciences. He was hired a year later as principal of a seminary at Augusta, Kentucky, and three years after that, appointed president of a women's college in Tuscumbia, Alabama. In 1830, he returned to Cincinnati and opened a drug-manufacturing business with his son George Merrell and grandson Charles G. Merrell. With the encouragement of Beach and Morrow at the E. M. Institute, he prepared medicines for botanic practitioners, introducing the preparations of sanguinaria and hydrastis canadensis and King's resin of podophyllum. The elder Merrell quickly brought these medicines into the fold of eclectic practice and won adherents among the faculty of the institute and among reform physicians in general, who designated them concentrated remedies, essential tinctures, and positive medicine.[22] Merrell also propounded a law of organic chemistry, which stated that pure alcohol, in its power as a solvent, extracted and separated those elements in vegetable and animal bodies that were medicinal or poisonous from those that were nutritive or inert. With this as a foundation, he developed a series of concentrated fluid medicines considered superior to all other herbal preparations. These solutions, or tinctures, retained the active principles of the plants from which they were prepared and were not prone to decomposition.[23]

Before Merrell, reform physicians had prepared most of their own compounds, teas, and decoctions; rolled their own pills; and mixed their own salves and plasters. This practice proved inconvenient and cumbersome for many physicians, and patients frequently objected to their bulk and unpleasantness. Merrell's concentrated remedies, made from the whole plant, came as a welcome stimulus to reform medicine, which believed that it had discovered an armamentarium equal to the alkaloid pharmaceuticals of the allopaths and the infinitesimal triturations of the homeopaths.[24]

Other pharmaceutical companies soon sought to benefit from the lucrative new industry. They included H. M. Merrell Co. of Cincinnati (later Lloyd Brothers Pharmacists, Inc.); Hosea Winchester of Missouri; F. D. Hill and Co. of Cincinnati (1852); American Chemical Institute, better known as B. Keith and Co. of New York City (1854); William H. Baker and Co., St. Louis (1854); T. C. Thorpe, Cincinnati (1854); Dr. I. Wilson, Cincinnati (1854); Tilden and Co., New York (1856); George M. Dixon, Cincinnati (1856); H. H. Hill and Co., Cincinnati (1862); and T. L. A. Greve, Cincinnati (1862). These firms listed their products as alkaloids, resinoids, resins, and concentrated medicines. But, observed one manufacturer and critic, "no attempt was made to distinguish between useful agents and those questionable, or between the unworthy and those entitled to a systematic position, by legitimate scientific nomenclature." As a result, "the odium of it all rested, unfortunately, on the eclectic school of medicine, by reason of the origin of the first of these products, the Resin of Podophyllum, and a few other worthy members, introduced by Dr. King." Enthusiastic eclectics found themselves "entrapped in the craze," and business rivals, bitterly antagonistic and viciously personal in their claims, embroiled the reform medical practice in their competitive struggles.[25]

William Elmer of Auburn, New York, formed a partnership with Stephen H. Potter of Syracuse Medical College. Together with John T. Goodin of Utica, New York, Dwight Russell, Sears Crosby, and Alexander Wilder, they opened the American College of Pharmacy in 1851 to teach general and pharmaceutical chemistry, theoretical and practical pharmacy, materia medica and therapeutics, as well as to prepare and dispense a scientific materia medica based on reform principles. Another objective of the college was more mercenary in intent, that is, they wished to supply the profession with pure and reliable drugs, both crude and concentrated, thereby avoiding the dangers of impure and imported medicines.[26] Wilder later withdrew from the college to join B. Keith and Co., which successfully manufactured concentrated remedies for reform physicians. Dr. B. Keith owed much of his success to his affiliation with Dr. Grover Coe, an ex-president of the National Eclectic Medical Association, who drew upon his reputation and professional contacts to advertise and sell the company's products. Coe also authored _Positive Medical Agents_ (1855) to market the products manufactured by B. Keith and Co.[27]

The concentrated medicines disappointed eclectic practitioners, who turned gradually to the more popular alkaloid pharmacy of the regulars. The decline in popularity of these drugs stemmed from allegations of adulteration and, equally important, the schism within the E. M. Institute that resulted in the formation of Joseph R. Buchanan's rival school, the Eclectic College of Medicine, which criticized the institute's endorsement of the drugs manufactured by B. Keith and Co.[28] Robert S. Newton and Zoheth Freeman, along with Lorenzo E. Jones and Alexander H. Baldridge, supported B. Keith and Co. and represented one side, while Charles H. Cleaveland, William Sherwood, John King, John Wesley Hoyt, and Buchanan represented the opposition. The hostility between these two camps reached such a pitch that one man reportedly kicked an adversary down a stairway at the institute.[29] Besides these internal feuds, noted scientists and pharmacists attacked the loose nomenclature and lack of original work in the eclectic's materia medica. This criticism also extended to eclectic practice itself, and practitioners were forced to defend themselves and their system from barrages made on the basis of the tarnished reputations of their pharmaceutical manufacturers. Although supporters of reform medical practice boasted that many of their plant drugs had passed into regular practice, having entered the _U.S. Pharmacopoeia_ and the _National Formulary_, this claim proved false on closer scrutiny. The success of plant drugs actually resulted more from increasing interest by scientists and regulars in the effectiveness of indigenous plant medicines than from claims made by the eclectics themselves.[30]

Disgusted with the mercenary aspects of eclectic pharmacy, King refused to be affiliated with the aggressive marketing campaign that grew out of his original discoveries. "A resinoid craze arose," observed drug manufacturer John Uri Lloyd, "similar to other professional distempers and fanaticisms, such as the American elixir craze of the early seventies, and similar fads that from time to time have risen to plague over-zealous enthusiasts." While

King endorsed only those derived from podophyllum and macrotys, and those called irisin and leptandrin, other concentrated remedies had entered the market without sufficient investigation, including baptisin (from baptisia, or wild indigo); caulophylline (from caulophyllum, or blue cohosh); cornine (from dogwood); corydaline (from corydalis, or turkey pea); cypripedin (from cypripedium, or lady's slipper); dioscorein (from dioscorea, or wild yam); eryngine (from eryngium, or corn snakeroot); eupatorine (from eupatorium, or boneset); geranine (from geranium, or cranesbill); jalapin (from jalap root); myricin (from bayberry); lobeline (from lobelia herb); juglandin (from juglans, or butternut bark); phytolaccin (from phytolocca, or garget or pokeweed); prunine (from prunus, or wild cherry); sanguinarin (from sanguinaria, or bloodroot); trillin (from trillium, or birthroot); and xanthoxylin (from xanthoxylum, or prickly ash bark).[31]

King, appalled by the adulterations attributed to his original discovery, wrote a trenchant criticism of the concentrated preparations in the *Worcester Journal of Medicine* in 1855. "I now wish to call [the] attention of all classes of physicians to a most stupendous fraud which is being perpetrated upon them in relation to concentrated preparations," he wrote. He believed that these remedies tarnished the cause of eclecticism and condemned them as quackery. Already, old-school physicians were manifesting an interest in concentrated medicines, and if "we permit such trash to be foisted upon them as pure agents," they would soon attribute this pharmaceutical junk to eclecticism itself.[32] Simultaneously came remarks from Edwin S. Wayne, a Cincinnati pharmacist and a chemist affiliated with the Ohio Medical College. In the *American Journal of Pharmacy*, he challenged the purity of the alkaloids, resinoids, and concentrations made by B. Keith and Grover Coe, claiming that, of the eighteen drugs manufactured by the company, only jalapin, podophyllin, sanguinarin, and hydrastine were true representations. The remainder were "mixtures of inorganic bodies, such as magnesia, and traces of vegetable extractives." Wayne attacked the entire class of substances not only for impurities but for the dogma of a single principle paralleling the plant as a whole.[33]

For reasons not entirely altruistic, John M. Scudder entered the fray, arguing that the so-called concentrated medicines were nothing but "unmitigated humbug" and that reform practice had

been cursed with "poor medicines" because of the misrepresenta-
tions of manufacturers. With the exception of the resin of podophyllum and the alkaloidal salts of hydrastis and sanguinaria, the
rest were best forgotten and replaced with a "kindlier" system of
medication.[34] Scudder exhorted his colleagues to return to "office
pharmacy" or to purchase their drugs from reputable drug houses
that guaranteed the quality of their medicines.[35] In an editorial in
1867 in the *American Eclectic Medical Review*, coeditors Robert S.
Newton and P. Albert Morrow reinforced Scudder's view by explaining that the *Eclectic Dispensatory* denied any relationship with
the "indefinite and unauthoritative manner" in which unskilled
manufacturers had prepared eclectic remedies. In particular, they
disavowed responsibility for the concentrated medicines manufactured in the absence of uniform standards.[36]

Concentrated medicines continued to be manufactured despite
criticism, and the list of items "enlarged by leaps and bounds."
According to one of the most constant critics, legitimate resinous
precipitates were "crowded into a corner," while a succession of
concentrations appeared "as parasites to plague the school." The
work of Merrell and of King, lost amid products masquerading
under the plant names and eclectic medicine, became saddled with
the alkaloidal-resinoidal fad that discredited their most earnest
efforts.[37]

Specific Medicine

Throughout the first three-quarters of the nineteenth century,
therapeutic specificity meant that practitioners had to relate such
idiosyncratic variables as sex, constitution, temperament, diet, oc-
cupation, climate, race, and age to their rationalistic systems. While
the principles of medicine were immutable, physicians learned the
practice of medicine in the context of these variables. Here was
the truly "artful" part of the art of medicine. The regulars regarded
this concept of therapeutic specificity as distinct from disease-spe-
cific treatment, which, during this same period, was decried as the
property of the quacks and charlatans whose medical "cookbooks"
matched each disease with a specific drug.[38] Specific medicine also
referred to the specific in nosology, in etiology, and in therapy.
Originating in ancient medicine, it was revived during the Renaissance by Paracelsus (called by some historians "the Nestor of the
specific in medicine") and remained popular through the seven-

teenth century. Thomas Sydenham viewed diseases as entities that, like botanists' plant specimens, could be observed, described, and classified. Indeed, for Sydenham, specificity in medicine meant specific nosology and specific etiology, as was true for treatment. And although he could point only to cinchona, he held that other therapeutic specifics would be discovered.[39]

Attempts to identify morbid entities meant relying on clinical observations classified by various taxonomic lists. The best example of this thinking appeared in *Nosologia methodica* (1768) by François Boissier de Sauvages de la Croix (1706–67), a follower of George Ernst Stahl. Sauvages identified the soul as the activator of the body and classified twenty-four hundred different diseases as though they were specimens in natural history. The very magnitude of these lists enraged opponents, who argued that the supposed entities were simply names given to combinations of symptoms. This criticism allowed men like Benjamin Rush, William Cullen, and John Brown to deny the actual existence of disease entities. Yet, as Richard H. Shryock noted, the doctrines of these system builders were "more misleading than were the nosologies they repudiated." Not until Giovanni Morgagni (1682–1771) of Padua sought to demonstrate disease entities by correlating symptoms with postmortem pathology did medicine find a way out of this nosologic confusion.[40]

In 1824, Gottlieb M. W. Ludwig Rau (1779–1840) of Hesse published a treatise, *Ueber den werth des homeöopathischen Heilverfahrens* (*The Value of the Homeopathic Practice of Medicine*), which urged fellow homeopaths to acquire more thorough scientific and technical knowledge of disease processes. Years later, in his *Organon of the Specific Healing Art* (1847), Rau saw himself as perfecting the work of Samuel Hahnemann by picking out the "particles of truth in whatever system he may find them, and by means of the Specific principle, arranging them into one harmonious whole."[41] His system of specific medication (*spezifischen heilkuntz*) consisted of not so much the means and the medicines used as it did the rules by which they were employed.[42]

Rau criticized the physiological theories then in vogue as pretentious and uncertain and deprecated the trend in pathology as little more than gross materialism, believing that pathologists had overlooked the existence of a vital activity. Finally, he declared that knowledge in regard to the cause of disease was scarcely more than speculation and that healing required a careful study of the external phenomena as well. Understanding these two principles enabled the physician to select the proper remedy. In an effort to improve Hahnemann's method, Rau proposed to analyze the two agencies involved in the production of disease: the external, or morbific, cause; and the internal cause, meaning the organism itself. In other words, disease was not just a juxtaposition of symptoms; it was also a physiological disturbance of the organism that served as a basis for pathological facts and symptoms. A drug, to be effective, had to invade the organism in the same manner as the morbific principle. "The similarity," wrote Alexander Wilder, "which is the essence of the Homeopathic dogma, should not pertain merely to the outward resemblance of the drug-symptoms to the symptoms of the disease. It must go deeper and apply to the drug-disease reflected by its pathogenic symptoms and likewise to the morbid conditions or pathologic state of the organism."[43]

Dr. Charles J. Hempel (1811–79), one of the earliest American converts to the doctrines of Hahnemann, published *Organon of Specific Homeopathy* (1854) in which he sought to clarify the incomplete system of Hahnemann. Adopting the sentiments of Rau, he argued that the phenomena of disease were as definite and as logical as the phenomena of health and that physiological functions served as a basis of pathological facts and symptoms. And borrowing from Emanuel Swedenborg's contention that a "correspondence" existed between all things spiritual and physical, Hempel argued that the principle of "similarity," which represented the essence of homeopathic dogma, went beyond the outward resemblance of drug symptoms to symptoms of disease and applied as well to the pathologic state of the organism. The principle, he concluded, implied "a PERFECT CORRESPONDENCE between the drug disease and the natural pathological disturbance; and in order to leave no doubt that this compound similarity or perfect correspondence is the import of the formula, a more adequate expression thereof would be: CORRESPONDENTIA CORRESPONDENTIBUS CURANTUR."[44]

Eclectic medicine emphasized the importance of simplicity in prescribing therapeutic agents singly or in comparatively simple combinations, with definite ideas about the purpose and effect of each medicine. Although single remedies were a characteristic of homeopathic practice, eclectics carried the concept one step further, believing that disease "should not be treated by routine methods, according to disease names, but that the treatment should be specifically adapted to the particular symptom-complex under observation." This doctrine, elaborated on and systematized by John M. Scudder in *Specific Medication and Specific Medicines* (1870) and *Specific Diagnosis* (1874), theorized that a fixed relationship existed between drug force and disease expression and recommended the use of a simple medication as a direct remedy for a specific pathological condition. Put another way, Scudder suggested applying empiricism and experimentation to form the foundation of knowledge concerning each specific medicine.[45] This meant using *Asclepias tuberosa* for pleurisy; *Cereus bonplandii* in angina pectoris and palpitation; belladonna for scarlatina (scarlet fever) and pertussis (whooping cough); *Drosera rotundifolia* for the cough of measles; lobelia for the spasmodic attacks of asthma; phosphorus and nux vomica in typhoid conditions; cimicifuga in rheumatism; and ergot for uterine hemorrhage.[46]

Unlike homeopaths, Scudder did not recognize a "law" of cure. While he did prescribe according to symptomatic expression (which resembled homeopathic practice), he did "not prejudge the effect of his medicines because it has produced a certain action in health." Scudder believed his system differed as well from allopathy, which used such specifics as mercury and arsenic for syphilis and other spirillum-based diseases; thymol and oil of chenopodium for hookworm; quinine for malaria; sulfur for the itch (psoriasis); salicylates for rheumatism; and numerous serums and vaccines for diseases due to infections.[47]

Scudder's advocacy of specific medication and specific diagnosis initially made him a pariah in his own school. But those students who sat in his lectures were impressed with the logic of his statements and with the forcefulness of his convictions. His colleague Eli G. Jones objected to the term *specific medication*, preferring instead the term *definite medication*, meaning the definite action of drugs for definite results and definite indications. Scudder's defenders, however, considered the terms synonymous. Indeed, Scudder's works contained frequent reference to direct medication and the direct action of drugs. One apologist attributed much of the confusion and misunderstanding to the old idea of specifics for diseases. "This was never the idea of Professor Scudder—that there were specifics for diseases. He emphasized the statement, more than once, that he rejected such an idea in his scheme of therapeutics. His doctrine was, specific medication for specific conditions; direct medication for special requirements, as indicated by specialized symptoms; definite medication for definite states as individually indicated."[48]

To paraphrase, the cardinal principles of specific medication included:

1. Disease is to be regarded as an impairment of the life of the creature. It may be of the structure in and by which he or she lives or of the forces that give life; but it is the life that is to be regarded in medicine.
2. Disease has distinct expressions, as has health; and they may be recognized by those who train themselves to undertake accurate observation. The expression "language of disease" is not a poetic allusion but a statement of fact.
3. There are certain forces in nature, locked up in substances called medicines, that act directly upon the living body, enabling it to resist disease and aiding in a restoration of normal functions and structures.
4. The action of such substances has been determined by observation in the past and is being further known by experiments and observations of the present. Even now our knowledge of the power of drugs is sufficient to enable us to apply them with certainty in a very large number of diseased conditions.
5. We have proven that special drugs meet special conditions of disease. As these conditions of disease have distinct expressions and may be recognized by the physician, we say that these disease expressions become drug indications.
6. Lastly, if these drug indications be followed, the action of remedies will be certain and curative, and the practice of medicine will have a scientific basis, which will ensure a continued improvement year by year.[49]

Eclectics considered the first four principles self-evident, while the fifth proposition became a distinctive feature of specific medication and of eclectic practice in the late nineteenth century. It required learning the language of disease and the specific actions of drugs and applying them in a rational way. For example, if the tongue exhibited a deep red color, the physician knew there was an excess of alkali, requiring the use of an acid. If, on the other hand, the tongue appeared white, this meant an excess of acid and the physician prescribed an alkali, perhaps sulfite of sodium. It did not matter if the physician diagnosed typhoid fever, pneumonia, or dysentery. The condition of the disease mandated the type of remedy. "Thus we learn to prescribe to conditions of disease, not names," remarked W. S. Turner in 1902. "We treat the patient, not the disease."[50]

Clearly, elements of Scudder's ideas existed earlier in the writings of Charles J. Hempel, Gottlieb M. W. Ludwig Rau, and Johann Martin Honigberger, all of whom belonged to the homeopathic school; some even claimed it was part of physio-medical doctrine. Nevertheless, Scudder diverged from homeopathic and physio-medical antecedents when he called the new doctrine *specific medication*, meaning "certain well-determined deviations from the healthy state will always be corrected by specific medications."[51] When he became professor of theory and practice of medicine and pathology at the E. M. Institute, Scudder drew to his ideas the attention of the profession and turned to John Uri Lloyd to manufacture his preparations. Lloyd copyrighted the labels of Scudder's specific medicines to maintain uniform standards and to protect physicians from the proliferation of imitations that had earlier damaged the reputation of John King's concentrated medicines.[52]

As the administration of violent ultimates gave way to Scudder's "kindlier methods," the motto *vires vitales sustinete* (sustain the vital forces) became the watchword of reform practice. "Small doses of kindly remedies, established by clinical study in disease, administered for curative action, not systemic shock, now universally prevail," wrote Lloyd. "The non-poisonous remedies, made of innocuous drugs, are now sought and are administered with a degree of therapeutic satisfaction unknown in past heroic dosage."[53] From Scudder's point of view, eclectic medicine had achieved its early reform goals. With the introduction of specific medication, he hoped to begin a second revolution in the materia medica, eliminating many of the polypharmaceutical compounds current in the multitude of balsams, pills, powders, and syrups that dominated therapeutic practice. Instead, Scudder and Lloyd offered specific medicines gathered at the right season and from the right locality. These were simple tinctures made by percolation, with one troy ounce of drug to one fluid ounce of tincture. For the eclectic physician, the art and science of pharmacy had progressed from roots, barks, and herbs to decoctions, infusions, solid extracts, tinctures, fluid extracts, and finally to specific medicines.[54] Lloyd Brothers, Pharmacists, Inc., manufactured the specific medicines, supplying them in four-, eight-, and sixteen-ounce square bottles, each labeled with the indications for the remedy and the recommended dosage. Each specific medicine was made from a certain part of the plant supplying its name (i.e., bark, root, leaf, catkin, gum, wood, seed, flower, fruit, or stem). In some cases, Scudder preferred the green drug; in others, the dried form.[55]

The concept of specific medication was initially a source of criticism and acrimony among eclectics. Eventually, however, most eclectic schools and their faculties adopted specific medication as the principal tenet of their faith. "And now," observed Herbert T. Webster, M.D., "we realize that specific medication, direct medication, or definite medication, is really all there is, that is of much worth therapeutically, to medical practice." With the barriers down, only "the most stupid practitioners of medicine now stand aloof of the generally accepted doctrine that the proper method of treating disease is by the direct method—the direct action of remedies for definite conditions."[56] Specific medications in effect transformed eclectic practice in the second half of the nineteenth century, giving it a level of scientific exactness that enabled it to compete with the synthetic pharmacy of the regulars. "Scudderism," wrote Otto Juettner of Cincinnati, became "a synonym for advanced eclecticism."[57]

Even though specific medication contained certain well-defined principles, it could not be categorized as a universal practice among eclectics. John Buchanan of the Eclectic Medical College of Philadelphia called it a "gigantic fraud" foisted upon suffering humanity by a gang of eclectics eager to divide the spoils of their deceit.[58] "I would use specific medication just as any other—just as far as it will go, and no farther," wrote E. Younkin in 1895.[59] Similarly, when Andrew Jackson Howe was asked if he believed in specific medication, he replied that he always advocated the application of remedies specifically prescribed to symptoms when the causes of disease were not understood. Howe was appointed demonstrator and professor of anatomy at the E. M. Institute in 1859, and in 1861, he succeeded Zoheth Freeman as chair of surgery, which he occupied until his death in 1892.[60] He believed in a well-devised system of nosology and preferred not to quibble over the difference between nosology and symptomatology. "If bacteriology means anything," he wrote in 1892, "it leans toward specific pathology." He saw the drift of pathology throughout the scientific world as a move in the direction of specific medication. "All practitioners of medicine are in search of a remedial hammer which will hit the morbid nail on the head ... [and] there is less and less shot-gun practice; less firing in the bushes; less and less mixing and compounding; and more and more rifle practice—aiming at the bull's eye."[61]

The Lloyd Brothers

When eclectic pharmacists began their investigations into the American materia medica, indigenous drugs were generally limited to a few examples, which were unsightly in appearance, bulky in dosage, nauseating in taste, of indefinite quality and strength, and uncertain in action. As demands increased, pharmaceutical firms, such as Merrell, Thorp, and Lloyd; Lloyd Brothers; W. S. Merrell; and B. O. and G. C. Wilson, began supplying American botanic and herbal remedies.[62] John Uri Lloyd (1849–1936), dubbed the "wizard of American plant pharmacy and chemistry," whose investigations into the colloidal conditions of plant-drug constituents opened a whole new field of pharmacology, stood heir to W. S. Merrell and B. Keith and Co. as the principal manufacturer of eclectic medicines and foremost among the pharmaceutical manufacturers of reform medical practice in the late nineteenth and early twentieth centuries. He regretted that pharmacists had only superficially scrutinized the vegetable world for remedial agents and that Americans preferred to import increasing amounts of medicinal plants while doing little to advance their own native materia medica. He challenged physicians and pharmacists to be "as fair, as discriminative, as patriotic, as have been the Eclectics in their work of the organic vegetable field," claiming there were twelve thousand plants west of the Mississippi yet to be examined for potential medicinal properties.[63] The possibilities locked up in this plant life promised a wealth of information for the future materia medica.[64]

John Uri, eldest of the Lloyd brothers, suffered from asthma when young and supposedly cured himself with a course of lobelia pills supplied by his grandfather, John Lloyd, and prepared according to the formula of Samuel Thomson.[65] At age fourteen, he entered pharmacy as an apprentice, working with J. W. Gordon at Eighth Street and Western Row (Central Avenue) in Cincinnati. Two years later, he completed a second apprenticeship with German pharmacist George Edger in 1865. During that time, he also attended lectures on chemistry given by Dr. Roberts Bartholow at the Ohio Medical College and matriculated both at the Cincinnati College of Pharmacy and at Miami Medical College, in Miami, Ohio. He became a clerk at Gordon's Pharmacy in 1869, and a few months later, his brother Nelson Ashley Lloyd (1852–1926) joined him there by working as an apprentice. In 1870, John Uri took the position of chemist with H. M. Merrell and Co., and at the suggestion of John King (and against the advice of Bartholow), he undertook a systematic study of the eclectic materia medica. Thus affiliated with reform medical practice, he carried the stigma of "irregular" with him the remainder of his life.[66]

John Uri and Nelson Ashley opened a laboratory for the study of the plant materia medica in 1876. A short time later, T. C. Thorp, the senior member of H. M. Merrell and Co., proposed that the two firms consolidate. With the merger of Merrell, Thorp, and Lloyd, John Uri took charge of the laboratory, while Nelson Ashley became a traveling salesman for Reakirt, Hale, and Co., wholesale druggists of Cincinnati. H. M. Merrell retired in 1881, and the firm changed to Thorp and Lloyd Brothers until 1885, when the brothers bought out the Thorp interest and changed the name to Lloyd Brothers, Pharmacists, Inc. John Uri had, through all of these years, attended the eclectic societys meetings, as well as those of the American Pharmaceutical Association and the Ohio State Pharmaceutical Association. Despite his connection with reform medicine, he was elected president of the American Pharmaceutical Association in 1887, after having served for many years as chair of the Committee on Queries and Papers.[67]

The youngest brother, Curtis Gates Lloyd (1859–1926), joined the drug establishment of Reakirt, Hale, and Co. (with whom Nelson Ashley was still associated), and he and John Uri published the first issue of a quarterly entitled *Drugs and Medicines of North America* (1884). Curtis became a partner in the firm with his brothers in 1886, with Nelson Ashley managing the business, John Uri supervising the laboratory, and Curtis devoting himself to the accumulation of books and the study of fungi.[68]

According to John Uri Lloyd, the American people's anger toward the abuses of medicine came from both educated and uneducated alike. "It was a combination of the unorganized, unprofessional majority, assisted by an inside, rebellious, self-sacrificing, professional minority. It was a home-to-home crusade, that needed no outside witnesses, no argument from afar, because in every American household pleaded the face of a tortured loved one, or lingered the memory of one who had failed to withstand the physician's inhuman ordeal." Out of this travail evolved the remedies of the botanics, whose preparations were the simple and compound syrups, tinctures, acetates, juices of plants both fresh and dried, as well as powders, infusions, and decoctions. Because many reform physicians could not disengage themselves from the fallacies of the day, the doses of these early preparations were often large and distressingly nauseating. "Even those in rebellion against dominant methods too often imagined that a medicine, to be useful, must be disagreeable, and that the depleting action of both the cathartic and the emetic was a necessity, in the simplest ailment." Thus, many of the reform practitioners' substitutes were themselves "viciously energetic" and dreadful to take.[69]

In his address before the Ohio State Pharmaceutical Association in 1895, John Uri Lloyd urged physicians to turn over the manufacture of medicines to experienced pharmaceutical companies. "I would not go back if I could to the medicines of thirty years ago. I would not change from the present to the past," he wrote. "I would not want my children to take the nastiness I used to prepare, and considered excellent medicine. While possibly our young men will regret, perhaps oppose, the changes that must come during the next twenty-five or thirty years, I believe that at the end of the time they will not be willing to go back to the position we are in now."[70]

With the outbreak of the First World War, American physicians found themselves embarrassingly dependent on foreign synthetics and serum products. Regulars had, in effect, neglected their own country's long-established plant materia medica. Not only were the sheet anchors of the materia medica (which by then came from German synthetics) cut off but drugs from India, Madagascar, Australia, and southern Africa were also affected by the war and by the disruption of shipping. The price of carbolic acid increased 1,125 percent from August 1914 to November 1915. Salicylic acid and sodium salicylate increased 825 percent, creosote 700 percent, and potassium permanganate 1,233 percent over their former values in the same time period.[71] In contrast, Lloyd took patriotic pride in the eclectic medicines, which "in an altruism that is truly American, resisted these synthetic innovations." By comparison, prices of eclectic drugs remained relatively inexpensive during the war years, with arnica flowers increasing 133 percent, senna leaves and belladonna leaves 200 percent, cannabis indica 20 percent, buckthorn bark 150 percent, dandelion root and kamala 100 percent, and ipecac 90 percent. The decision to hold the line on prices earned for eclectic medicine the secondary title "the American school of medicine."[72] During the war years, Americans turned to alternatives, finding gelsemium a substitute for monkshood (aconite); passiflora for Trional and vernal; and crataegus, cactus, and convallaria as replacements for digitalis and strophanthus.[73] Eclectics employed monkshood (aconite), gelsemium, bryonia, macrotys, varatrine, eupatorium, lobelia, asclepias, and ipecac during the influenza epidemic of 1918; and in treating pneumonia, they prescribed bryonia, monkshood, veratrine, lobelia, ipecac, and sanguinaria. External applications consisted of Libradol, compound emetic powder, turpentine applications, antiphlogistics, mustard drafts, camphorated oil, onion poultice, iodine applications, and on occasion flaxseed poultice, quinine inunction, snuff, and black pepper.[74]

Eclectics received unexpected praise from regulars because of their efforts to replace foreign drugs with those grown in the United States. William Pepper of the University of Pennsylvania acknowledged that eclectics deserved credit for establishing native botanical products. Similar praise came from Roberts Bartholow and Charles Rice, chair of the Committee of Revision of the *U.S. Pharmacopoeia*.[75]

John Uri Lloyd became a frequent speaker at reform medical colleges following the war. Esteemed as one of the "Fathers of Eclecticism," his articles were printed and reprinted in many of the eclectic journals. Most articles in the 1920s and 1930s were actually simply reprintings of writings from the turn of the century. Despite his age, Lloyd remained an active cheerleader for reform medicine, encouraging students to be proud of their minority status and staunch in their commitment to eclectic theory. Anyone could become a member of the majority school, he observed. But while the majority captured the greater numbers, the minority appealed to ideals. "It is the minority that, wedging into new fields, moves

men onward and upward. . . . Out of the minority come the ideal-
ists, who finally take advantage of opportunities that are in turn
seized upon by the majority, to benefit the people at large. . . . The
majority too often follow a leader, stepping duck-like, one after
the other."[76]

By the 1930s, nearly two hundred specific medicines were used
in eclectic practice. Some of the more popular eclectic medicines
included colocynthis, *Conium maculatum*, cypripedium, digitalis,
ergot, euonymus, gaultheria, gelsemium, geranium, gossypol (cotton root bark), grindelia (gumweed), hydrastis, ipecac, lappa, leptandra (Culvers root), lobelia, myrrh, nux vomica, and phytolacca.
Eclectic physicians never opposed legitimate drug combinations
that fortified each other or compounds of invaluable qualities possessed by no single drug. And even though eclectics opposed the
use of mercurials, John M. Scudder, Andrew Jackson Howe, and
John King prescribed both Donovan's Solution and Fowler's Solution (each an arsenical compound), biniodide of mercury, ammoni-
ated chloride of mercury, and chloride of gold. To their credit,
they avoided the heroic doses that regulars routinely prescribed.[77]

Lobelia, the time-honored Thomsonian remedy, used in infusion, decoction, powder, and fluid forms, also stood the test of
eclectic therapeutics. Eclectics prescribed it as late as the 1930s for
inflammatory conditions of the respiratory organs and in bronchi-
tis, pneumonia, and pleuropneumonia. As a stimulating expecto-
rant, they applied it for its relaxing influence in chronic cough;
and with the discovery by a Dr. Jentsch of Chicago of the specific
action of subculoyd lobelia administered hypodermically in diphtheria, its application expanded even further.[78]

With the demise of eclectic schools in the twentieth century,
numerous botanical drugs were dropped from the *U.S. Pharmacopoeia*. The 1900 revision omitted eleven; the 1910 revision, another
twenty-two; and the 1920 revision, yet another seventeen. Preparations chiefly affected were the so-called blood remedies, or alteratives, along with rheumatism, kidney, female, and nerve
remedies.[79]

Bacteriology

Since ancient times, doctors had viewed illness as an internal
imbalance of the body, expressed by disturbances in the secretions
(sweat, urine, phlegm, etc.) and implicit in the terms *isonomia* and

eukrasia. The idea of disease as a discrete clinical entity with its own distinctive natural history challenged this integrated view of the body—a challenge felt acutely in medical orthodoxy and among sectarians. Physicians in both camps found it difficult to give up long-held theories about the nature of the body and its illnesses. Nevertheless, achievements in surgery, anesthesiology, and pharmaceutical chemistry and in the theory of self-limited disease went far in compromising age-old ideas and in paving the way for the acceptance of germ theory, the reduction of diseases to definite and distinct species, and the corresponding need for therapeutic discreteness and specificity.

The concept of contagious and infectious diseases originating from microorganisms was certainly not new; Athanasius Kircher (1601–80) advanced it in the seventeenth century, as did Antoni van Leeuwenhoek. Italian Agostino Bassi (1773–1856) studied silkworm disease (muscardine) and demonstrated a causal relationship between the mold found on dead silkworms and the specific disease that killed them. Jacob Henle (1809–85), who announced the theory of a *contagium animatum* in 1840, recognized in Bassi's work an explanation for the "miasmatic-contagious" diseases, which spread by direct contact between individuals or indirectly through the air or through some other medium.

The discovery of muscardine was important because it was a disease caused by a living organism transmitted from one host to another by means of "germs." (Often the terms *virus, organism,* and *bacterium* were used synonymously with *germ.*) The study of molds visible under the microscope led directly to the study of bacteria and microscopic granules and their relationship to each other. Joseph Lister (1827–1912), through his antiseptic treatments, focused on ways to eliminate the presence of these germs from wounds.[80]

The gains made by chemists in the development of alkaloids in the early decades of the nineteenth century and the later synthesis of organic and synthetic molecules "opened the era of chemical agents consciously designed to act with molecular and cellular specificity." When Louis Pasteur and Robert Koch (1843–1910) demonstrated that specific microorganisms were the cause of certain illnesses, the stage was set for an era of immuno- and serotherapy that gave the bedside practitioner a tool whose precision equaled that of the surgeon's knife. "Disease is now seen as discrete entities," wrote Edmund D. Pellegrino, "with discrete causes; medication is selected for specific, not generic actions; therapy is aimed at removing causes, if at all possible, and genuine cure is, in many diseases, a very realistic objective; the measure of effectiveness, as it was in the nineteenth century, is not a predictable physiological response, but a predictable alteration of the expected evolution of the disease."[81]

Koch's work on anthrax, published in 1876, proved conclusively that a bacterium could be a specific infectious agent. He found that bacilli and micrococci existed for each specific complaint and urged the cultivation of such bacilli in order to apply them by inoculation as remedies and prophylactics.[82] Koch demonstrated the direct causal relationship between bacteria and disease by showing with meticulous skill and logic that different diseases were clinically distinguishable and associated with different specific microorganisms. Different pathogenic bacteria, despite morphological similarities, represented distinct species and produced diseases that were specific.[83]

An extensive literature grew out of Koch's discovery and helped elevate laboratory medicine to the rank of an exact science. Doctors consequently saw such diseases as measles, scarlet fever, diphtheria, leprosy, tuberculosis, cholera, and fevers in the context of bacteria and tribes of microbes. On the basis of this hypothesis, they revived several previously obsolete drugs, including mercury and antimony, to act as germicides—a revival that understandably came as a challenge to eclectics, who favored the milder vegetable materia medica.[84]   The shape and character of medicine's mind-set underwent profound change in the last quarter of the nineteenth century with the rise of Listerian antisepsis and pathogenic specificity, as well as the new serum regimens. Of all the sciences, bacteriology was the most successful in getting at, understanding, and attacking the *causes* of disease; it altered the conceptual foundations of medicine. And while this period opened new vistas, it also threatened the way physicians habitually thought about disease and treated patients, particularly those with tetanus, typhoid, malaria, and yellow fever. It made practitioners feel in jeopardy, wrote Russell C. Maulitz, by suggesting that scientific values, so promising of enhanced efficacy and legitimacy, might remove them from the bedside to the bench."[85] Laboratory science increasingly made inroads into the art and science of medicine. Chemistry, pathology, bacteriology, and physiology now required extensive laboratory work. Indeed, Koch's bacteriological achievements in the 1880s and 1890s brought laboratory research directly to the patient's bedside and, with it, a view of disease that was demonstrably distant from the disease theories of former times. The identification of specific pathogens for anthrax, diphtheria, tuberculosis, and cholera was the beginning of a revolution that threatened the very basis of the practitioner's status and armamentarium.

The work of Robert Koch and that of other pioneer bacteriologists in Europe had little impact on medicine in the United States before the 1880s. With the exception of E. P. Herd, who found evidence of germ theory untenable and suggested instead a chemical origin of contagion, American scientists and physicians were relatively indifferent to the early years of European debate on the issue, particularly since they saw little direct application to therapeutics. This changed when Koch announced his discovery in March 1882 of the tubercle bacillus by special culture and staining methods. Now, for the first time, physicians had an exact method of diagnosis that could differentiate the disease from the more common catarrh. Many hoped that the discovery of causation would result in a therapeutic advance as well.[86]

In 1883, William T. Belfield recounted in the New York *Medical Record* the history of the debate, including the many fallacies and conflicting claims that dominated much of the discussion.[87] Three years later, James T. Whittaker expressed his belief that practitioners might benefit from this research by finding a "specific therapy" for infectious disease.[88] The breakthrough came in 1884 with the work of Friedrich August Löffler (1852–1915), the identifier of the specific bacillus of diphtheria, and the parallel work of Pasteur, of Emil von Behring (1854–1917), and of Shibasaburo Kitasato (1852–1931), who promoted the study of immunology. The first human patients received the diphtheria antitoxin in 1891, and by 1895 the *Journal of the American Medical Association* recommended laboratory testing and the importance of serum injections in the therapeutic practice of the physician. By the 1890s, American researchers were publishing their findings in U.S. medical journals and were contributing regularly to the canon of antitoxin literature and the specificity of disease.[89]

The *American Journal of Pharmacy* continued to publish nongerm and antigerm theories of disease as late as 1885, while at the same time, advertisements in the journal touted the importance of sterile hypodermic solutions; antiseptic powders, gauzes, solutions, sponges, phenols and their derivatives; inorganic salts; antiseptic mouthwashes and tooth powders. The debate over germ theory had all but disappeared from its pages in the 1890s; instead, the journal routinely published articles on the public-health applications of the germ theory of disease. Also at this time, pharmacy took seriously the use of the microscope in bacteriological assays and in detecting adulteration in drugs.[90]

Certain practitioners confidently *opposed* germ theory, attacking much of the research as unscientific. Edinburgh gynecologist Sir Lawson Tait (1845–99) was so settled on its error that he even offered to apply microorganisms to surgical wounds to demonstrate his conviction. Eclectics accused allopaths of uncritically turning to serotherapy and attenuated or modified virus as a means of treating disease. This, they argued, made them akin to the homeopaths and their principle of *similia similiabus curantur* and to the allopaths and their earlier reliance on salivating and bleeding.[91] In years to come, remarked William E. Bloyer, M.D., president of the National Eclectic Medical Association in 1896, the regulars would still be hunting for the fountain of youth, the philosopher's stone, a universal germicide, or something else just as unlikely. Allopathy had become a "school of fancy, of fads, of vague theories, of much speculation—a close corporation of erratic dreamers, or hypothetical speculators—of theorists, and of slaves to the synthetic and coal tar products of German laboratories—in short, to the foreign patent medicine vendor."[92]

Other eclectics, many of whom were armed with the notoriety that befell Koch when his lymph cure failed, served notice that "germ-crazed theorists" and their high regard for every new form of serum therapy had actually increased the prevalence of cancer and consumption by disseminating the products of diseased animal tissue among humans. "The fact that statistics show a greater death rate from [cancer and tuberculosis] since the wonderful discovery of the germ theory," J. W. Hodge argued, "is strong evidence of the injury wrought by this monstrous medical fallacy." Essentially, germ theory had no scientific basis upon which to rest its claims. "It is," he reasoned, "a mere fantasy of fussy microscopists who know little or nothing of the real nature of disease." Hodge particularly objected to doctors who upheld the germ theory of disease and urged people to boil the water they drank. "The deluded guardians of the public health," he observed, "seem to be entirely oblivious of the fact that the large majority of the people who have suffered from typhoid fever have been victims of boiled water."[93]

Although an eclectic occasionally attempted to come to terms with germ theory, the *Eclectic Medical Journal* published a series of articles in 1905 poking fun at microbiology as the new religion and Pasteur as its god. Pasteurian medicine, one author predicted, "will go down in the future history of medicine as the most cruel deception ever practiced on the public by men calling themselves doctors."[94] In a similar vein, Vincent A. Baker, once president of the National Eclectic Medical Association, complained in an address that Lister had departed from common sense in his desire to kill spores and thus prevent suppuration.[95] Scudder was equally critical. In the *Eclectic Medical Journal*, he accused the majority school of directing its investigations almost wholly to bacteriology and not to validating the means of cure. As new remedies made their appearance, they fell by the wayside with the same rapidity. Eclectics, on the other hand, had escaped the stampede to this new and unknown form of medicine, including not just the patented synthetic remedies but also the "poisoned animal serum and gland juices." Reform medicine uniformly condemned Charles-Édouard Brown-Séquard's juice of testicles, and the countless "toxines" and serums of animals.[96] "The solid, practical part of the study of medicines as therapeutic agents is simply being neglected," Scudder wrote, so that "someone may have his name attached to that of some bacillus." In contrast, eclectic practice promised a more stable platform for medicine: "A good old medicine or method," avowed the editor, "is not quickly thrown over for a new and untried one."[97]

Scudder's views aside, some eclectics insisted that the doctrine of specific medication was compatible with bacteriology. "Biological facts," commented George H. Knapp of Cincinnati, "are not the peculiar property of any school, but are of universal application and not open to controversy."[98]

It may be said that it is not mandatory for one who practices specific medication to maintain an attitude of hostility toward bacteriology or to be abnormally incredulous in admitting evidence from this field of investigation. The incomplete, fragmentary evidence adduced to the argument of the opponents of the

germ theory has in no way refuted the fundamental facts of
bacteriology, but a redeeming feature of the animal versions
sometimes cast at the germ theory by its detractors has been a
restraining, leavening influence on the assertions of certain
over zealous enthusiasts whose statements have at times bor-
dered closely on the absurd and ridiculous. Many points in bacteriology are still obscure, fact and theory not always clearly
delimited, and the opinions of bacteriologists are frequently at
variance, yet when the germ theory is considered in its entirety
the overwhelming burden of evidence forces one to believe that
the central idea of a contagium vivum is correct. But there is
no immediate danger of the great work which has been done
by the Eclectic school in the development of its Materia Medica
being abrogated by serum therapy.[99]

In a paper delivered before the California Eclectic Medical
Society, Charles Clark, M.D., of San Francisco, pressed his colleagues to overcome their prejudices against the use of vaccines
and serums. "I am sorry to say that the suggestion of such material
to the average Eclectic is almost equivalent to raising a red flag
before the proverbial bull," he stated. "If we are truly what our
name implies we should thoroughly investigate before we
condemn."[100]

Retrospect

By the late nineteenth century, the eclectics had developed a
distinctive pharmacy, in that their use of plants indigenous to the
United States represented a significant challenge to allopathy and
a decided effort to establish a therapeutic arsenal that could stand
alongside the claims of medical orthodoxy. The young physician
starting out in reform practice in the 1880s carried in his medical
bag a number of drugs basic to eclectic practice. Foremost among
them was monkshood (aconite) for the initial stages of a chill and
croup. Next came bryonia, indicated in pleurisy, pleuropneumonia, and articular rheumatism, followed by belladonna for capillary
congestion, blue skin, dullness, dilated pupils, and stupor. Other
essential drugs included nux vomica for abdominal pain and atonic
diarrhea, nausea, and general lack of innervation; colocynthis in
dysentery and pains in the bowels, even in colic from cold or other
causes; gelsemium for infantile spasms, neuralgia, and in nervous
tension during parturition; phytolacca for sore throat; *Rhus toxico-*

dendron (poison ivy) for restlessness; jaborandi in heart pains; macrotys in muscular pain and uterine inertia in labor; bromide of ammonia with gelsemium in convulsions; bichromate of potassium for hoarseness and sore throat; hamamelis tincture as a specific in hemorrhage of the bowels; tincture of cinnamon for postpartum hemorrhage; and apomorphine as an emetic in cases of poisoning when a stomach pump could not be used. Eclectics prescribed camphor, capsicum, and morphine for cholera; bayberry bark, ginger, macrotys, and capsicum for smallpox; triturated belladonna, sulfate of cinchona, and triturated leptandra (Culvers root) for measles; and dwarf elder, Indian hemp, and marshmallows for enuresis and incontinence. In addition, they recommended compound pills of camphor for cholera, compound pills of leptandra in liver affections, compound pills of black cohosh in cholera and derangements of the nervous system, compound powder of pleurisy root (butterfly weed) and spearmint in febrile diseases, and compound powder of jalap for all febrile, inflammatory, and chronic diseases.[101]

In a questionnaire on the more popular remedies used by eclectics at the turn of the century, all respondents reported using monkshood and belladonna; 90 percent used cimicifuga, gelsemium, cactus, ipecac, nux vomica, veratrum, thuja, and pulsatilla; and 75 percent listed apocynin (from dogbane), baptisia, bismuth, bryonia, chionanthus, chloroform, digitalis, dioscorea (wild yam), eryngium (corn snakeroot), ergot, hydrastis, jaborandi, lobelia, opium (and its salts), passiflora, phytolacca, podophyllum, quinine, *Rhus toxicodendron* (poison ivy), and viburnum. In all, 70 percent of the eclectic school of medicines practitioners routinely depended upon one hundred forty different remedies.[102]

Some of the many drugs introduced into regular medicine by the eclectics included *Podophyllum peltatum* (mayapple, mandrake root) and iris versicolor as cathartics; *Gelsemium sempervirens* (yellow jessamine) for tetanus, gonorrhea, headaches, and fevers; and *Caulophyllum thalictroides* (blue cohosh) for "female complaints" and as an emmenagogue. Others included *Rumex crispus* (yellow dock), barberry, *Apocynum cannabinum* (Indian hemp), *Euonymus atropurpureus* (wahoo), cimicifuga, or black cohosh, lobelia, hydrastis (goldenseal), baptisia (wild indigo), sanguinaria (bloodroot), and spotted wintergreen.[103]

Many reformers objected to using tablets. The so-called tablet mania threatened the eclectics' independence, making them reliant on the competence of pharmaceutical manufacturers. Those who had given up their concentrations for the convenience of tablets faced problems of drug impurity because few drugs could be processed through tablet machines without contamination. Moreover, the makers of machine tablets used a variety of substances not indicated on the labels, including powdered acacia, starch, glucose, bicarbonate of soda, tartaric acid, citric acid, white Vaseline, powdered talcum, and a solution of Vaseline in ether.[104]

For the eclectic, however, the vegetable materia medica did not constitute the whole armamentarium of medicine. Reform practitioners, drawing from Joseph R. Buchanan's earlier theories, appreciated the influence of the mind over the body—the patient's mind over his or her own body and the physician's mind over the patient. Sometimes called *mental therapeutics, psychotherapy*, or *suggestive therapeutics*, eclectics distinguished their beliefs from those of magnetic healers and Christian Scientists. They recognized that the mental states of grief, joy, anger, and melancholy greatly influenced the functions of life and that these states were produced by suggestions received through the sympathetic nervous system; reformers therefore believed it important to associate the relationships of mental states to the functions and energies of the body. "All doctors believe that drugs can heal; that water can heal; that electricity can heal—in fact, that any force, properly applied, which can influence the blood stream, flush capillaries or remove congestions can heal," observed W. R. Fowler of Texas. "We ought to believe, for we must know, if we stop to think, that suggestion is equally endowed with healing powers."[105]

"The Eclectic of fifty years ago was no more like the Eclectic of today than the Allopath of that period was like the advanced educated physician we see at the present time," said H. M. Campbell in his address before the Eclectic Medical Association of West Virginia in 1896. "We have advanced all the way from the crude decoctions, mixtures and syrups of our fathers . . . and prescribed according to the commonly accepted nosology of the time, to the specific medication of the present day."[106] Perhaps the most striking change in the eclectics' attitude came with the renewed use of mercury, opposition to which, as noted, had been the source of eclecticism's early strength. By 1902, partly in response to germ theory, the eclectic journals recommended using mercury, particularly for syphilis. References to calomel and other forms of mercury carried cautions regarding salivation, but reform medicine had resurrected mercury from the dustbin of eclectic medical practice.

In May 1893, eclectics assembled at the Hall of Columbus in the Memorial Art Palace in Chicago to open the first and only World's Medical Congress of Eclectic Physicians and Surgeons. The congress was organized into eight divisions: general medicine and surgery; homeopathic medicine and surgery; eclectic medicine and surgery; medical jurisprudence; dentistry; pharmacy; medicoclimatology; and public health. Only three—eclectic medicine and surgery, medicoclimatology, and homeopathic medicine and surgery—met during the convention; the others were postponed to a later date or were canceled. Despite this, convention speakers urged their colleagues to comprehend intelligently all -pathies. "Whatever will prevent or relieve human suffering, from whatever school or source it may be obtained, is worthy of the diligent study, attention, and candid acknowledgment of the individual whose vocation it is, by the Practice of Medicine, to administer to human needs."[107]

E. Younkin, in the *American Medical Journal* in 1895, enlarged upon this theme when he denied that eclectics should be designated *sectarian* because that term applied to those adhering to exclusive doctrines. There was nothing sectarian in the name *eclectic*. "Its meaning is too far reaching," Younkin argued. "It is as wide as the universe, and deep as the earth." The only manner in which eclectic practice could be construed as a sect was in the decision by regulars to refuse any association with them. Younkin did not deny the successes of allopathy. "I counter-irritate to relieve congestion and pain," he wrote. "I would put on a blister, or create an issue, to counter-irritate; to draw blood from diseased organs to another part; to eliminate peccant matter. I give a cathartic often for its revulsive effect—to revert disease from one part to another. Thus we divert the morbific matter into eliminative channels. Yet I am not an Allopath by any means." Similarly, he sometimes relied on the law of *similia similiabus curantur*, believing that certain drugs that cured disease were also capable of producing symptoms in a healthy body, and it was on this basis that he prescribed quinine, strychnine, *Rhus toxicodendron* (poison ivy), and colocynthis. Nevertheless, argued Younkin, the laws of allopathy and homeopathy were limited, "and it was never intended by the Creator of all laws that either or any of them should be made universal in the cure of disease." The eclectic physician had to determine the "fitness of things, and to appropriate whatever experience has shown to be good."[108]

7
Challenges, 1875–1910

Throughout the nineteenth century, American medical education suffered whenever it was compared with the European system, which insisted on a strong preparatory education, demonstrated by rigorous examination. European medical schools offered more disciplines for study and four years of schooling, with each year's program lasting nine months. Individual educators in the United States often lamented the comparison, but most medical schools and their faculties ignored the contrast; nor did they see the need for extending courses from four months to six; for graded courses, with basic disciplines taught before the clinical subjects; for more clinical teaching and hospital experience; for greater emphasis on dissection and examinations; or for separating the diploma from the license to practice.[1]

Unlike medical colleges in Great Britain and France, which existed as departments of universities, the majority of American medical schools proudly defended their independence from any college or university. By 1877, fewer than twenty of the sixty-five medical schools had any connection with institutions of higher learning. But as Kenneth M. Ludmerer explained in *Learning to Heal*, the modern medical school was well under way long before the Carnegie Foundation published Abraham Flexner's landmark report in 1910. The modern university emerged as a real presence in American higher education beginning in the mid-1880s. The signs of this phenomenon were evident in the revival of state and federal regulatory authority, the dedication of millions of dollars in gifts from industrial barons for the construction of laboratories and teaching hospitals, the employment of full-time faculty, the gradual elimination of proprietary schools, and the increasing function of research. Academic medicine became a real force within the field of medicine, driven by individuals whose goals were to professionalize their respective disciplines and specializations.[2]

Biting the Bullet

Only a few schools willingly tempted fate by implementing their own early reforms. The newly established Medical Department of Lind University in Chicago in 1859 initiated a five-month sequential program with an optional graded curriculum as an alternative to the standard fare of two four-month terms of lectures, with the second identical to the first. Nathan Smith Davis, one of several architects of this reform effort, left the faculty of Rush Medical College and joined the new school (Chicago Medical College) to repair what he felt were shortcomings in the medical-education system. Unlike other medical schools, Chicago Medical College required entering students to be college graduates or to undergo a rigorous examination to ascertain the presence of a sound preliminary education. The college enrolled far fewer students than did Rush Medical College but persisted in maintaining its higher standards. In 1869, Lind University affiliated with Northwestern University; and in 1891, Chicago Medical College became Northwestern University Medical School.[3]

Soon after the reforms at Chicago Medical College, the faculty at St. Louis College of Medicine and Natural Sciences, the College of Physicians and Surgeons in St. Louis, and the Women's Medical College of the New York Infirmary for Women and Children adopted graded courses. But not until 1871, when Charles W. Eliot (1834–1926), president of Harvard University from 1869 to 1909, took a personal interest in academic reform, did more systemic change take place. Eliot, a longtime admirer of German education, made the Harvard Medical School an integral part of Harvard University, placing faculty on regular salaries, independent of student fees. This accomplished, academic quality in the school rose, and with it came a graded curriculum, higher admission standards, and new subject matter. The academic year was lengthened to nine months, with three years of required classroom instruction. For Henry J. Bigelow (1818–90), Oliver W. Holmes, Edward H. Clarke (1820–77), and a few other stalwarts who opposed these reforms, Harvard functioned to train physicians and not necessarily to educate scientists. Indeed, only 20 percent of Harvard's medical students at the time of Eliot's reforms had college degrees. The enmity between Eliot and some of the older medical faculty reflected the intellectual tension that separated two different generations of educators—the advocates of the French clinical school and the emerging laboratory tradition of German education. This was a reform that Eliot, who had trained as a chemist, would win because the empiricism of the laboratory had already won adherents among a generation of younger faculty schooled in German postgraduate work. Among some of Eliot's strongest supporters were James Clarke White, David Cheever, and Calvin Ellis—all of whom had studied in Germany and Austria. Eliot presided over nothing less than a wholly new philosophy of education.[4]

What, in many ways, began as a drive for the professionalization and acceptance of the sciences in American universities evolved into a general overhaul of medical education, the need for a stronger laboratory-based curriculum, and a better-prepared matriculant. As certain schools (e.g., Harvard, Yale, Columbia, Pennsylvania, Michigan, Syracuse, and Cornell) caught the spirit of reform, they transformed academic medicine from an anomaly to a desired form of pedagogy and, in doing so, forced second- and third-tier schools, as well as those in the backwaters of education, to join in the reform or face the consequences of obsolescence. Proprietary schools, which for decades had served society with low-cost, didactic education, could no longer meet the demands of the new age. Recognizing that salaried teachers, laboratories, affiliated hospitals, dispensaries, and scientific equipment entailed costs far greater than could be financed through student tuition and fees, schools saw the wisdom of affiliating with universities to secure private endowments, as well as tax dollars. Those that resisted these changes fell quickly from sight—which is not to say they closed: rather, they provided an increasingly marginal education and, tempted on occasion to augment their incomes, sold fraudulent degrees as a means of existence.[5]

While integration of medical schools with universities occurred with some regularity in the 1880s, the relationship was still often nominal, with the medical faculty surrendering little autonomy. Many retained a separate board of trustees and maintained unrestricted control over the finances, faculty appointments, standards of admission and graduation, and other critical aspects of school governance. And, all too often, the schools' geographical separation from the parent institutions only exacerbated the nature of the relationship. Sometimes the only visible evidence of any connection existed in announcements and letterheads and the annual appearance of the university president, who conferred degrees at commencement. According to John M. Dodson, M.D., of Chicago, writing in the *Journal of the American Medical Association* in 1902, medical schools would never gain the full measure of the relationship unless they became "an intimate, integral part of the university," with financial management turned over to trustees who would derive no pecuniary advantage from the relationship. This also meant that the basic medical sciences (the first two years of the curriculum) would have to be provided by the university physics, chemistry, anatomy, zoology, physiology, and bacteriology departments. Such offerings would eliminate unnecessary duplication of resources; moreover, argued Dodson, "the transfer of the teaching . . . to the halls and laboratories of the university proper, will do more toward the creation of a strong and influential profession than any other plan that has yet been tried."[6]

Reform in medical education principally derived from academic scientists seeking recognition for their respective disciplines and their research and from such men as Eliot of Harvard, Seth Low and Nicholas Murray Butler of Columbia, James Angell of Michigan, and William Pepper of Pennsylvania, whose leadership heralded the authority and influence of the modern university. All had come to believe that a more scientific medicine was both necessary and overdue. It meant a more practical instruction and a shift away from didactic teaching. It meant laboratory work, new curricula, new equipment and, in keeping with the newer trends in university education, the adoption of German-based pedagogy. It meant the replacement of student fees with university salaries, the strengthening of clinical arrangements with neighboring hospitals, the expectation of premedical academic achievements, the abandonment of apprenticeships in the 1870s and 1880s, and the insistence on graded and lengthened curricula. It meant the recognition of research as a partner in teaching and practice, the establishment of state boards to provide licensing, and the strengthening of professional societies. It meant, in essence, transforming American medicine and its educational system. Some of these changes reflected long-standing concerns of the AMA; other reforms represented pedagogic issues that went far beyond the traditional viewpoint of the AMA. For one thing, tighter standards as encouraged by the AMA did not encompass the need for rigorous laboratory science. Yet both objectives moved forward, while marginal schools found themselves increasingly unable to keep step with expectations. The model that emerged was, as Thomas N. Bonner explained, "an amalgam of advanced German medical training, British bedside and clinical traditions, and a homegrown philosophy of learning by doing."[7]

The founding in 1876 of the American Medical College Association by twenty-two schools represented a significant event in the advancement of medical education. The association disbanded in 1883 but revived again in 1890 as the Association of American Medical Colleges following a call from Baltimore physicians Aaron Friedenwald and Eugene F. Cordell representing the Maryland medical colleges. Nathan Smith Davis, who had been an active reformer of medical education since the 1840s, was elected president of the association. By 1896, fifty-five of the nation's 155 medical schools had become members. The association later joined with the National Confederation of State Medical Examining and Licensing Boards to encourage the exchange of information and improve the leverage that boards eventually exerted over inferior schools. Together, they recommended a minimum three-year program, graduation from high school, and a uniform curriculum.[8]

Added impetus to improved medical education came with the creation of scientific societies and groups of specialists, such as the American Surgical Association (1880), the Association of American Physicians (1886), the American Physiological Society (1887), the American Association of Anatomists (1888), the Pediatric Society (1888), and the American Association of Pathologists and Bacteriologists (1900). Members of these organizations, many of whom were educated in Germany, Austria, England, and France, recognized the need for improved training and enhancement of their specialties against the claims and practices of less educated physicians.[9]

Not all organizations were so dedicated. The American Association of Physicians and Surgeons formed in 1894 with members drawn principally from Indiana. Claiming to be "nondenominational," it welcomed members from many different schools, including regular, homeopathy, eclectic, physio-medical, hygienic, hydrotherapeutic, and electrotherapeutic. The association also formed the American Medical College in Indianapolis, whose students could elect to take courses in regular, homeopathic, eclectic, or physio-medical areas.[10] John M. Scudder condemned the association for having succeeded in gathering into its fold "the queer of all schools."[11]

In a report to the thirteenth annual meeting of the American Academy of Medicine in Chicago in 1889, the academy's education committee once again acknowledged the inadequacy of premedical education and urged that every matriculant have a degree of bachelor of arts, science, or philosophy. After comparing information from official announcements of medical schools with annual reports of the Illinois State Board of Health and with statistics compiled by W. G. Eggleston, M.D., of Chicago, the committee complained of discrepancies in the self-reported statistics, as well as the "lack of candor on the part of some of the deans or secretaries of the medical schools." Too many schools existed to enhance the professional reputation of their faculties and, given their continued dependence on fees, had little or no incentive to insist on high standards. J. E. Emerson, M.D., writing in the *Journal of the American Medical Association*, stated, "No appeal to higher motives can successfully antagonize the purely selfish and mercenary motive that dictated their origin and governs their policy."[12]

Medical education in the 1880s entered an era of self-assessment and introspection. The Illinois State Board of Health, empowered by the Illinois Medical Practice Act of 1877 to maintain lists of recognized doctors, issued reports between 1883 and 1889 on schools in "good standing" both inside and outside Illinois. The board's criteria included moral character and premedical education, a curriculum of ten subjects, the expectation of two courses in dissection and two terms of clinical instruction, and a minimum of three years of training. The board examined fifty-seven institutions, including forty-three regular, ten homeopathic, three eclectic, and one physio-medical schools. Of those, only fifteen schools (fourteen regular and one homeopathic) had qualifications for matriculation. The remaining forty-two schools required no preliminary education for students. In addition, thirty of the forty-three regular schools, eight of the ten homeopathic, and three eclectic schools conferred an M.D. degree after two years of study and attendance upon two annual courses of lectures of twenty-six weeks. Only thirteen regular and two homeopathic schools required three annual courses of lectures and three years of study before graduation.

On the basis of these reports, the board announced that, after the sessions of 1882–83, no college that did not subscribe to specified requirements would be accepted in "good standing." Although it is unlikely that a direct correlation exists between the Illinois board's schedule of minimum requirements and the subsequent closing in 1884 of four regular and three eclectic schools, the fact remains that the board's decree reflected a growing clamor for more rigorous and expanded curricula, tighter entrance requirements, lengthened terms, and the replacement of the lecture mode of instruction with laboratory and clinical teaching. Not surprisingly, the number of eclectic schools fell from fifteen in 1883 to eight in 1893.[13] Said J. Collins Warren, M.D., speaking before the Pan-American Medical Congress in 1894, these reports exerted "a more powerful influence on the movement in education than any other publication which our medical literature has produced."[14]

With the implementation of its rating system, the Illinois State Board of Health asserted significant influence over American medicine. However tentative its methodology, the system became the touchstone of future reform and self-regulation and, coincidentally, the hallmark of the influence of the AMA in a later decade. Separate examining boards admittedly did continue to operate, and some states persisted in accepting either diplomas or examinations as the basis for licensing. Proprietary schools continued to flourish, and students could still obtain degrees and begin practice after attending only two courses of lectures of less than five months' duration. Even in many so-called good schools, the marginal student could obtain a degree with a minimum of effort.[15] "Comparing the requirements of the Canadian with those of the American medical schools," observed critic J. E. Emerson, "one feels a humiliating sense of inferiority."[16] Nevertheless, the force of reform became clear: by the mid-1890s, twenty-two states required both a diploma and the successful completion of a state examination as the prerequisite to practicing medicine.[17]

Homeopaths and eclectics, the two largest sectarian groups, noticeably began to blend their medical education with that of allopathy. Along with this mainstreaming of medical education came a greater attention to research and scientific medicine and a growing intolerance toward discredited schools, inferior medical training, and cheapened standards. Educational reform measures still required concerted effort, but the gradual move to lengthened terms, graded courses, three-year curricula, and annual testing made sense to a nation well on its way to becoming a world power. As noted earlier, the incentive for much of this reform came from outside the AMA, which was years away from displaying the power it would eventually carry. Its membership—both individual and institutional—continued to divide on the fundamental issues of intellectual elitism in a nation of democratic values.

The nation's medical schools were not immune to the pressures of self-regulation and quality control. By 1893, all of the nineteen homeopathic colleges and the eight eclectic schools, as well as 104 of the 109 regular colleges, required some form of preliminary education before admitting students to lecture classes. In addition, the percentage of schools requiring attendance of three or more courses of lectures before graduation increased from 26.8 percent in 1880 to 96.3 percent in 1893. In fact, forty-five regular, seventeen homeopathic, and six eclectic schools required four or more full years of study before graduation.[18]

From 1845 to 1878, the E. M. Institute required three years' reading in an apprenticeship, with attendance at two sessions, or four years' practice in lieu of one session; after 1871, the institute awarded no honorary degrees. The term increased to twenty weeks, including nineteen weeks of lectures and one of examinations, in 1879. Thus, in two twenty-week sessions, a student attended 1,368 lectures, replacing the earlier sixteen-week session of 558 lectures. These requirements were not unlike the early recommendations made by the American Medical College Association in June 1876 that students study medicine for three years and that they attend two full courses of instruction on anatomy (including dissection), physiology, chemistry, materia medica and therapeutics, obstetrics, surgery, pathology, and practice of medicine. In 1890, the E. M. Institute lengthened the term again, requiring three full courses of lectures for graduation. The requirements tightened even further in 1893: students matriculating on or after September 11, 1893, would "be required to have read medicine for four years, including attendance upon three annual courses of lectures and not less than six months each, the last of which, at least, must have been in this institute. No two sessions within one twelve-month period will fill this requirement." In May 1895, the institute announced that one session would be held each year and continue for eight months. The institute until then had held two sessions each year. Here again, the changes approached the 1894 recommendations of the newly constituted Association of American Medical Colleges for a four-year program of at least four courses of lectures of not less than six months each.[19]

Not until the reorganization of the AMA in 1901, which brought local medical societies closer to the national organization, did the profession feel the full weight of AMA power. Much of the real reform had previously come from individual schools, their faculties, and their enlightened administrators. The AMA concluded that its greatest strength lay in the county-level society since it furnished every physician the opportunity of membership, fellowship, scientific advancement, and political influence. United together, the county groups constituted the state society, and the state societies formed the national organization. There was a "unity in this trinity and a trinity in the unity, each dependent on the other, but all making one complete organization."[20] Membership was like having "a postgraduate school at one's door," in that members could, with the mutual help of one another, continue the education begun in medical college. In contrast, the physician who worked alone day after day without associating with his colleagues would, in spite of himself, "become narrow, get into a rut, and his professional horizon will soon extend only to the narrowed confines of his own narrowed views and medical life."[21] The failure of the profession in former years had been due to its dependence on voluntary efforts and self-sacrificing work done by a few individuals. Not having applied business principles to their efforts, they had accomplished little that had stood the test of time.[22]

At the recommendation of delegates at the Atlantic City, New Jersey, meeting in June 1900, a committee formed to consider and develop a plan of reorganization for the AMA. Its report, brought forward at the St. Paul, Minnesota, meeting in June 1901, included a revised constitution in accord with the changes suggested by the committee. The first significant modification provided for a reapportionment of delegates to better reflect the total population, with each affiliated society (state, district, county, and local) entitled to one delegate for each ten, or a major fraction of ten, of its members. Under the new constitution, the state societies alone would be represented at the national meetings, with other societies represented through their state organization. Each state or territorial society was entitled to one delegate for each five hundred active members. The second change gave the legislative body a name: the House of Delegates. While the old delegate body had averaged fifteen to seventeen hundred members, the new body had its number of delegates limited to 150 and included not only representatives from the affiliated state and territorial societies but also representatives from the medical departments of the army, navy, and the marine hospital services. The strength of the newly organized AMA depended ultimately on the federation of county or district societies, which in turn constituted the membership of the respective state societies.[23]

Following its reorganization and a revision of its code of ethics, the AMA deliberately set out to absorb the eclectics and the homeopaths. One could argue that the AMA was being magnanimous in its goodwill and liberal in its spirit to accept these sectarians as bona fide members. But looks alone were deceptive because the conditions of membership required eclectics and homeopaths to drop their special designations. "How peaceful the regular lion will look, after swallowing the innocent eclectic and homeopathic lambs, 20,000 in number," remarked one skeptic. For strong partisans of reform, there was nothing to be gained by union. Eclectics and homeopaths had everything to lose—including their names— while regulars gave up nothing.[24] According to Herbert T. Webster, M.D., in the *Eclectic Medical Journal* in 1909, the offer by the AMA reminded him of the man who "in driving his ass to market tried to please everybody, pleased nobody, and lost his ass in the bargain." Despite warnings from a number of outspoken sectarians, the strategy of the AMA proved effective.[25]

In general, eclectics were openly critical of the association's reorganization because it not only made all allopathic medical societies subsidiary to it but enticed sectarians with the prospect of legitimacy and a more promising financial future. This "powerful political machine," wrote the editors of the *California Eclectic Medical Journal,* "is now being used to wrest from the people the right of each citizen to employ the physician of his choice." This power, originally vested in the states, had been turned over to the "American Medical Trust." Putting aside these protests, the fact is that numerous homeopathic and eclectic physicians chose this opportunity to merge into the mainstream of regular medicine.[26]

Eclectic Societies and Schools

By the 1870s, most eclectic physicians were convinced that they had become a fixed alternative to regular practice. Firm in their independence, guarded in their relations with regulars and homeopaths, they followed a course roughly parallel to medical orthodoxy in terms of educational requirements and standards. In keeping with this idea of themselves, eclectics tried (albeit not too successfully) to avoid public criticism by establishing the legitimacy of what they thought of as their more practical methods and approaches. In an environment of regular schools' taking the lead in advocating curricular reform and in developing hospital affiliations and extramural programs to supplement didactic instruction, the eclectics found it difficult to maintain the status quo.

Aside from their own assertions of having found a niche in American medicine, eclectic medicine was far from secure—as was evident in the lack of strong local, state, and national organizations. For example, the Eclectic Medical Society of the State of New York, chartered in 1865, claimed numerous auxiliaries; yet only two, the Eclectic Medical Society for the City of New York and the Central New York Eclectic Medical Society, reported fifty or more members; the remainder functioned with ten or fewer. Rhode Island reported ten eclectic practitioners and no association. There did exist, however, a society whose members styled themselves as liberals and contained three known eclectics. Eighty-three practicing physicians in Rhode Island were not connected with any society; one-third of them had never graduated from medical school or from college.[27]

In the (then) Northwest, Wisconsin boasted two hundred eclectic practitioners, most of whom graduated from the E. M. Institute or from Bennett College of Eclectic Medicine and Surgery in Chicago.[28] However, the Wisconsin Eclectic Medical College, a Milwaukee diploma mill, put these numbers in doubt by having offered diplomas for thirty-five dollars to all with aspirations of practicing medicine. The school's owner, Fred Rutland, advised holders of diplomas to practice only in Wisconsin, Michigan, Indiana, Kansas, Idaho, Nevada, Wyoming, and Oklahoma (these states required no licensing exams).[29] In Illinois, the advocates of reform medical practice lamented that any "traveling nostrum-vendor who wanted to could call himself an eclectic, much to the disgust of every member of the profession." True eclectics referred to these interlopers as "a fungus growth on our school of practice" and urged their expulsion by "excision" and by "caustic" means.[30]

Reformers elsewhere also felt tarnished "in consequence of the number of uneducated men practicing quackery, under the name eclectic." In a concerted, state-level effort to regulate practice and to unite behind higher standards and qualifications, reform physicians met at Kalamazoo, Michigan, in 1876 to adopt a constitution that would set forth the principles of their practice. Organized as the Michigan State Eclectic Medical and Surgical Society, they intended to enforce standards of professional education, as well as to offer mutual recognition and fellowship. They limited membership to

> practitioners of Medicine and Surgery in the State of Michigan, who shall have received the degree of Doctor of Medicine from a Medical School or College legally empowered to confer such a degree, and such other persons as have sustained a reputable practice as physicians and surgeons for ten years, with previous study, and no others; all of whom shall be elected by vote of a majority at any regular meeting of the society, their eligibility being previously reported upon by the Board of Censors.[31]

Dr. J. W. Marmon reported to the National Eclectic Medical Association that there had been approximately one hundred twenty-five "respectable" eclectic physicians practicing medicine in Iowa in 1875. He used the term *respectable* to distinguish from "those parasites who claim to be eclectics, but who have none of the qualifications that make true eclectics." Marmon noted that practitioners from the state had sent twenty-five students to different eclectic colleges and that the Iowa State Eclectic Medical Society consisted of forty-five members who held annual meetings in Des Moines.[32] In Ohio, where the National Eclectic Medical Association first formed in 1849, two district organizations (the Miami Valley Eclectic Medical Association and the Clermont Eclectic Medical Association) claimed membership of approximately fifty each. Numerous eclectics practiced in other parts of Ohio, but none had formed themselves into associations.

In Pennsylvania, the general Corporation Act of 1874 granted a charter to the Eclectic Medical Association of the State of Pennsylvania in September 1875. In addition, the Susquehanna Eclectic Medical Society organized in 1872, followed by the Eclectic Medical Society of Northwestern Pennsylvania and the Central Eclectic Medical Society of Pennsylvania in 1875, and the Allegheny County Eclectic Medical Society in 1877. In all, 132 eclectic physicians registered in either the state society or its auxilaries.[33]

West Virginia had neither an eclectic medical society nor, for that matter, any physicians practicing as eclectics. This condition resulted from state law, which required the West Virginia State Board of Medical Examiners to accept only diplomas from medical colleges in good standing. In 1886, F. M. Dent, M.D., a graduate of the American Eclectic Medical College of Cincinnati (organized in 1876 and declared not in good standing by the Ohio State Medical Board in 1896), was indicted and fined for practicing medicine. After his appeal to the United States Supreme Court on the grounds that the statute violated the Fourteenth Amendment, Associate Justice Stephen J. Field stated for the majority that the constitutional provision did not interfere with the authority of the states in such matters.[34]

Reform medicine remained popular in the southern states. Tennessee reported eclectic practitioners in every city and in nearly all of the towns and villages and chartered a state organization of eclectics in 1887. According to F. H. Fisk of Nashville, Tennessee became known as the home of eclecticism in the South, claiming such pioneers as Robert S. Newton, Zoheth Freeman, and G. W. Morrow.[35] Texas reported nearly two hundred practicing eclectics in the 1880s, and its medical association, formed in 1887, sought to minimize damage done by the old-school society by maintaining a standing committee to lobby the legislature. The Texas State Medical Association (regular) recommended that both homeopaths and eclectics be recognized but insisted that this not be construed as an endorsement of their beliefs. "We stand by the code of the American Medical Association and will expel any doctor of the Texas State Medical Association who will so lower the dignity of regular medicine as to meet them in consultation."[36] Like many other states, Texas created an examining board to license practitioners; however, much to the dismay of regulars, it had no power to enforce its actions. Irregular physicians thus had only to register their diplomas, "and those without any [could] proceed to ply their vocation without fear of molestation."[37]

In 1887, Alabama placed all standards of medical qualification in the hands of the Boards of Medical Examiners of the Medical Association of the State of Alabama. No one could practice medicine without first passing an examination before one of these authorized boards. The authorized boards were those boards of censors of the county medical societies holding charters from the state medical association. There were sixty-six of these county societies and therefore sixty-six county boards of medical examiners. Neither the state board nor the state association could reverse a decision of any county board; they could, however, issue a reprimand and even a censure. County boards examined none but graduates of reputable medical colleges, but the state board reserved the right to examine nongraduates.[38] Because Alabama law did not recognize sectarian differences among doctors, eclectics and homeopaths had to pass the same examination as regulars. If an irregular doctor passed the examination and demonstrated his fitness to practice medicine, he was entitled to join the county society. In doing so, however, he also pledged to abide by the ethical code of the AMA since it was incorporated into the constitution of each of the county societies. By this action, the eclectic ceased to be an irregular.[39]

Eclectics called the Alabama statute *class legislation*, designed to rid the state of alternative systems of medicine. A "Witches' Kitchen," it was devised by those who had raped the constitution, disgraced the statutes, and betrayed the trust of the people. "We know that the Medical Statute of Alabama is an utter barbarism and contrary to the genius of free American institutions," commented

J. W. R. Williams, M.D., "that it outrages the rights of citizens—
the liberty, property and reputation of the physician; that it dishon-
ors and degrades a worthy profession, and obstructs progress in
Medicine."[40]

The greatest numbers of eclectics practiced in California, Illinois, Indiana, Missouri, New York, and Ohio.[41] In fourteen states,
however, there were fewer than twenty-five eclectics. Moreover,
thirteen states had no reform organizations of any type; and, in
fifteen states, no eclectic practitioners registered as members of
the National Eclectic Medical Association. In fact, there were only
508 physicians registered with that national body in 1896, causing
frequent editorials in the *Eclectic Medical Journal* lamenting the
weak state of the national association. "In numbers there is
strength," argued D. Maclean, M.D., of San Francisco. But "a strag-
gling army is easily routed. A corps of well-disciplined men, with
earnestness of purpose, can resist the aggressions of a horde."[42]

The National Eclectic Medical Association, which was overly
generous in its estimates, guessed the number of eclectics to be
between eight and ten thousand at the end of the nineteenth century. Other records suggest a considerably smaller number, with
fewer than four hundred belonging to the association. Apologists
explained these discrepancies by saying that state restrictions
caused many eclectics to practice under the banner of old-school
medicine. In addition, a number of eclectics, particularly those
practicing in cities and in wealthier communities, preferred to be
called homeopaths or regulars as it guaranteed a healthier annual
income.[43] Finley Ellingwood, however, said that most eclectics had
become "too lethargic" and "too self-absorbed" and lacked the
reform spirit found in those of earlier decades. The homeopaths,
in contrast, touted an almost equal number of physicians, with
nearly 20 percent of their rank and file belonging to their national
association. In truth, of course, new forces—industrialism, urban-
ization, immigration, unionization, and economic conflict—consumed those energies that had earlier formed the basis of sectarian
medicine's crusade, and the regional divisions and loyalties that
had predominated in the decades before the Civil War were less
intense following Abraham Lincoln's assassination.[44]

Estimates by Finley Ellingwood, secretary of the National Eclectic Medical Association, indicated that 8,244 eclectic physicians
practiced in the United States in 1902. Ellingwood's tabulation

was likewise generous and probably included many graduates of eclectic colleges who had chosen to conceal their sectarian status.[45]

Table 7.1
Practicing Eclectic Physicians, 1902

State	Number	State	Number
Alabama	65	Montana	9
Arizona	7	Nebraska	215
Arkansas	216	Nevada	6
California	491	New Hampshire	29
Colorado	65	New Jersey	57
Connecticut	93	New York	656
Delaware	7	North Carolina	13
Dist. of Columbia	9	North Dakota	9
Florida	58	Ohio	879
Georgia	339	Oklahoma Territory	64
Idaho	22	Oregon	61
Illinois	903	Pennsylvania	273
Indiana	690	Rhode Island	13
Indian Territory	90	South Carolina	7
Iowa	294	South Dakota	43
Kansas	340	Tennessee	167
Kentucky	245	Texas	250
Louisiana	27	Utah	16
Maine	39	Vermont	39
Maryland	14	Virginia	18
Massachusetts	118	Washington	62
Michigan	342	West Virginia	99
Minnesota	88	Wisconsin	158
Mississippi	31	Wyoming	9
Missouri	499		

In the September 6, 1902, issue of the *Journal of the American Medical Association*, the editors reported 156 medical colleges in the United States, with 6,776 instructors, enrolling 27,501 students, and graduating 5,002. Of the total number of graduates, 4,498 were regulars; 335, homeopaths; 138, eclectics; and 31 belonged to miscellaneous groups. For the eclectics, the statistics of graduates for 1902 were as follows:[46]

Table 7.2
Eclectic Medical Colleges Graduates, 1902

Institution	Students	Graduates
E. M. Institute, Cincinnati (1845)	142	36
Bennett College of Eclectic Medicine and Surgery, Chicago (1868)	104	21
Eclectic Medical·College of the City of New York (1865)	100	7
Lincoln Medical College, Lincoln, Nebraska (1889)	98	21
California Medical College, San Francisco (1879)	84	6
American Medical College, St. Louis (1873)	69	14
Georgia College of Eclectic Medicine and Surgery, Atlanta (1866)	58	21
Eclectic Medical University, Kansas City, Missouri (1897)	49	12
American College of Medicine and Surgery, Chicago (1901)	36	—
Eclectic Medical College of Indiana, Indianapolis (1900)	25	—

At the annual meeting of the National Eclectic Medical Association in 1894, members created the National Confederation of Eclectic Medical Colleges, which was composed of two delegates from each college recognized by the National Eclectic Medical Association and formed to promote the interests of the colleges, establish uniform minimum requirements and curriculum, and further the cause of higher medical education. By 1904, the confederation included the American Medical College, St. Louis; Bennett College of Eclectic Medicine and Surgery, Chicago; the California Medical College, San Francisco; the Eclectic Medical College of the City of New York; the Eclectic Medical Institute, Cincinnati; Georgia College of Eclectic Medicine and Surgery, Atlanta; Lincoln Medical College, Lincoln, Nebraska; and Eclectic Medical University, Kansas City, Missouri. Membership in the confederation required maintaining minimum standards for college admission, including a good English education "to be attested by (a) first grade teacher's certificate; or (b) a diploma from a graded high school, or literary or scientific college or university; or (c) regent's medical student's certificate; or (d) entrance examination covering a good English education including an elementary knowledge of natural history, physics and Latin." In addition, the program had to offer a four-year, graded course of study or its equivalent, including four sessions of six months each, in four different calendar years.[47]

The declining number of eclectic medical schools and the concomitant decrease in graduates resulted in a demand by regulars for greater control of hospitals and patients. Cook County Hospital in Chicago had instituted a policy in which its patients were distributed among regular (63 percent), homeopathic (20 percent) and eclectic (17 percent) services. This apportionment, originally based on the numbers of students registered in the city's medical schools, caused considerable rancor among regulars. An editorial in the *Journal of the American Medical Association* in 1900 stated that eclectic students in Chicago numbered 101, or 3 percent; homeopathic, 659, or 19 percent; and regular, 2,648, or 78 percent. These statistics represented a decline in eclectic students, a slight growth in homeopathic students, and a steady increase of students in regular schools. Demanding reapportionment on the basis of the newer figures, the editor recommended a 1:5:26 ratio, which would more accurately represent the numbers of medical students in each of the schools. For future adjustments, the editor suggested that a committee of four (one eclectic, one homeopathic, two regulars) examine graduates of all medical schools in Cook County and that the number of successful candidates from each "school" determine the ratio of patients assigned for that particular year.[48]

Eclectics were hard-pressed to fight the implications of their declining numbers. Nevertheless, they continued to espouse their sectarian differences into the twentieth century. "We acknowledge that in several fields of work we have not come up to their [regular] standard," remarked J. D. McCann in his presidential address before the National Eclectic Medical Association in 1903. "We learned medicine, not so much as a matter of laboratories [but] as an art of discerning disease and treating it properly with remedies."[49] In other words, while eclectics identified ideologically with the Paris clinical school, they did not extend the same recognition to the newer emphasis on experimental laboratory investigation.

German medical science did not appeal to the medical protestants. The cell theory of Matthias Jakob Schleiden (1804–81) and Theodor Schwann (1810–82), the work of Johannes Müller (1801–58) and Emil Heinrich Du Bois-Reymond (1818–96) in physiology, the cellular pathology of Rudolf Virchow (1821–1902), and the eventual bacteriological investigations of Robert Koch each represented an excursion into biology and experimental science that held out little to the eclectics and offered little for the eclectics to do; they were trapped within the confines of Scudder's specific medicines. It seemed to many of the stalwarts of reform medicine that the art of medicine had succumbed entirely to the excitement of the laboratory. The medical migration to Germany found few sympathizers among eclectics, who emerged in the twentieth century unschooled and unable to respond to the challenges of advanced clinical study and research. Few, if any, of the thousands of American students who studied in Germany between 1870 and World War I were eclectics.

Mother Institute

Of the reform schools, the E. M. Institute remained the mecca of eclectic thinking. Its strength in botany, pharmacy, and materia medica added to the already-established reputation of the school as a source for plant drugs.[50] Known as the mother institute of reform medicine, the school described itself to prospective students: "We will give a full explanation of what is known as 'specific' or 'direct' medication," noted the college catalog. "We teach Specific Medication, and we propose to present it in such form that the student can make use of it. The remedies are to be pleasant in form, small in dose, certain in action, relieving the unpleasantness of disease, shortening its duration, and saving life."[51]

By 1902, the institute's faculty had written more than one hundred books and had graduated 3,743 students.[52] Admission and graduation requirements remained generally the same as those recommended by the Homeopathic College Association and by the National Confederation of Eclectic Medical Colleges, as well as those of most state boards of medical registration. Students unable to furnish appropriate admissions credentials were tested in English, higher arithmetic, geography, elementary physics, Latin prose, and United States history. Once admitted, they received instruction in the form of lectures and daily quizzes. No private classes were allowed. Each matriculant studied medicine for four years and enrolled in four annual courses of lectures of at least six months each. Students daily received two hours of clinical experience (observation only) in the Cincinnati General Hospital and also received daily clinical instruction on diseases of the eye, ear, nose, and throat; diseases of the skin; medical and surgical diseases of women and children; general surgery and medicine; and physical diagnosis.[53]

Unfortunately for the faculty at the E. M. Institute, the full potential of using a hospital for clinical teaching and research remained unrealized, underutilized, and no more than a distant wish, if that. Indeed, the more basic prospect of using hospital wards to help teach clinical subjects, utilizing group instruction, continued to challenge the institute's trustees because none of the faculty held staff appointments at the Cincinnati General Hospital. Only the Sisters of Charity made Seton Hospital available to demonstrate to students eclectic medicine and surgery. With the 1910 decision by the Council on Medical Education (which had formed in 1904) of the AMA to grade schools on their access to and use of hospitals for teaching purposes, the pressure on the E. M. Institute began to rise dramatically.[54]

These impediments did not deter the faculty at the institute from seeking additional educational reforms. In particular, the school sought a common set of entrance, curricular, and graduation standards for all of the nation's medical schools. "The root of the great evil in our present system," wrote John King Scudder, "is the non-recognition and non-requirement in all the medical schools of a well-understood, ubiquitously and permanently established entrance examination—an examination that shall require the applicant to be possessed of knowledge of such a character as will ensure his being a proper and suitable person to undertake medical study." According to Scudder, who took over from his father the editorship of the *Eclectic Medical Journal*, medical education had failed due to a lack of common examinations, common curricula, and common methods of securing a degree. Only the enforcement of uniform standards would remove the barriers erected by municipal, state, and collegiate bodies. The evils endemic to the present educational system were the "lack of uniform and competent national entrance examinations for all medical schools" and the "unrestricted multiplication of medical schools."

An advocate of change, the younger Scudder recommended a national law limiting the number of medical schools and, equally important, the establishment of national standards for medical-school teachers. Those standards should prohibit "personal ambitions or aims outside of the school" and would eliminate the destructive tendencies inherent in "the pernicious competition of inferior schools."[55]

Because of the bifurcated nature of medical education, the states to protect themselves began in the 1870s to create licensure boards with the power to rule on medical diplomas and thereby control access to the practice of medicine. Some states even refused to accept a diploma from a regularly chartered college as sufficient grounds to practice. Instead, they imposed additional obligations, typically in the form of examinations. These licensure laws resulted in the elevation of standards, but as many physicians complained, they also led to a lack of uniformity. This was in part due to genuine ambivalence within and outside medicine regarding the appropriateness of endorsing established medical practice. In some states, nearly all candidates passed the examinations, irrespective of the college they attended, while other states rejected up to 30 percent of those examined. Problems resided not in the examinations but in the fact that each state had a method and a standard of its own. To further complicate matters, states found themselves attempting to account for differences among the various philosophical schools of medicine. Some states thus established separate boards for homeopaths, eclectics, and regulars, while others chose to create proportionately mixed boards in accordance with their numbers in the state.[56]

Owing to the inequality that existed among the states in their licensing laws, John King Scudder recommended the establishment of a national examining board with the power to examine physicians and grant certificates to practice in any part of the United States. The board would have the power to endorse the certificates of state boards, rendering them universally valid without further inquiry. This, the editor explained, would effectively regulate the practice of medicine, abolish quackery, and elevate the standard of medical education in the United States. National control and regulated entrance and graduation examinations, supervised by disinterested individuals, would ensure the "survival of the fittest" among schools—the natural and safest way to address the defects of the medical-education system.[57]

Although certain faculty and friends of the E. M. Institute feared that the college would suffer as a result of higher entrance standards, the school continued to maintain a record number of matriculants. The higher standards frightened away some potential students, but the institute's bold stand led to a greater number wishing to prepare themselves to face the state examining boards of the future. In fact, the increased class size forced the institute to cancel its proposed practitioners' course for lack of space.[58] "Some of our friends," remarked Scudder, "are beginning to be alarmed and to say that the eclectic school is in more danger of destruction in our present prosperity than we were in our adversity because others are adopting us and our methods; we fail to see where the danger lies."[59]

The higher standards supported by the E. M. Institute did not include a similar commitment to laboratory research, equipment, and support staff. For the eclectic, modern medicine extended as far as the bedside but not to the experimental laboratory; the practitioner of the future could learn all there was to know in the teaching environment of the hospital ward. Laboratory or full-time medical research held little appeal for the advocates of practical medicine.

The Flexner Report

In 1903, Nathan Smith Davis, M.D., remarked in the *Journal of the American Medical Association* that the profession had yet to determine the ideal entrance requirements for medical school. Existing requirements ranged from completion of the eighth grade to a complete college of arts and sciences curriculum, with the mean for most good schools being satisfactory completion of a four-year high school. Davis believed that graduates of high schools and preparatories "have as much general education as need be demanded" but that only courses offered by colleges of arts and sciences furnished "the kind and grade of instruction which is requisite for an understanding of portions of a modern medical curriculum." He therefore argued that a student should have completed at least part of a college curriculum before being allowed entrance to medical school. His ideal curriculum included courses in inorganic chemistry and qualitative analysis; mechanics, light, heat, and electricity; general biology; some comparative anatomy; German and French; experimental psychology and logic; and an acquaintance with botany. Davis urged medical students to seek a combined B.S. (or B.A.) and M.D. in six years. Programs offered at Michigan, Northwestern, and Chicago required students to spend three years in a college of liberal arts, during which most or all of the freshman courses in medicine were completed; this was then followed by three years in a medical school. At Chicago, two years were spent in the arts and four in the medical college; while at Harvard and Cornell, the faculty introduced a seven-year combination.[60] In surveying these schools, George H. Simmons discovered that nearly forty schools required an eight-month course; a like number required seven; and twenty-six required only six months for the college year. But the lack of calendar uniformity was not nearly as serious as the variability in curricula—evinced in the time given to specific subjects, the omission of certain topics, and the lack of consistency in sequencing course work. Anatomy, for example, varied from 200 to 1,248 hours; physiology, 96 to 450; chemistry, 176 to 652; histology and embryology, 70 to 450; bacteriology, 45 to 364; and pathology, 54 to 512. Surgery varied from 64 hours to 1,168; medicine, from 140 to 1,232; and obstetrics, from 67 to 320.[61]

With the Council on Medical Education's recommendations for improved clinical training, full-time preclinical chairs, and endowments, the AMA, in effect, endorsed a progressive medical-education system that closely paralleled that of Johns Hopkins University Medical School, which had opened in 1893 and required for admission not only a bachelor's degree in liberal arts but also a year's work in biology, physics, and chemistry and a reading knowledge of French and German.[62] Johns Hopkins also insisted that medical research become an integral part of medical education. The council concluded that, unless proprietary schools could provide an equally strong education at a profit, they should close their doors and turn their responsibilities over to university-affiliated medical schools supported by endowments, tuition, and state dollars—a recommendation that came as no surprise since every member of the council was a noted researcher with appointments in university-affiliated medical schools. The members included Victor C. Vaughan, dean of the University of Michigan Medical

School; William T. Councilman, professor of pathology at Harvard Medical School; Charles H. Frazier, professor of surgery at the University of Pennsylvania Medical School; J. A. Witherspoon, professor of medicine at Vanderbilt, Nashville; and Arthur D. Bevan, professor of surgery at Rush Medical College.[63]

In 1906, the council published the results of state examinations, thereby giving notice to inferior schools that the reputation and future of each was at risk. The council conducted a survey of all 162 medical schools a year later and graded each on a set of criteria: the success of graduates before state boards; entrance requirements, curricula, facilities, laboratory instruction, dispensary facilities and instruction, hospital facilities and instruction; the quality of faculty; the fiscal organization of each school; and the libraries and other learning resources, including equipment. The council sent the results to state licensing boards but did not make them public.[64]

Concerned about the potential impact of the AMA classification system, the E. M. Institute sought legal advice to determine if the classification violated any constitutional rights, particularly if the effect of the action compelled a college to close its doors. The advice proved disappointing. "If the Eclectic Medical College [sic] maintained an institution which complied with the requirements set forth by the AMA, it would probably be considered an abuse of discretion, remediable by action at law, not to rate the college as one in good standing. Needless to say, no action could be brought against the AMA as it is an unofficial body."[65]

In addition to its own assessment of medical colleges, the Council on Medical Education also recommended extensive independent on-site evaluation of each of the nation's medical schools. Given the anticipated cost of the evaluation, the council sought financial assistance from the Foundation for the Advancement of Teaching, funded by the Carnegie Foundation. The foundation's president, Henry S. Pritchett, former president of the Massachusetts Institute of Technology, selected Abraham Flexner (1866–1959), a teacher and graduate of Johns Hopkins in 1886, and brother of Simon Flexner, pathologist and director of laboratories of the Rockefeller Institute of Medical Research, to undertake the survey. Dr. Nathan P. Colwell of the Council on Medical Education collaborated with Flexner on his site visits.[66]

In 1910, the Carnegie Foundation for the Advancement of

Teaching published Abraham Flexner's study on *Medical Education in the United States and Canada*. Beginning with the assumption that "amongst the thousand institutions in English-speaking North America which bore the name college or university there was little unity of purpose or of standards," the trustees of the foundation directed Flexner to ascertain the facts concerning medical education through an on-site examination of medical school facilities, resources, and methods of instruction. The trustees intended that Flexner include *all* schools in the study, visiting all 155 of them regardless of sectarian bias, and that he bring together all records.[67] In addition, the trustees concluded that, even though many educational institutions were private, the public was entitled to know the facts—whether financial or educational—because these institutions operated, in effect, as "public service corporations." Pritchett believed that "only by such publicity can the true interests of education and of the universities themselves be subserved. In such a reasonable publicity lies the hope for progress in medical education."[68]

Flexner first recounted the history of medical education in North America, explaining the development of the commercial medical school as a distinctly American phenomenon, the eventual integration of medical education into the university environment, and the efforts to raise standards. Following this historical overview, Flexner reported on each medical school, using a common set of indices: entrance requirements, attendance, teaching staff, resources available for maintenance, laboratory facilities, and general considerations.

The results of Flexner's report to the Carnegie Foundation confirmed that medical education had been so commercialized that the public could not make "any discrimination between the well-trained physician and the physician who has had no adequate training whatsoever."[69] Of the 155 schools that Flexner visited, sixteen required two years of college education, six demanded only one year, and fifty required only a high school education or its equivalent.[70] Flexner reported first that there had been an overproduction of uneducated medical practitioners in callous disregard for public welfare; second, that the overproduction stemmed from the activities of commercial schools, which—through questionable advertising and marketing methods—recruited students unprepared for the study of medicine; third, that medical education had long been sustained as a for-profit business, which for efficiency focused on didactic instruction rather than on costly laboratories and clinical experience; fourth, that, while in recent years colleges and universities had annexed medical schools, they had failed to recognize the cost of medical study or the standards essential for professional practice; and fifth, that medical schools required the opening of wards in hospitals for teaching.[71] He ended his study by advocating that there be articulation between medical education and the university and its general system of education and urged consolidation, even elimination, of many existing schools. This meant fewer but better-trained and better-educated physicians.

Flexner maintained that scientific medicine made "all historic dogma" obsolete; and, for this reason, sectarian medicine, which had begun with a prepossessed formula or doctrine, no longer served as a defensible alternative. If sectarians taught pathology, bacteriology, and clinical microscopy, they committed themselves to the scientific method; they could not, therefore, apply the scientific method to the laboratory and not allow it to permeate their educational processes as well. No compromise existed between objective science and dogmatic belief.[72] Indeed, the era of scientific medicine had made allopathy just as untenable as homeopathy and eclecticism had become: modern medicine demanded facts, not dogma.

> Medicine is a discipline, in which the effort is made to use knowledge procured in various ways in order to effect certain practical ends. With abstract general propositions it has nothing to do. It harbors no preconceptions as to diseases or their cure. Instead of starting with a finished and supposedly adequate dogma or principle, it has progressively become less cocksure and more modest. It distrusts general propositions, a priori explanations, grandiose and comforting generalizations. It needs theories only as convenient summaries in which a number of ascertained facts may be used tentatively to define a course of action. It makes no effort to use its discoveries to substantiate a principle formulated before the facts were even suspected. For it has learned from the previous history of human thought that men possessed of vague preconceived ideas are strongly disposed to force facts to fit, defend, or explain them. And this tendency both interferes with the free search for truth and limits the good which can be extracted from such truths.[73]

Eight eclectic, eight osteopathic, one physio-medical, and fifteen homeopathic schools existed at the time of Flexner's report.

Of the fifteen homeopathic institutions, only five required a high school education for entrance; the remainder had virtually no admissions standards. While homeopathic educators readily admitted the importance of laboratory science, few of their schools showed any evidence of "progressive scientific work." Only the Boston University Homeopathic College, the New York Homeopathic College, and the Hahnemann Medical College of Philadelphia possessed equipment for effectively teaching anatomy, pathology, bacteriology, and physiology.[74] Flexner found a certain inevitability in the evidence. "The ebbing vitality of homeopathic schools is a striking demonstration of the incompatibility of science and dogma," he observed. "One may begin with science and work through the entire medical curriculum consistently, exposing everything to the same sort of test; or one may begin with a dogmatic assertion and resolutely refuse to entertain anything at variance with it. But one cannot do both." The options for homeopaths were clear: they could either "withdraw into the isolation in which alone any peculiar tenet can maintain itself," or "put that tenet into the melting pot."[75]

The eight eclectic schools of medicine were located Kansas City; St. Louis; Lincoln; Cincinnati; New York City; Atlanta; and Los Angeles, California. Flexner's visits to these schools did not occur in an environment of conviviality. Like many marginal schools—both regular and sectarian—faculty and administrators feared (and objected to) the elitist biases of both the Carnegie and Rockefeller Foundations. The editors of the *California Eclectic Medical Journal*, for example, accused these foundations of being "conceived under circumstances which made them inimical to a republican form of government." Nonetheless, the schools cooperated, albeit grudgingly, with the on-site visits.[76]

While the New York City school required a four-year high school education and the E. M. Institute required a preliminary education necessary to meet standards in Ohio, the criteria for the others were less clear. Only the New York and Cincinnati schools provided adequate buildings, and neither had sufficient equipment, books, or models; and of the eight schools, none offered adequate clinical opportunities for their students. The New York school sent three students twice each week to Sydenham Hospital, while the E. M. Institute affiliated with Seton Hospital, with twenty-four beds (almost all of which were surgical), and also sent students to observe the public clinics at City Hospital. St. Louis students observed one day a week at the City Hospital, while the other five schools claimed affiliation with private infirmaries or private hospitals. Flexner castigated the eclectics for boasting equipment and scientific instruction when, in reality, they had neither. None of the schools had laboratory equipment even remotely resembling the claims in the catalogs. "They talk of laboratories, not because they appreciate their place or significance," he wrote, "but because it pays them to defer thus far to the spirit of the times." Even worse, they failed to uphold their own tenets. "The eclectics are drug mad," Flexner wrote, "yet, with the exception of the Cincinnati and New York schools, none of them can do justice to [their] creed. For they are not equipped to teach the drugs or the drug therapy which constitutes their sole reason for existence." Flexner saw little future for the eclectic schools. Enrollment, 1,014 in 1904, had shrunk to 413 in 1909; and the combined number of graduates of all eight schools numbered only 84 in 1909.[77]

The results of Flexner's undertaking became evident even before he completed his survey, as medical colleges closed, merged, or reorganized along lines recommended by the Council on Medical Education. Few medical colleges existed without university affiliation. And reform came swiftly: from 1910 to 1930, changes included requiring a B.A. for admission, adding graded curricula, and improving clinical facilities. By 1928, only five sectarian colleges were left. The remainder, along with a great number of regular schools, had closed their doors, had merged, or had undergone reorganization.[78]

The stockholders of the E. M. Institute, recognizing as early as 1908 the inevitability of reform, surrendered their shares to allow for a reorganization of the college. In 1910, the institute changed its official name to the Eclectic Medical College. The college became with reorganization a strictly educational, nonprofit institution, having no stock or stockholders. A perpetual board of trustees, comprised of fifteen members, five of whom belonged to the alumni association of the college, administrated its properties (grounds, seven thousand dollars; six-story brick and stone building, forty-five thousand; equipment and furniture, five thousand), along with its financial and educational interests. By 1910, its graduates numbered 3,978, of whom 1,842 actively practiced medicine.[79]

Eclectic medical schools continued to matriculate students, but they seemed unable to captivate many disciples—either as students or as patients. The National Eclectic Medical Association inaugurated a recruiting drive in response to this malaise to increase membership and to demonstrate a stronger defense against the seductive absorption tactics of the AMA. However laudable these objectives, the association lacked the stamina to sustain its efforts, and by the time the progressive era ended, only the E. M. College remained of the eight schools. By then, however, the sectarian movement's recruitment abilities had all but disappeared, and its system of specific drug therapy had fallen before the onrush of serum and vaccine therapies.

8

Malaise, 1910–1939

However significant Abraham Flexner's report on medical education, its conclusions detailed changes that had already come with modern pathology and bacteriology and with the subsequent advances in pharmacology, in physiology, in anatomy, and especially in histology and embryology. Laboratory medicine had forced new expectations for medical schools. Not surprisingly, marginal and sectarian schools closed or merged in the wake of these raised expectations, and American public opinion showed little sympathy for their plight. The development of scientific medicine made any rational basis for the perpetuation of sectarian dogmas irrelevant or inappropriate. Being sectarian no longer carried the same righteous appeal it had garnered in the nineteenth century. Ever anxious to stretch their claims in the world of ideas, machines, and empires, the people of the United States had come to realize, however late, that *reformed*, *sectarian*, *cultist*, and *irregular* were terms that really implied substandard quality, misplaced objectives, and idiosyncratic reasoning. Thus, the public soon distinguished between the University of Chicago and Northwestern on one hand and Bennett College of Eclectic Medicine and Surgery, Jenner Medical College, Chicago (formerly Harvard Evening Medical College, Chicago), and Hering Medical College (homeopathic), Chicago, on the other.[1]

The Meaning of Medicine

If by the term *regular* society implied that medicine should be governed by a set of rules or that a certain coterie should dictate all lines of treatment, the eclectic at the start of the twentieth century responded that definitions of this type had no place in medicine. "Until medicine becomes an exact science," argued G. W. Johnson, M.D., in 1903, "we are perfectly justified in holding different views upon subjects medical." Eclectics thus continued to defend both their therapeutic and their organizational individuality. Their principle of physiological law, expressed in a study of direct action for direct effect, distinguished them from the members of all other schools of therapeutic thinking and placed them on record as opposed to "synthetic prescribing for disease." Reform medicine rested on the twin pillars of scientific diagnosis and specific medication, which included the purity of its medical products. Johnson approved of bringing eclectics and regulars together for "social and scientific benefit," but he objected to any unification effort designed to renounce the system of reformed practice. "When it comes to showing the white feather for the privilege of being dictated to and ruled by any clique that is in direct opposition to my belief," he wrote, "I reserve the right to most humbly decline."[2] Eclectics agreed that anatomy, physiology, chemistry, and histology should be the same when taught in the various philosophical schools; nevertheless, this sameness did *not* extend to the application of remedies. The differences among allopaths, homeopaths, and eclectics lay in their particular therapeutic *means*. In applying remedies, eclectics judged other schools as "helplessly at sea without a chart or compass."[3]

By the turn of the century, however, eclectic reformers were showing greater tolerance than ever before. "If we are to be eclectics in spirit and in truth," commented H. C. Smith, M.D., of Los Angeles in 1913, "we must investigate every therapeutic measure which promises relief to suffering humanity, and must accept and use what is of value in each and every one." This policy meant putting a stop to "roasting the regulars" and "speaking sneeringly" of osteopaths, naturopaths, and Christian Scientists. Instead, eclectics were urged to add whatever was useful from their techniques to the therapeutic armamentarium of reform medicine.[4] At the annual meeting of the National Eclectic Medical Association in San Francisco in June 1915, a Dr. Miller, president of the American Institute of Homeopathy, recommended merger of their two medical systems. According to Miller, only trifling differences separated their methods of practice, especially since Samuel Hahnemann's doctrine of specific medication had been adopted by John M. Scudder and the new leaders of reform medical practice. He believed that a union of the two schools would advance therapeutic knowledge and "not magnify the importance of scientific branches at the expense of the therapeutic art."[5] Similarly, in the issues of the *California Eclectic Medical Journal* for 1916, editor O. C. Welbourn, M.D., published several articles on homeopathic practice that urged "mutual recognition." The schools differed in theory, "yet in practice they approach one to the other quite closely, and their use of many drugs may be said to be identical."[6]

These feelings derived, however, more from internal weaknesses and fear of extinction than from any carefully articulated ratiocination. Those who looked for amalgamation with homeopathy, wrote the editor of the *Eclectic Medical Journal* in 1903, "have mixed a little fire of moral sentiment with personal heat, with gross exaggeration and the blindness that prefers some pet measure, some eccentricity of action, to justice or truth." In pursuing this cause, proponents of merger failed to catch the true spirit of the age, having confused combination with unity, idealism with practicality; and more importantly, they forgot the traditions and beliefs that had led to the development of their distinct philosophies.[7]

As for the offer by the AMA to open its membership to sectarian physicians, loyal eclectics at the time of the First World War likened the offer to that of the Hohenzollern family seeking to extend its influence over Austria and Hungary. "They have their von Hindenburgs and their Ludendorffs ever ready to lay the schemes and give orders to their numerous lieutenants all over the country to scatter the 'medical Hun' propaganda and aid in carrying out their plans of destruction." Unfortunately, wrote O. S. Coffin, a member of the Council of Medical Education of the National Eclectic Medical Association, the Hohenzollerns had captured some of the good men and carried them away into their ranks. "Are we going to throw up our hands and surrender to this 'Potsdam gang' of the AMA? or are we going to stand by our rights of freedom to practice medicine according to the teachings of our Eclectic college." It was as important to "lick the medical Huns" of America as it was to "lick the enemies of freedom across the seas."[8]

John Uri Lloyd eventually suggested that the medical profession eliminate the term *regular* from its lexicon, as well as the terms *irregular* and *sectarian*. In their place, he offered *dominant section* or *majority section* for the regular wing while retaining the term *eclectic* for the reform wing of medicine. These appellations should represent separate family designations rather than attitudes of derision.[9] "To accept the term Regular in the sense that all outside is irregular, and needs to be suppressed," he wrote, "is to paralyze investigation, prohibit free thought, circumscribe the individual's opportunities and retard the world's advancement."[10]

Abiding Principles

Throughout more than a century of practice, the eclectics exhibited certain shifts in emphasis in response to changes in conviction, determination, historical circumstances, personality, and laboratory science that brought larger perspectives and newer thinking into the marketplace of ideas. Despite their full share of eccentricities, controversies, and internal convulsions, eclectics maintained a denominational resilience that earned them grudging respect in medical circles. "Many of the principles professed by the eclectics are quite admirable," wrote John B. Nichols, M.D., in 1913 in the *Journal of the American Medical Association*, "but they have nothing to offer in the way of resources, methods or principles that regular medicine does not possess." Nichols suggested that their continued existence simply perpetuated the eclectic name and organization "after the reasons that may have originally called it into being have ceased to operate."[11] Regardless of this opinion, eclectics redoubled their determination to discredit the majority party, claiming that the regulars had achieved questionable popularity through their fortuitous alliance with germ theory, serotherapy, and newer scientific theories. The eclectics in contrast drifted into a position increasingly contemptuous of change, truculent, slow in accepting new knowledge, and comfortable in musing about the past. Having become overly cautious in disposition and argument, the reformers propounded a dialectic that was apologetic in its defense of traditional medicine—a role reversal that occurred without fanfare and without critique.

Eclecticism through time marshaled to its side a set of principles that represented the authentic experience of the reform practice of medicine. From 1825, when Wooster Beach first started teaching students in his home, until the introduction of Scudder's specific medicines in 1869, these principles had included a commitment to utilizing vegetable medicines as the safest remedies for disease; an opposition to antiphlogistics, to bloodletting, to radical doses of mercury and antimony, and to the unnecessary use of opiates; a retention of the conservative approach to surgery; a belief in sustaining the vital forces, advocating single remedies, and wherever possible using simple combinations; a predilection for kindly medication and kindly treatment; an objection to continuous use of unpleasant remedies, drastic cathartics, harsh diuretics, and diaphoretics; a refusal to accept that physiologic actions of drugs upon animals correlated to the same actions in humans; a special emphasis in their colleges upon courses of materia medica and drug therapy; a preference for dispensing their own medicines; as well as a tendency to be risk takers by practicing independent, rational medicine. But the abuses and practices that had originally called forth the denunciations of the pioneer eclectics had ceased to exist in the 1890s except in the memories of those who had witnessed them half a century earlier.

What did still separate eclectics from regulars was the concept of specific diagnosis and the direct application of a specific remedy to a single disease condition. This—rather than enlightened empiricism—became the watchword of reform practice in the late nineteenth century. Derived from the combined labors of John King, Ichabod Gibson Jones, and John M. Scudder, specific medication gave new meaning to the philosophy and methods first laid down by Beach. Instead of the doctrines of contraries and similars, or even of the medium system of therapeutics, specific medication became the distinctive doctrine and keynote of eclectic practice. "Any medication other than specific is medication at random and unworthy" of the name "science or . . . art," commented one eclectic in 1895. Specific medication, he argued, is certainty in medicine, something that old-school medicine could never achieve.[12]

Following the elder Scudder's introduction of specific medication, eclectics added to their original principles by their refusal to combine toxicity and therapeutic efficiency; their refusal to view medicine as simply a poison in small doses (therefore, an agent without poisonous quality must be devoid of medicinal quality); their belief that disease should not be treated by routine methods, according to disease names, but adapted to the particular symptom complex under observation; their recognition of the relationship between certain drug actions and specific disease expressions; their renewed identification with vitalistic principles; their opposition to the continuous use of coal-tar preparations; and their decided affinity for general practice rather than for specialization.[13] Eclectics also supported increased emphasis on physical culture; believed in the therapeutic effects of X rays in treating phthisis, carcinoma, lupus, eczema, and neuralgia; attacked Christian Science as neither Christian nor scientific but explainable on the basis of suggestion; campaigned for pasteurized milk; fought drug adulteration; and advocated conservatism in gynecology, thereby condemning much of the radical surgery then in high fashion.[14]

But all was not well in eclectic practice. Of the old-timers of the E. M. Institute and other schools, only John Uri Lloyd remained to carry on the cause of reform medicine. Age and ill health had taken its toll upon the others. Storm Rosa, Charles Thomas Hart, George Washington Lafayette Bickley, Charles H. Cleaveland, and William Byrd Powell died in the 1860s; followed by Benjamin L. Hill, William Sherwood, and Lorenzo E. Jones in 1871; Alexander H. Baldridge and John French Judge in 1874; Robert S. Newton in 1881; Horatio P. Gatchell in 1886; Edwin Freeman in 1887; Andrew Jackson Howe in 1888; John King in 1893; John M. Scudder in 1894; Zoheth Freeman in 1898; Frederick John Locke in 1904; and Alexander Wilder in 1908. Howe, King, and Scudder had represented the "Great Eclectic Trinity."[15] As this older generation of reformers passed away, eclectic medicine lacked an infusion of new blood, renewed commitment, and staunch defenders. The same applied to its medical texts. With a few exceptions— Alexander Wilder, *History of Medicine* (1904); Albert F. Stephens, *The Essentials of Medical Gynecology* (1907); Kent O. Foltz, *Diseases of the Nose, Throat and Ear* (1906) and *Diseases of the Eye* (1909); Eli G. Jones, *Cancer, Its Causes and Treatment* (1911); John M. Scudder, *Specific Medication and Specific Medicines* (1913); John W. Fyfe, *Specific Diagnosis and Specific Medication* (1914); Rolla L. Thomas, *The Eclectic Practice of Medicine* (1922); Harvey W. Felter, *The Eclectic Materia Medica, Pharmacology and Therapeutics* (1922); and Charles Woodward, *Pathological Alkalinity* (1926)—not many works remained in print. And with future editions of John King's *American Dispensatory* in question, eclecticism no longer represented a viable botanico-medical movement. The 1909 reprint of the earlier revision served little purpose in furthering a specialized formulary on eclectic drugs. In effect, the younger generation of physicians had begun to merge with the majority school rather than carry the stigma of sectarian beliefs.[16]

Licensure Laws and Scandals

As noted earlier, state licensing boards took renewed interest in their responsibility for certifying schools and examining applicants for medical practice in the 1870s. This effort remained mired in politics for many states because of improperly constituted boards, lax requirements, and reluctance to countenance governmental regulation; and there was a continued desire to resist an elitist educational system. Within this context, Flexner's report of 1910 served as a principal catalyst for action. The report, in keeping with other progressive reform literature of the day, became the incentive for significant new state legislation that focused on licensing as a legitimate and proper role for government in the regulation of medical education. Here, too, the Association of American Medical Colleges, the Council on Medical Education of the AMA, the Federation of State Medical Boards, and the National Board of Medical Examiners played important roles by urging uniform licensing standards across the states.[17]

California law before 1913 required applicants for a medical license to undergo an examination before a mixed, or composite, examining board (five allopaths, two homeopaths, two eclectics, and two osteopaths) appointed by the governor. Applicants from each of the four schools of healing took the same examination on ten subjects, or fundamentals. Because two board members were doctors of osteopathy (D.O.), not doctors of medicine (M.D.), the examination excluded questions about materia medica and therapeutics, surgery, and practice of medicine. The standards nevertheless remained those of the dominant school. According to eclectics, the majority school had ensured that, besides having to file credentials and testimonials of good character, applicants for licensure had to have a diploma issued by a legally chartered medical school whose requirements were no less than those prescribed by the Association of American Medical Colleges (AAMC) for that year.[18] The California examining board had, in effect, accepted the criteria dictated by the "Medical Trust" (AMA) of Chicago. Equally distressing to eclectics, the California law provided no reciprocity for a physician holding a license legally issued in another state. Without further examination, no individual could receive a license to practice in California. "It strikes one as rather strange," wrote Henry Ford Scudder (youngest son of John M. Scudder) in 1913, "that here in California, one of the most progressive states in the Union, with [a] liberal legislature, that the ... medical colleges of our state, and the fitness of our own graduates in medicine and surgery, should have to be determined by the Medical Trust located in Chicago."[19]

Henry Ford Scudder, who had graduated from the E. M. Institute in 1893 and had practiced in San Diego, opposed the organizational makeup of the board of examiners because of its preponderance of allopaths. However, with revision to the legislation passed in 1913, reformers lost even more ground. The new law gave no recognition to sectarian medicine and, further, gave no assurance that the governor would even appoint sectarian representatives to the board.[20] Actually, neither the allopaths nor the eclectics found comfort in the bill's final wording. Regulars criticized it openly in the *California State Journal of Medicine*; and eclectics, though victorious on several points, expressed concern with its long-term implications. An important victory for the eclectics included the reciprocity aspect of the proposed new law, which gave a physician licensed elsewhere the right to obtain a license in California. Equally important, California no longer based its licensing standards on those set by the AMA. Finally, the law recognized two classes of practitioners (the drug and drugless) with separate examinations.[21]

California's tribulations with its examining boards reflected a common theme across America. State legislatures had created approximately ninety-six separate and independent boards to control medical licensure. As many as six different boards exercised this licensing power in some states and applied just as many different standards of educational qualification.

It was out of this confusion that the licensure scandal of 1922–23 arose, in which eclectics played a prominent role. The AMA acted as catalyst when, in 1918, it protested the manner in which eclectic boards in Arkansas and Connecticut licensed graduates of low-grade medical colleges. Through successive issues of the *Journal of the American Medical Association*, the AMA accused the Arkansas State Board of Eclectic Examiners of being in collusion with the Kansas City College of Medicine and Surgery in Missouri and warned Connecticut that it harbored a similar relationship with its eclectic board.

In a halfhearted response to these complaints, the Missouri State Legislature substituted "legally chartered" for "reputable" in its medical practice act of 1921. This change in wording removed from the licensing board the authority to refuse examinations to graduates of notoriously inferior medical schools. Faced with mounting criticism from within and without the state, however, Missouri revised its standards again in 1923 with a bill restoring the word *reputable* to the medical practices act.[22]

In 1922, the Kansas City *Journal-Post* and the St. Louis *Star* reported that the Connecticut Eclectic Licensing Board had licensed seventy-one physicians, sixty-one of whom had graduated from marginal medical schools and three of whom came from California institutions that had never been recognized. Only twenty-five of those licensed were graduates of eclectic medical colleges; the remainder were from regular colleges of low standing. In its investigation, the *Star* learned that the board had arranged licenses for both in-state and out-of-state graduates of marginal schools, including noneclectic schools, thus giving them legal entrance into medical practice. The Connecticut Eclectic Licensing Board had not limited itself to graduates of eclectic colleges, as prescribed by law, but had accepted for examination any medical graduate. One individual, having failed the examination given by the (regular) Connecticut Board of Medical Examiners on eight separate occasions, passed the eclectic board's examination with high marks. William P. Best, recording secretary for the National Eclectic Medical Association, reported in a letter to the *Journal of the American Medical Association* that Dr. Ralph A. Voigt of Kansas City and Dr. D. R. Alexander of the Kansas City College of Medicine and Surgery (the real masterminds behind the Connecticut scandal) had never been members of the National Eclectic Medical Association. Best deplored the action of the board, calling it "a discredit to the profession in general and to . . . Eclectics in particular."[23] The state eventually revoked 167 (granted over multiple years) of the questionable licenses. On the basis of this scandal, the AMA urged each state to create a single board of medical examiners with minimum standards of qualification, which *all* applicants must meet regardless of medical affiliation or practice.[24]

Licensing boards were involved in a seemingly continuous string of scandals throughout the 1920s. (In the files of the E. M. College in Cincinnati, newspaper clippings reporting these embarrassments are prominently included among other memorabilia.) The licensure frauds and diploma-mill trials, unfortunately for the eclectics, seriously eroded efforts to raise endowment funds to assist the the E. M. College in its plan for reorganization. Even when it was demonstrated that a given eclectic board had been taken over by noneclectics, the various bogus licensing schemes simply enraged the public and opened the way for tough new regulations. One obvious outcome of these new regulations was the closure of proprietary schools and, with them, the final method of providing a "practical" medical education. The age of corporate medicine had arrived.[25]

The Appeal to Eclectics

"There is more need for Eclecticism now than there ever was," argued a physician in the *Eclectic Medical Journal* in 1903, "and what Eclecticism needs today is not a council to prepare a funeral oration, but a genuine old-fashioned Methodist revival, wherein backsliders shall be reclaimed, the feeble strengthened, and the lukewarm set on fire."[26] A decade later, eclectics continued their appeal to wayward members. "In this age of medical nihilism, brother, the world needs Eclectics and we need you," wrote M. F. Bettencourt, M.D., of Texas. "We want you in our ranks. Don't be ashamed of our numbers, brother—a tenth of the medical profession of the United States in three-quarters of a century is not a bad showing. Come back, brother, be faithful to your trust; stand for what you believe right and show the world what you are. Eclecticism has nothing to be ashamed of, but, rather, much of which to be proud." This appeal in the pages of the *California Eclectic Medical Journal* reflected the preoccupation of the California Eclectic Medical College, Los Angeles, with surviving as an alternative to the majority school. Reform medical practice clearly faced a crisis of identity; surrounded by so many marvels in medical science, the public ignored eclecticism, concluding that its schools would close within a few years.[27]

In 1908, the National Confederation of Eclectic Medical Colleges identified its eight member institutions: American Medical College of St. Louis, in Missouri; Bennett College of Eclectic Medicine and Surgery, Chicago; California Eclectic Medical College, Los Angeles; Eclectic Medical College of the City of New York; Eclectic Medical Institute, Cincinnati; Georgia College of Eclectic Medicine and Surgery, Atlanta; Lincoln Medical College, Lincoln, Nebraska; and Western Eclectic College of Medicine and Surgery, Kansas City, Kansas. Left off the list because of their questionable quality were the Eclectic Medical College of Indiana, in Indianapolis, and the Eclectic Medical University in Kansas City, Missouri.

In the decade following Flexner's report, all but one of these schools closed outright or merged with university-based medical colleges. The Bennett College of Eclectic Medicine and Surgery had dropped "eclectic" from its title in 1909—a change that failed to impress Flexner. Unenthusiastic in his estimation of the newly named college, Flexner described it as commercial, as a stock company "practically owned by the Dean."[28] A year later, Bennett absorbed two Chicago schools—the Illinois Medical College and the Reliance Medical College—and became, by affiliation, the School of Medicine of Loyola University. Not until 1916, however, did Loyola University of Chicago assume full control of the school.[29]

The *Journal of the American Medical Association* in 1913 listed the Georgia College of Eclectic Medicine and Surgery, Bennett College of Medicine and Surgery, the American Medical College in Indianapolis, the Eclectic Medical College of the City of New York, and the Eclectic Medical College in Cincinnati as having more than 20 percent failures before state boards.[30] Only the E. M. College in Cincinnati succeeded in obtaining a "Class B" status; the other schools required a complete reorganization to make them acceptable.[31]

The California Eclectic Medical College organized in 1879 in Oakland, moved to San Francisco in 1887, suspended operations in 1906, and then reorganized in Los Angeles in 1907. The announcement for the college's thirty-fifth annual term (1913–14) informed applicants that, for matriculation, they had to possess a California high school diploma or its equivalent or pass a satisfactory examination to enter the college. The college also announced its support of coeducation, its commitment to Scudder's method of specific medication, its curricular focus on the medicoclimatology problems of the Southwest, and its combination of didactic and clinical teaching. The announcement explained to the prospective student that eclectic practice represented "the liberal doctrine of choice," meaning "freedom and independence and a square deal for all." With many different systems of healing in vogue, each containing something of value, eclecticism intended to "get good results" with "whatever will relieve and cure the patient . . . no matter what its source."[32] The announcement went on to explain that eclectic medicine had taken the lead in plant-drug investigation, with nearly two hundred proven remedies prepared in fluid form and known as specific medicines. Moreover, Lloyd Brothers, Pharmacists, Inc., of Cincinnati had provided the college with "a full line of their specific medicines in a handsome glass cabinet for the use of its students in studying materia medica and therapeutics." The college also maintained a three-acre botanical garden near Compton, between Long Beach and Los Angeles, where students would learn practical pharmacy by growing their own plants, making tinctured medicines in the laboratory, and administering the products of these field and classroom investigations in the college's clinics.[33]

Notwithstanding these claims, the college failed to provide students with adequate laboratories and instruction. According to Flexner, the institution had led "a roving and precarious existence" and occupied "a few neglected rooms on the second floor of a fifty-foot frame building." Its equipment, "dirty and disorderly beyond description," consisted of a few bones, a few bottles of reagents, a rusty incubator, a single microscope, and a "few unlabeled wet specimens." Having neither a dispensary nor access to hospital facilities, it was "a disgrace to the state whose laws permit its existence." The college closed its doors in 1915.[34]

By that same year, the total number of students attending nonsectarian (regular) medical schools was 13,914, with only 736 at homeopathic and 241 at eclectic schools. The attendance at homeopathic colleges represented a decrease of 61.4 percent from its numbers in 1900, when 1,909 were enrolled. Eclectic colleges in 1915 enrolled twenty-nine fewer students than they had in the previous year and 773 (76.2 percent) fewer than in 1904, the year in which the greatest number had enrolled (1,014). Eclectic colleges graduated fifty-five, or fifteen fewer than in the previous year and

166 (75.1 percent) fewer than in 1890, when 221—its greatest number of physicians—graduated.[35]

The American Medical College of St. Louis, which had organized in 1873, had twenty-eight students at the time of Flexner's visit. In his report, he stated that the college had meager equipment, with little indication of its being used, a weekly clinic held at the City Hospital, and a poorly attended dispensary. The college dropped its eclectic affiliation in 1910 and, a year later, absorbed the Barnes Medical College to become the Medical Department of the National University of Arts and Sciences. It finally suspended operations in 1918.[36]

The Eclectic Medical College of the City of New York, with ninety-six in attendance at the time of Flexner's visit, closed in 1913, as did the Georgia College of Eclectic Medicine and Surgery in Atlanta in 1914. Flexner said the Georgia college occupied a building that, "in respect to filthy conditions, has few equals, but no superiors, among medical schools." Its anatomy room contained a single cadaver "indescribably foul," and its chemical laboratory consisted of little more than a few old tables and "a few bottles, without water, drain, lockers, or reagents." He noted that "nothing more disgraceful calling itself a medical school can be found anywhere."[37]

In Kansas City, Missouri, the Western Eclectic College of Medicine and Surgery organized as the Eclectic Medical University in 1898, moved to Kansas City, Kansas, in 1907, and then returned to Missouri in 1909. At the time of Flexner's visit, there were twenty-one students in attendance and a teaching staff of thirty-two. Owning little in the form of laboratory equipment and offering almost no clinical opportunities for students beyond a dispensary that averaged three patients daily, this stock company had little resemblance to a real medical school. It was reorganized as the Kansas City College of Medicine and Surgery in 1915 and suspended operations in 1918.[38]

As a result of the classification of colleges by the AMA, the West Virginia State Legislature amended its medical law by recognizing only graduates of AMA "Class A" colleges. In response, John King Scudder wrote to eclectic physicians around the state urging them to lobby the legislature to ensure that the "Class A" status be given not only to medical schools classified by the Council on Medical Education of the AMA but also those classified as "Class A" by the American Institute of Homeopathy and the National Eclectic Medical Association.[39] Although the National Eclectic Medical Association judged its institutions to be "Class A" medical schools and furnished this information on request to various boards of medical examination and licensure, there was little correlation between their classifications and those defined by the Council on Medical Education of the AMA.[40]

As for Lincoln Medical College in Lincoln, Nebraska (which had affiliated with the Medical Department of Cotner University), Flexner found few laboratory facilities and no clinical opportunities, not even a dispensary. In 1911, the college was renamed the Cotner University Medical College. It canceled its affiliation with the university in 1915 and resumed the Lincoln Medical College title, closing permanently in 1918.

In Cincinnati, the E. M. College *Bulletin* carried a special notice in June 1926 stating that, as the plans for the reorganization of the college were incomplete, the trustees had decided not to matriculate a freshman class in 1926–27; instruction of the 110 students in the three upper classes would continue as usual. With no new students enrolled, the college graduated in May 1929 what appeared to many observers to be its last class. Outsiders speculated on the future of the "extinct" school, but in June, the college announced a successful reorganization, including the creation of a Building and Endowment Committee and a report on modern methods of medical education. The college renovated its building and laboratories, salaried its professors, and hired additional support staff, so that the curriculum and facilities would compare favorably with other medical institutions. In addition, the college extended the length of its semesters to meet the requirements of other states. The trustees in January 1931 stated that the fate of reform medicine was in the hands of forty-eight hundred eclectic physicians in the United States. Having sent a booklet to each of these physicians concerning the position of the college, the trustees appealed to affiliated members to support the last bastion of reform medical education in America. "By intelligent enthusiasm is meant your own sincere informed belief, coupled with such equally sincere presentation of it as you are capable of giving." Implied in these words was the hope that each physician would support the college with a minimum two-hundred-dollar pledge.[41] In appealing to honor and patriotism, the trustees claimed that the E. M. College was "an American institution, American in origin, American in concept, and American in practice."[42] Many contributions did come from reform practitioners around the country, but the college's chief benefactor during these years was John Uri Lloyd, who pledged ten thousand dollars annually and then increased the amount to fifty thousand. Although greatly appreciated by the college, the amount did not compare to the millions of dollars channeled from large and small foundations to the elite schools. Ernest V. Hollis estimated that the larger foundations directed $150 million into medical education between 1910 and 1932, while smaller donors—as a group—gave three or four times that figure.[43]

The trustees of the E. M. College from 1929 on considered the possibility of closure. In a March 28, 1931, meeting, a "free and general discussion" took place on the topic of the college's future, with some members actively urging closure. The president of the board said the trustees had no legal right to terminate the college at that meeting, noting the necessity for calling a special meeting and notifying all board members of the issue. The majority of voting members, after prolonged discussion, resolved that "an effort should be made to rehabilitate the institute, independent of any dictation, of the Council on Medical Education of the American Medical Association."[44] Following two years of "rest," the college reopened its doors on September 21, 1931, with a freshman class only. The session lasted until June 11, 1932, with twenty-eight of the original thirty-five freshmen enrolling in the sophomore class.[45] The decision to resume active operation of the college stemmed from requests by several state medical societies, the alumni association of the college, the National Eclectic Medical Association, and the Building and Endowment Committee of the college.

Following instructions from the trustees at its May 1932 meeting in Chicago, bids were taken and contracts let for renovating the college. The work was completed in September 1932 and provided the college with new lecture halls; four special prosecting rooms; laboratories for pharmacology, pathology, neurology, and bacteriology; and new teaching equipment. While the remodeling program was under way, the faculty revised the curriculum; the Eclectic Education Loyalty Fund struggled to meet the college's financial needs; and administrators arranged an affiliation with Union Bethel Clinic, where a complete outpatient department was organized for junior-year instruction. Even with these changes, the college made little pretense at claiming to be an advanced research center, nor could they. Pasteur's dictum, that "men of science without laboratories are as soldiers without armies," had become all too real to the faculty and the trustees.[46]

The trustees in 1932 approved the college's effort to apply for membership in the AAMC. Specifically, the trustees urged the college to seek approval for the new freshman courses of instruction by the Committee on Inspection of Medical Colleges of the AAMC. This decision was not unanimous: some board members believed that AAMC approval would cause the college to lose its distinctiveness. The dean, however, pointed out that members of the faculty were reluctant to teach for any length of time unless the college received a positive rating. Moreover, having discussed with the dean of the University of Cincinnati's School of Medicine the use of its professors to provide adjunct instruction at the college, he informed the board that the professors were unlikely to agree to teach until the college received an acceptable rating.[47] The application for AAMC membership, however, was held back because the school subsequently learned that it could not expect a review until completion of at least two years of the new freshman program.[48]

In December 1932, Rolla L. Thomas, dean first of the E. M. Institute and then of the E. M. College after its name change, died, leaving the school without leadership. From Thomas Vaughan Morrow (1845–50) to Joseph R. Buchanan (1850–56), Robert S. Newton (1856–61), John M. Scudder (1861–94), Frederick John Locke (1894–1904), and Rolla L. Thomas (1904–32), the college had been led by men of strong personality who insisted that eclecticism was not so much a scientific system as it was a comprehensive mass of science embracing everything connected with the healing art. Though reality often proved disappointingly different, these men had dedicated their lives to the principle of eclecticism.

After Thomas' death, the college turned to Dr. Byron H. Nellans (1892–1949), who served as dean until 1939, working at improving the organization and administration of the college and guiding curriculum and accreditation efforts. Nellans had graduated from the E. M. College in 1914, had served his internship in Seton Hospital, and from 1918 to 1934 had held the post of professor of physical diagnosis and medicine at the college.

Under Nellans' guidance, the college fought to retain its place in American medical education. In 1934, the Council of Medical Education of the National Eclectic Medical Association approved the school, giving it a "Class A" rating. Eben B. Shewman, president of the association (and head of the Department of Surgery at the college), stated that students in the college wrote the same final examination as the students from the University of Cincinnati, "thus offsetting any criticism from [other] Rating Agencies."[49] By 1935, the college boasted approval by the Council of Medical Education of the National Eclectic Medical Association, by the Ohio State Board of Medical Registration and Examination, and twenty-six other state boards as well.[50] The E. M. College reported that its students had access to the Lloyd Library's sixty thousand books and thirty thousand pamphlets, the Cincinnati General Hospital Library, the Cincinnati Public Library, and the college's own library of four thousand books. Operating under its reorganization plan of 1931, the college graduated its first class of twenty in June 1935. There were then 133 students (31 seniors, 23 juniors, 35 sophomores, and 44 freshmen) enrolled.[51]

The secretary of the Ohio State Board of Medical Registration and Examination informed the college in January 1935 that certain additional improvements had to be made "at the earliest possible moment." The secretary urged construction of a new building, noted the need for better supervision of students at the Cincinnati General Hospital, and warned that in 1938 the board would take under consideration the progress of the E. M. College in relation to the results of a survey made by H. G. Weiskotten, M.D., on behalf of the Council of Medical Education, the AAMC, and the Federation of State Medical Boards. In March 1935, Harold Rypins, M.D., secretary of the New York State Board of Medical Examiners, made a three-day visit to the college. His report, dated May 7, 1935, was ominous.

> In view of the fact that a thorough inspection of the Eclectic Medical College shows that it does not have adequate equipment and resources, that it does not have suitable hospital and clinical facilities, that it does not maintain an adequate medical library and that it does not have a sufficient number of full-time salaried instructors giving their entire time to professional instruction, and thus does not meet four of the seven requirements . . . for the recognition of a medical school . . . it is recom-

mended that the application of the Eclectic Medical College be denied.[52]

On June 21, 1935, the college received an official letter from William D. Cutter, M.D., secretary of the Council on Medical Education and Hospitals of the AMA, which detailed the council's findings based on Rypins's survey. The council made note of the improper organization of the board of trustees (three of the department heads were members of the board), insufficient hospital and clinical facilities, too few salaried instructors and laboratory assistants, and lack of research. Most serious was the "farming out" of its students at the Cincinnati General Hospital to faculty of other schools because no member of the eclectic faculty held a position on the hospital staff.[53]

The college failed, even with the heroic efforts of Nellans, to survive the death in 1936 of its chief benefactor, John Uri Lloyd. With his passing, the college lost not only Lloyd's generous contributions to the alumni fund but the manufacture of Lloyd's specific medicines. The *National Eclectic Medical Association Quarterly* expressed the hope that the firm of Lloyd Brothers, Pharmacists, Inc., would continue to prepare specific medicines. But the future looked bleak.[54] In a revealing confession, R. O. Hoffman wrote,

> We have no new books nor have we had, even in our own beloved Materia Medica a complete revision in several years. We have few outstanding men, even in our own estimation, so why fight a losing game? . . . We are no longer a new school, pioneering in a promising field, but we are losing in numbers and prestige as a school as the years go by and I suggest, if I may, a course that still has a modicum of possibility. . . . The last Old War Horse [John Uri Lloyd] is gone, so the sentiment that attached to the Old Guard of the Old College may now be laid aside, even if it does pull at the heart strings of some of us if by so doing we may perpetuate the good that has been gained.[55]

Dean Nellans called in January 1936 for a special meeting of the board of trustees. In reporting to Reverend Louis G. Hoeck, president of the board, Nellans reminded him of the changes that had been made in the composition of the board, the revisions made in the curriculum, and the efforts under way to comply with the suggestions of Drs. Cutter and Weiskotten. Indeed, the three department heads (Eben B. Shewman, Charles W. Beaman, and Byron H. Nellans) had resigned from the board, and Nellans became a full-time administrator. Nellans had also negotiated better arrangements for students at Cincinnati General Hospital. However, the financial condition of the college had prevented it from hiring additional full-time salaried instructors and assistants. Nellans then reported that the Council on Medical Education and Hospitals had gone on record as stating that "the advances of the medical sciences have been and should be independent of any sectarian point of view, and medical education should not be handicapped or directed by a dogmatic attitude toward disease." After July 1, 1938, the council had resolved to carry no sectarian schools on its approved list.[56]

In recognition of the inevitable, the board of trustees decided in 1936 to prohibit the continued admission of new students, a decision that left the college's educational mission limited to graduating its remaining thirty-two seniors and thirty-six juniors. Nellans then labored to dispose of all medical apparatus owned by the college. To ensure that students would receive proper instruction, he negotiated arrangements for junior-year instruction with Union Bethel Clinic, while senior-year instruction was arranged in consultation with the dean of the University of Cincinnati Medical School and with the heads of departments at Cincinnati General Hospital. Nellans also sought a waiver from the Council on Medical Education and Hospitals of the AMA of its ruling that prevented the college's graduates from interning in council-approved hospitals.[57] Unfortunately for the college, the AMA was prepared to credit the graduates of the college for their work but *only* after an official order of dissolution of the college was made by the trustees to Secretary of State John E. Sweeney of Ohio. In the meantime, representatives of the college, including the Reverend Hoeck, attempted unsuccessfully to negotiate an affiliation with the University of Cincinnati.[58]

In 1938, two years after John Uri Lloyd's death, the S. B. Penick Co. of New York City purchased Lloyd Brothers, Pharmacists, Inc., promising to continue the ideals, plans, and products of the brothers, as well as to take up chemical research on all of the drugs in the eclectic materia medica.[59] But the S. B. Penick Co.'s production of the specific medicines declined as it became apparent that fewer and fewer eclectics were choosing to remain within the fold of botanic medicine. To complicate matters, John Uri's drug-formula books disappeared about the time of S. B. Penick Co.'s purchase. The trustees of Lloyd's estate (Nellans, Charles R. Campbell, and John Thomas Lloyd) seem not to have turned over the formula books for specific medicines to the new company. When Lloyd's son, John Thomas Lloyd, a former entomologist at Cornell University, set up his own company to continue his father's medicines (under the new name Lloydson Medicines), the S. B. Penick Co. sued, suspecting that he may have taken the formulas. After litigation, John T. Lloyd Laboratories, Inc., maker of Lloydson Medicines, was forced to note in its advertisements that the company had "no connection with Lloyd Brothers Pharmacists, Inc., which was the sole successor to the pharmaceutical business established in 1885 under the name Lloyd Brothers." The ads had to state further that, after being sold to S. B. Penick Co., "no member of the Lloyd family retained any connection with it." Whether son John took the formulas is unclear, but in all probability he did. In any case, the whereabouts of the drug formulas for Lloyd's specific medicines remain a mystery, even today.[60]

On June 7, 1939, Dean Nellans presided over the eighty-eighth commencement exercises of the E. M. College as thirty-six students received the doctor of medicine degree. Upon conclusion of the ceremony, the ninety-four-year career of the college came to an end. Yielding to the "almost prohibitive cost" of privately conducted medical education, the college passed into history, having graduated a total of 4,666 students, including 440 women.[61] The National Eclectic Medical Association issued a statement saying that the college surrendered its charter to the state because it was "no longer an economic or scientific necessity to maintain a separate school of medicine since the curricula in all American medical colleges were well standardized and the advances in therapeutics and practice originated and contributed by the Eclectic section of medicine was generally well accepted."[62] Actually, this rationalization was more fiction than truth. A more accurate statement by George C. Porter, president of the association in 1939, noted that too many eclectics had failed to keep their "distinctive faith," trading it away for a mere "Doctor of Medicine." They thereby relinquished an "enduring truth" for a "contaminated fiction."[63] Porter, a 1903 graduate of the college, admitted that eclecticism had "failed to keep the pace of time" and became "somewhat neglectful of scientific advancement."[64]

When the E. M. College closed, various eclectics made plans for the creation of an eclectic research foundation. Dr. Eben B. Shewman, chair of the committee appointed to set up the foundation, gave no specific details, except to say that the college property would be sold and the money combined with other funds to initiate the foundation.[65] The foundation, however laudable the intention, never materialized. The small amount of money obtained from the sale of the college was insufficient to begin the project, so the trustees chose to divide the money equally between St. Mary's Hospital and Bethesda Hospital to be used for their nursing programs.[66] In 1942, the trustees empowered Byron H. Nellans, Dr. Charles R. Campbell, and John Thomas Lloyd to dispose of the college's library. Its books and periodicals, papers, board minutes, and scrapbooks became the property of John T. Lloyd Laboratories and were later turned over to the Lloyd Library and Museum.[67]

But the National Eclectic Medical Association continued to function on behalf of its members. In 1949, Ralph B. Taylor of Columbus, president of the association, noted that too many eclectic graduates had either "neglected or spurned" their origins. "Let's hang together, not fall apart."[68] The association continued to meet into the 1960s. The last record of the association and its quarterly journal was the September–December issue in 1965, which noted the coming 1966 convention for June 15–17 at the Aristocrat Hotel in Hot Springs, Arkansas. That these last stalwarts of reform medicine should have chosen the Aristocrat for their final meeting must have caused Clio, the Muse of history, to smile at the irony.

More recently, the traditions of eclectic medicine have undergone a revival with the establishment in 1982 of the Eclectic Institute Incorporated of Portland, Oregon, by naturopathic physicians Edward K. Alstat and Michael Ancharski. The research of this herb company focuses on analytical and clinical studies of botanical preparations, principally the medicines of John Uri Lloyd and John King. Alstat, company president and cofounder, who is also a pharmacist, reintroduced many of Lloyd's original specific medicines, but he has utilized the more advanced technique of freeze-drying (lyophilization) to capture the true properties (vital force) of the plants. The institute offers some thirty-five herbs in freeze-dried state and carries a line of herbal alcohol extracts and nutritional supplements, which are sold mainly to naturopaths and chiropractors. In addition, the institute publishes reprints of earlier eclectic texts (including works by Harvey W. Felter, Finley Elling-wood, John M. Scudder, William H. Cook, and David M. R. Culbreth) and retains a close association with the National College of Naturopathic Medicine, Portland, with which both Alstat and Ancharski were once affiliated. Like William S. Merrell, whose drug-manufacturing business maintained close ties with Beach and Morrow at the E. M. Institute, Portland's Eclectic Institute Incorporated is housed on the grounds of the National College of Naturopathic Medicine and "has played a very active role as a financial advocate for the school's success." And, like Lloyd's specific medicines, which were endorsed as the official medicines of the eclectic medical schools, the medicinal products of the institute are endorsed by the National College of Naturopathic Medicine.[69]

Looking Backward

The expansion of American civilization created a fertile ground for a new and distinctive system of reform medicine that in retrospect seems quite natural. The monopolistic hold that orthodox medicine maintained in Europe underwent a transformation in the United States, a nation in which accommodation and toleration prevailed. Orthodoxy gave way to multiplicity as dissenting medical sects developed into organizations, albeit less formal, that were strong enough to weather assaults on their existence. In a voluntary, freely competitive environment, the medical sectarians settled into what religious sectarians called *denominationalism* and politicians called *parties*. For typical Americans, the denominations, parties, and medical sects represented societies among which they were free to choose. A vital part of the motivation for that voluntarism grew from a disdain for past orthodoxies and a belief, however naive, that American creeds—political, religious, and medical—represented a break from European corruption.

American medical sectarians commonly believed that the historical development of medicine was not an accretion of valuable cures and practices but a process of corruption and degeneration in which the original purity and intentions of Greek and Roman medicine had been lost. For that reason, sectarians chose not to preserve the prevailing forms and practices but to recapture the purity of medicine's prelapsarian past. Many sought a return to the empiricism of early medicine; others appealed to private judgment in matters of health, hoping to break the bonds of historical beliefs and systems. In either case, they viewed their systems as good for the general welfare, returning medicine to simple, commonsense principles and beliefs. They in many ways succeeded where regular medicine failed, as the common people came back to medicine with simple ideas, voiced by forceful and persuasive leaders who avoided the complexities of overly rationalistic systems.

Those sectarians who subscribed to botanic medicine were never really a homogeneous group for, with the passing of the first generation and the enlargement of their numbers, they fragmented into competing idiosyncratic camps. The older botanics, especially those in the more remote and rural communities, clung hard to the original principles that their leaders had first announced, and they fought all efforts to mimic the educational pretensions of an upwardly mobile society. By the 1840s, however, there had also arisen a group of younger, more independent botanics, cosmopolitan in outlook, liberal in medical tendencies, and conversant with the latest medical influences. Tending to encourage greater tolerance and a broader pursuit of learning, they cultivated the sciences and exhibited less patience with the more truculent members of the older generation. As a group, this younger generation was more learned; however, its leadership was less effective at controlling members.

The eclectics, believing it important to hold fast to all that was good in medicine, found themselves borrowing from all medical systems and sects. Forging a place within the ambiguities of medicine, they asserted their openness to all of medicine's intellectual inheritance, provided that it worked. Their catholic approach, unlike the approaches of the Thomsonians and homeopaths, remained open and fluid through most of their history, never formulating a coherent therapeutic doctrine but, instead, choosing a deliberate course that relied on the purely empirical.

Most eclectics held that medicine would eventually find a way out of its balkanized, sectarian state and merge into a single school of scientific knowledge. They predicted a time somewhere in the future when medical practice would be based on sound empirical evidence, when nothing metaphysical would distract physicians from the art and science of their calling. The day would come when nothing but factual demonstration would satisfy medical minds. Those rationalistic systems, once they had claimed to have solved the riddle of disease, would then defer to a philosophy as positive as it would be unemotional, nourished continually by scientific discoveries—discoveries that, while variable and transient, while shaped to the changing trends of thought, would nonetheless be grounded in experience. Thus, in theory, eclecticism would never cease to enlarge its frontiers; each generation would rise above the scientific outlook of the previous one, with future generations carrying the process even further. Eclectics saw themselves as blazing trails through the unknown with new methods of research and discovery, achieving what their forebears only dreamed.

During the first fifty years of their history, eclectics tended to be opportunistic, hedging their bets with every new claim by noting that, while the truths of medicine were not to be swallowed whole, they had to be sifted until palatable bits and pieces were found. They viewed science and medicine as continually in transition and, recognizing that much would prove false, maintained a fervor for change and an openness to ideas. They reassured patients that the world was governed by an immutable law of progress, which although not always linear could be achieved through man's active pursuit of new knowledge. Every day and in every way, medicine had the capacity to become more refined and perfect. Eclectic practice also increased the faith of patients in medicine itself. Because it was freed from the bonds of orthodoxy, patients could adapt to change without being confronted by a crisis of values; Americans could adjust to the changes in therapeutics without losing faith in medical institutions. In an age of rampant change, reform medicine brought patients and practitioners together under a common roof that encouraged tolerance, community, sympathy, helpfulness, and cooperation.

The eclectics by the late nineteenth century had become strikingly similar in their beliefs to the modernists in religion. Both opened American minds to new ways of thinking. Yet the modernists made so many concessions to the age that they seemed to have abandoned the real substance of their beliefs. The same proved true for most eclectics who, in their liberalism and in their optimistic belief in progress and the need for continually adopting new ideas and techniques, failed to build anything lasting. In theory, eclecticism represented a willingness to adapt, accommodate, and adjust to the most contemporary scientific thinking (with the exception of germ theory). It began by taking the intellectual culture of early-nineteenth-century society as its criterion and adjusting eclectic practice to that standard. But here, too, shallowness and transience prevailed. Eclecticism, like modernism, arose out of a temporary crisis in faith and took a stance that for the time seemed both wise and correct. Yet, for all their openness to new ideas, eclectics were so busy adjusting themselves to the modern mind that they had no energy to explore on their own, to validate or challenge, or to restate the fundamentals of medicine. At best, they represented a heterogeneous group of practitioners who believed in all and in nothing and failed ultimately to provide meaning to their medical art. By the late nineteenth century, they held such a strong sentimental attachment to their earlier botanic ideas and to specific medication that they were never really able to accept germ theory without wondering if it would bring censure from colleagues.

Within the supporters of eclecticism was an authentic Americanism, with roots sunk deep in the wells of individualism and empiricism. Theirs was a system that, while open-minded and tolerant, believing doubt to be an essential part of the method of science, felt it possible to practice medicine without the infallibility or authority of Old World system builders. Nevertheless, only a minority of eclectics acquired the scientific habits of mind that allowed them to live the disinterested life science demanded. Most merely acquired odds and ends of information that, because they rejected the authority of inherited medical systems, fit into no plan and supported no consistent view of health and disease.

In theory, eclectics learned how to live without the support of any one particular creed, taking a position that was utterly self-sufficient and divorced from the claims of prior system builders. However, for most eclectic practitioners, such ideas made them feel insecure. Even an easy and tolerant skepticism proved impossible for most. They wanted ideas they could count on, sure cures, absolute promises, not situations with "ifs" and "perhapses." The faith of the patient was always hard, practical, and definite. Yet, in the end, eclectics found themselves unable to extricate themselves from similar expressions.

Notes
Selected Bibliography
Index

Notes

Introduction

1. Raymond T. Bond, *The Man Who Was Chesterton* (Garden City, N.Y.: Doubleday Image Books, 1960), 131. Sidney E. Mead used the phrase for the title of his book, *The Nation with the Soul of a Church* (New York: Harper and Row, 1975), 48–77.

2. Martyn Paine, "A Lecture on the Improvement of Medical Education in the United States," *New York Journal of Medicine*, I (1843), 367–78; Henry J. Bigelow, *Medical Education in America* (Cambridge: Welch, Bigelow and Co., 1871), 16.

1. The American Landscape

1. Richard H. Shryock, *Medical Licensing in America, 1650–1965* (Baltimore: Johns Hopkins University Press, 1967), 9.

2. John B. Blake, "Early American Medical Literature," *Clio Medica*, XI (1976), 152; Eric H. Christianson, "The Medical Practitioners of Massachusetts, 1630–1800: Patterns of Change and Continuity," in Colonial Society of Massachusetts, *Medicine in Colonial Massachusetts, 1620–1820* (Boston: The Colonial Society of Massachusetts, 1980), 51–54.

3. Richard D. Brown, "The Healing Arts in Colonial and Revolutionary Massachusetts: The Context for Scientific Medicine," in *Medicine in Colonial Massachusetts, 1620–1820*, 37.

4. Cotton Mather, *A Letter about a Good Management under the Distemper of the Measles, at This Time Spreading in the Country* (Boston: n.p., 1713). The quote is from the subtitle of the book. David E. Stannard, *The Puritan Way of Death: A Study in Religion, Culture, and Social Change* (New York: Oxford University Press, 1977), chapter 4.

5. Francisco Guerra, "Medical Almanacs of the American Colonial Period," *Journal of the History of Medicine*, XVI (1961), 234–55; Brown, "The Healing Arts in Colonial and Revolutionary Massachusetts," 42.

6. Richard H. Shryock, *Medicine and Society in America, 1660–1860* (New York: New York University Press, 1960), 16; Lester S. King, *The Medical World of the Eighteenth Century* (Huntington, N.Y.: Robert E. Krieger Publishing Co., 1971), 37–38; R. S. Neiman, "Medical Thought in Colonial New England," *Tufts Folia Medica*, VIII (1962), 69; H. Thoms, *The Doctors of Yale College, 1702–1815, and the Foundation of the Medical Institution* (Hamden, Conn.: Shoe String Press, 1960); Harold Y. Vanderpool, "The Wesleyan-Methodist Tradition," in Ronald L. Numbers and Darrell W. Amundsen (eds.), *Caring and Curing: Health and Medicine in the Western Religious Traditions* (New York: Macmillan, 1986), 321, 323; John Cule, "The Reverend John Wesley, M.A. (Oxon.), 1703–1791: 'The Naked Empiricist' and Orthodox Medicine," *Journal of the History of Medicine*, XLV (1990), 41–63.

7. Charles E. Rosenberg, "Medical Text and Social Context: Explaining William Buchan's *Domestic Medicine*," *Bulletin of the History of Medicine*, LVII (1983), 22–42; Neil Hultin, "Some Aspects of Eighteenth-Century Folk Medicine," *Southern Folklore Quarterly*, XXXVIII (1974), 199–209.

8. Wyndham B. Blanton, *Medicine in Virginia in the Seventeenth Century* (Richmond: William Byrd Press, 1930), 81; Anthony P. Wagner, "The Adaption of the Ancient Philosophy of Medicine to the New World by Jean-Francois Coste," *Journal of the History of Medicine*, VII (1952), 10–12; Christianson, "The Medical Practitioners of Massachusetts, 1630–1800, in *Medicine in Colonial Massachusetts, 1620–1820*, 57–58.

9. Wyndham B. Blanton, *Medicine in Virginia in the Eighteenth Century* (Richmond: Garrett and Massie, 1931), 76.

10. Josiah Bartlett, "A Dissertation on the Progress of Medical Science in the Commonwealth of Massachusetts," *Medical Communications*, III (1810), 240; Blanton, *Medicine in Virginia in the Eighteenth Century*, 76; Blake, "Early American Medical Literature," 147–60; George W. Corner, "Apprenticed to Aesculapius: The American Medical Student, 1765–1965," *Proceedings of the American Philosophical Society*, CIX (1965), 249–58; C. Helen Brock, "The Influence of Europe in Colonial Massachusetts Medicine," in *Medicine in Colonial Massachusetts, 1620–1820*, 106–8.

11. Shryock, *Medicine and Society in America*, 7, 9.

12. John Parascandola, "What Kind of Therapy Was Employed to Treat the Colonials?" *Pharmacy Times*, XLI (1975), 68–71.

13. Whitfield J. Bell, Jr., *The Colonial Physician and Other Essays* (New York: Science History Publications, 1975), 41–42; James Tait Goodrich, "The Colonial American Medical Student: 1750–1776," *Connecticut Medicine*, XL (1976), 829–44; Francis R. Packard, "How London and Edinburgh Influenced Medicine in Philadelphia in the Eighteenth Century," *Annals of Medical History*, n.s., IV (1932), 219–44; Michael Kraus, "American and European Medicine in the Eighteenth Century," *Bulletin of the History of Medicine*, VIII (1940), 679–95; J. Gordon Wilson, "The Influence

of Edinburgh on American Medicine in the Eighteenth Century," *Proceedings*, Institute of Medicine of Chicago, VII (1929), 129–38; Whitfield J. Bell, Jr., "Philadelphia Medical Students in Europe, 1750–1800," *Pennsylvania Magazine of History and Biography*, LXVII (1943), 1–29; R. W. Innes Smith, *English-Speaking Students of Medicine at the University of Leyden* (Edinburgh: Uhuer and Boyd, 1932); A. Chaplin, "A History of Medical Education in the Universities of Oxford and Cambridge, 1500–1850," *Proceedings of the Royal Society of Medicine*, XIII (1920), 83–107.

14. Blanton, *Medicine in Virginia in the Eighteenth Century*, 83–84; A. C. Chitnis, "Medical Education in Edinburgh, 1790–1826, and Some Victorian Social Consequences," *Medical History*, XVII (1973), 174–78; Alexander Bower, *History of the University of Edinburgh* (3 vols. Edinburgh: Oliphant, Waugh and Innes, 1817–30); John D. Comrie, *History of Scottish Medicine* (2 vols. London: Bailliere, Tindall, and Cox, 1932); Douglas Guthrie, "The Influence of the Leyden School upon Scottish Medicine," *Medical History*, III (1959), 108–22.

15. Blanton, *Medicine in Virginia in the Eighteenth Century*, 86; Whitfield J. Bell, Jr., "Medicine in Boston and Philadelphia: Comparisons and Contrasts, 1750–1820," in *Medicine in Colonial Massachusetts, 1620–1820*, 170–74.

16. Daniel J. Boorstin, *The Americans: The Colonial Experience* (New York: Vintage Books, 1964), 209.

17. Shryock, *Medicine and Society in America*, 84; Otto T. Beal, Jr., and Richard H. Shryock, *Cotton Mather: First Significant Figure in American Medicine* (Baltimore: Johns Hopkins University Press, 1954), 46; Nicholas Culpeper, *The English Physician—Enlarged; With Three Hundred Sixty and Nine Medicines Made of English Herbs* (London: A. and J. Churchill, 1703); Francis R. Packard, *History of Medicine in the United States* (2 vols. New York: Hafner Publishing Co., 1963), II, 1228; George E. Gifford, Jr., "Botanic Remedies in Colonial Massachusetts, 1620–1820," in *Medicine in Colonial Massachusetts, 1620–1820*, 268.

18. Judith M. Taylor, "Early Botanists and the Introduction of Drug Specifics," *Bulletin of the New York Academy of Medicine*, LX (1979), 685. See also Virgil J. Vogel, *American Indian Medicine* (Norman: University of Oklahoma Press, 1970).

19. Order from Charles II, quoted in Blanton, *Medicine in Virginia in the Seventeenth Century*, 105, 100–101, 105–13; Wade Boyle, *Herb Doctors: Pioneers in Nineteenth-Century American Botanical Medicine and a History of the Eclectic Medical Institute of Cincinnati* (East Palestine, Ohio: Buckeye Naturopathic Press, 1988), ii.

20. Taylor, "Early Botanists and the Introduction of Drug Specifics," 684–85.

21. Catherine Wisswaesser, "Roots and Ramifications of Medicinal Herbs in 18th-Century North America," *Transactions and Studies*, College of Physicians of Philadelphia, XLIV (1977), 196; George E. Gifford, Jr.,

"Medicine and Natural History—Crosscurrents in Philadelphia in the Nineteenth Century," *Transactions and Studies*, College of Physicians of Philadelphia, XLV (1978), 139–40; Whitfield J. Bell, Jr., "Benjamin Smith Barton, M.D. (Kiel)," *Journal of the History of Medicine*, XXVI (1971), 197–203.

22. Wisswaesser, "Roots and Ramifications of Medicinal Herbs," 196.

23. Lyman H. Butterfield (ed.), *Letters of Benjamin Rush* (2 vols. Princeton, N.J.: Princeton University Press, 1951), II, 185.

24. Benjamin Rush, "Observations on the Duties of a Physician, and the Methods of Improving Medicine. Accommodated to the Present State of Society and Manners in the United States," in Benjamin Rush, *Medical Inquiries and Observations* (4 vols. 2d ed. Philadelphia: J. Conrad and Co., 1789), I, 406–7.

25. Alexander Wilder, *History of Medicine: A Brief Outline of Medical History from the Earliest Historic Period with an Extended Account of the Various Sects of Physicians and New Schools of Medicines in Later Centuries* (Augusta, Maine: Maine Farmer Publishing Co., 1904), 420.

26. George B. Wood, "Introductory Lecture to the Course of Materia Medica in the University of Pennsylvania, Delivered Nov. 3, 1840," *American Journal of Pharmacy*, n.s., VI (1841), 298–322.

27. Shryock, *Medical Licensing in America*, 13–15.

28. Elan Daniel Louis, "William Shippen's Unsuccessful Attempt to Establish the First 'School for Physick' in the American Colonies in 1762," *Journal of the History of Medicine*, XLIV (1989), 218–39.

29. William S. Middleton, "John Morgan, Father of Medical Education in North America," *Annals of Medical History*, IX (1927), 13–26; T. C. Moore and J. A. Shield, "Medical Education at America's First University," *Journal of Medical Education*, XLIV (1969), 241–48; W. Moll, "History of American Medical Education," *British Journal of Medical Education*, II (1968), 173–81; William F. Norwood, "The Mainstream of Medical Education, 1765–1965," *Annals of the New York Academy of Sciences*, CXXVIII (1965), 463–66; Joseph Carson, *A History of the Medical Department of the University of Pennsylvania, from Its Foundation in 1765* (Philadelphia: Lindsay and Blakistan, 1869), 52–55.

30. Boorstin, *The Americans: The Colonial Experience*, 235. See also George W. Corner, *Two Centuries of Medicine: A History of the School of Medicine, University of Pennsylvania* (Philadelphia: J.B. Lippincott, 1965), 15–31.

31. Shryock, *Medicine and Society in America*, 28.

32. Shryock, *Medical Licensing in America*, 16–17, 26.

33. Shryock, *Medical Licensing in America*, 23–24.

34. William F. Norwood, *Medical Education in the United States Before the Civil War* (Philadelphia: University of Pennsylvania Press, 1944), 223–41.

35. Saul Jarcho, "The Legacy of British Medicine to American Medi-

cine, 1800–1850," *Proceedings of the Royal Society of Medicine*, LXVIII (1975), 25; Martin Kaufman, *American Medical Education: The Formative Years, 1765–1910* (Westport, Conn.: Greenwood Press, 1976), 36–56.

36. F. Campbell Stewart, "Report of the Committee on Medical Education in the United States," *Transactions*, American Medical Association, II (1849), 257–352.

37. Charles E. Rosenberg, "The Therapeutic Revolution: Medicine, Meaning, and Social Change in Nineteenth-Century America," in Morris J. Vogel and Charles E. Rosenberg (eds.), *The Therapeutic Revolution: Essays in the Social History of American Medicine* (Philadelphia: University of Pennsylvania Press, 1979), 6, 8; see also Owsei Temkin, *Galenism: Rise and Decline of a Medical Philosophy* (Ithaca, N.Y.: Cornell University Press, 1973), chapter 4.

38. Francis Bacon, *The Advancement of Learning and New Atlantis* (London: Oxford University Press, 1969), 2:10:3; 2:10:5; Jeffrey Boss, "The Medical Philosophy of Francis Bacon (1561–1626)," *Medical Hypotheses*, IV (1978), 208–20.

39. J. R. Ravetz, "Francis Bacon and the Reform of Philosophy," in Allen G. Debus, *Science, Medicine and Society in the Renaissance: Essays to Honor Walter Pagel* (New York: Science History Publications, 1972), 97–117; Rudolph E. Siegel, "Galen's Concept of Bloodletting in Relation to His Ideas on Pulmonary and Peripheral Blood Flow and Blood Formation," in Debus, *Science, Medicine and Society*, 243–75; Lester S. King, "Rationalism in Early-Eighteenth-Century Medicine," *Journal of the History of Medicine*, XVIII (1963), 257–71; Lester S. King, "Medical Theory and Practice at the Beginning of the Eighteenth Century," *Bulletin of the History of Medicine*, XLVI (1972), 1–15.

40. F. Kraupl Taylor, "Sydenham's Disease Entities," *Psychological Medicine*, XII (1982), 243, 244.

41. Knud Faber, "Nosology in Modern Internal Medicine," *Annals of Medical History*, IV (1922), 3; K. Dewhurst, "Thomas Sydenham, Reformer of Clinical Medicine," *Medical History*, VI (1962), 101–8; R. R. Trial, "Sydenham's Impact on English Medicine," *Medical History*, IX (1965), 356–64; Gert Wallach, "The Mind of the Colonial Physician," *Connecticut Medicine*, XL (1976), 815–27.

42. G. A. Lindeboom, "Boerhaave's Concept of the Basic Structure of the Body," *Clio Medica*, V (1970), 203–8; Saul Jarcho, "Boerhaave on Inflammation," *American Journal of Cardiology*, XXV (1970), 244–46, 480–82; G. A. Lindeboom, "Boerhaave's Impact on the Relation between Chemistry and Medicine," *Clio Medica*, VII (1972), 271–78.

43. King, *Medical World of the Eighteenth Century*, 62–63.

44. Blanton, *Medicine in Virginia in the Eighteenth Century*, 5.

45. J. C. Reeve, "Some of the Latest Systems of Medicine," *Transactions*, Ohio Medical Society (1885), 34.

46. Quoted in Whitfield J. Bell, Jr., "Some American Students of 'That

Shining Oracle of Physic,' Dr. William Cullen of Edinburgh, 1755–1766," *Proceedings of the American Philosophical Society*, XCIV (1950), 275–81.

47. King, *Medical World of the Eighteenth Century*, 140–42; Guenter B. Risse, "Doctor William Cullen, Physician, Edinburgh: A Consultation Practice in the Eighteenth Century," *Bulletin of the History of Medicine*, XLVIII (1974), 348–49; Lester S. King, "The Debt of Modern Medicine to the Eighteenth Century," *Journal of the American Medical Association*, CXC (1964), 829–32; Esther Fischer-Homberger, "Eighteenth-Century Nosology and Its Survivors," *Medical History*, XIV (1970), 397–402.

48. Guenter B. Risse, "The Brownian System of Medicine; Its Theoretical and Practical Implications," *Clio Medica*, V (1970), 45–51; Guenter B. Risse, "The Quest for Certainty in Medicine, John Brown's System of Medicine in France," *Bulletin of the History of Medicine*, XLV (1971), 1–12; William Cullen Brown, *The Works of Dr. John Brown* (3 vols. London: J. Johnson, 1804), I, 190–91; II, 29–30, 145, 256, 369–72; III, 292–95; W. R. Trotter, "John Brown, and the Nonspecific Component of Human Sickness," *Perspectives in Biology and Medicine*, XXI (1978), 258–64; Thomas J. Bole III, "John Brown, Hegel and Speculative Concepts of Medicine," *Reports on Biology and Medicine*, XXXII (1974), 287–97.

49. Richard H. Shryock, "The Medical Reputation of Benjamin Rush: Contrasts over Two Centuries," *Bulletin of the History of Medicine*, XLV (1971), 510–12.

50. King, *Medical World of the Eighteenth Century*, 147–50; Richard H. Shryock, "Benjamin Rush from the Perspective of the Twentieth Century," *Transactions and Studies*, College of Physicians of Philadelphia, XIV (1946), 113–20.

51. Rush, *Medical Inquiries and Observations*, 276.

52. William Cobbett, "Comments," *The Republican Rush-Light*, I (1800), 49.

53. [Anonymous], "Doctors in Trouble," *Eclectic Medical Journal*, I (1853), 132.

54. John H. Warner, *The Therapeutic Perspective: Medical Practice, Knowledge, and Identity in America, 1820–1880* (Cambridge: Harvard University Press, 1986), 76; J. Worth Estes, "Therapeutic Practice in Colonial New England," in *Medicine in Colonial Massachusetts, 1620–1820*, 289–383.

55. Thomas Jefferson to Dr. Caspar Wistar, Jr., June 21, 1807, in Paul L. Ford (ed.), *The Writings of Thomas Jefferson* (10 vols. New York: G.P. Putnam's Sons, 1892–99), IX, 81–85. See also K. R. Crispell, "Medical Education—Jefferson and Flexner Revisited," *Transactions*, American Climatological Association, LXXXVII (1976), 247; Boorstin, *The Americans: The Colonial Experience*, 209; Alexander Wilder, "Eclectic Medicine; Its History and Scientific Basis," *Transactions*, National Eclectic Medical Association, XXI (1894), 56; George Rosen, "Political Order and Human Health in Jeffersonian Thought," *Bulletin of the History of Medicine*, XXVI

(1952), 32–44. Jefferson's comments were frequently quoted by medical reformers; see [Anonymous], "Opinion of Thomas Jefferson, on the State of Medicine," *Western Medical Reformer*, I (1836), 55–56; Wooster Beach, *The American Practice Condensed; Or, The Family Physician: Being the Scientific System of Medicine; On Vegetable Principles, Designed for All Classes* (New York: James M'Alister, 1847), 171–72.

56. Wilder, "Eclectic Medicine; Its History and Scientific Basis," 57.

57. E. H. Ackerknecht, *Medicine at the Paris Hospital, 1794–1848* (Baltimore: Johns Hopkins University Press, 1967), 5–12, 101; George Rosen, "The Philosophy of Ideology and the Emergence of Modern Medicine in France," *Bulletin of the History of Medicine*, XX (1946), 328–39.

58. Pierre Louis, *Researches on the Effects of Bloodletting in Some Inflammatory Diseases* (Boston: Hilliard, Gray and Co., 1836); Marshall Hall, *Researches Principally Relative to the Morbid and Curative Effects of Loss of Blood* (Philadelphia: E. L. Carey and A. Hart, 1830); Leon S. Burns, "Blood-letting in American Medicine, 1830–1892," *Bulletin of the History of Medicine*, XXXVIII (1964), 516–29; Terence D. Murphy, "Medical Knowledge and Statistical Methods in Early-Nineteenth-Century France," *Medical History*, XXV (1981), 301–9.

59. Warner, *The Therapeutic Perspective*, 43–57; E. H. Ackerknecht, "Elisha Bartlett and the Philosophy of the Paris Clinical School," *Bulletin of the History of Medicine*, XXIV (1950), 43–60.

60. Elisha Bartlett, *An Essay on the Philosophy of Medical Science* (Philadelphia: Lea and Blanchard, 1844), 245.

61. Bartlett, *An Essay on the Philosophy of Medical Science*, 306. See also Marie-François-Xavier Bichat, *Anatomie générale, appliquée à la physiologie et à la médécine* (4 vols.; Paris: Brosson, Gabon, 1801). The first English-language edition was published in 1822.

62. Russell M. Jones, "American Doctors in Paris, 1820–1861: A Statistical Profile," *Journal of the History of Medicine*, XXV (1970), 143–57; John H. Warner, "Remembering Paris: Memory and the American Disciples of French Medicine in the Nineteenth Century," *Bulletin of the History of Medicine*, LXV (1991), 301–25.

63. Bartlett, *An Essay on the Philosophy of Medical Science*, 300–301.

64. Jacob Bigelow, "On Self-Limited Diseases," *Medical Communications*, Massachusetts Medical Society, V (1830–36), 319–58. In England, Sir John Forbes, in *Nature and Art in the Cure of Disease* (New York: S.S. and W. Wood, 1858), favored the use of milder measures.

65. Worthington Hooker, "Rational Therapeutics," *Publications*, Massachusetts Medical Society, I (1860), 161–62, 183; Worthington Hooker, *The Present Mental Attitude and Tendencies of the Medical Profession* (New Haven, Conn.: T.J. Stafford, 1852), 15; Richard H. Shryock, "The Advent of Modern Medicine in Philadelphia, 1800–1850," *Yale Journal of Biology and Medicine*, XIII (1941), 715–38.

2. Every Man His Own Physician

1. The title of this chapter comes from Samuel Thomson, *New Guide to Health; Or, Botanic Family Physician, Containing a Complete System of Practice upon a Plan Entirely New: With a Description of the Vegetables Made Use of, and Directions for Preparing and Administering Them to Cure Disease* (Boston: J. Howe, 1831), 10. Thomson may himself have taken the phrase from John Theobald, *Every Man His Own Physician* (Boston: Cox and Berry, 1767).

2. For the history of the concept of progress, see J. B. Bury, *The Idea of Progress; An Inquiry into Its Origin and Growth* (New York: Macmillan, 1932), 1–7; J. E. Boodin, "The Idea of Progress," *Journal of Social Philosophy*, IV (1939), 101–20; Wilson D. Wallis, *Culture and Progress* (New York: McGraw-Hill, 1930); Lewis Mumford, *Technics and Civilization* (New York: Harcourt, Brace and Co., 1934); Arthur A. Ekirch, Jr., *The Idea of Progress in America, 1815–1860* (New York: Columbia University Press, 1944).

3. Abraham Flexner, *Medical Education in the United States and Canada; A Report to the Carnegie Foundation on the Advancement of Teaching* (New York: Carnegie Foundation, 1910), 156.

4. Norman Gevitz, "Sectarian Medicine," *Journal of the American Medical Association*, CCLVII (1987), 1636.

5. Thomson, *New Guide to Health*, 4.

6. Philip D. Jordan, "The Secret Six: An Inquiry into the Basic Materia Medica of the Thomsonian System of Botanic Medicine," *Ohio Archaeological and Historical Quarterly*, LII (1943), 350; Jacob Bigelow, *A Treatise on the Materia Medica: Intended as a Sequel to the Pharmacopoeia of the United States* (Boston: C. Ewer, 1822), 248–49.

7. Morris Mattson, *The American Vegetable Practice; Or, A New and Improved Guide to Health Designed for the Use of Families* (3d ed. Boston: Published for the Author, 1855), 171.

8. Thomson, *New Guide to Health*, 9–10.

9. Thomson, *New Guide to Health*, 13.

10. Frederick C. Waite, "The First Sectarian Medical School in New England, at Worcester (1846–1859), and Its Relation to Thomsonianism," *New England Journal of Medicine*, CCVII (1932), 984; L. F. Kebler, "United States Patents Granted for Medicines During the Pioneer Years of the Patent Office," *Journal of the American Pharmaceutical Association*, XXIV (1935), 485–89; E. P. Ford, "Who Are Eclectics, and What Are Their Principles of Medicine?" *Eclectic Medical Journal*, LVI (1896), 114; James M. Ball, "Samuel Thomson (1769–1843) and his Patented 'System' of Medicine," *Annals of Medical History*, VII (1925), 144–48.

11. Thomson, *New Guide to Health*, 44.

12. Quoted in Thomson, *New Guide to Health*, 57.

13. Alex Berman, "The Thomsonian Movement and Its Relation to American Pharmacy and Medicine," *Bulletin of the History of Medicine*, XXV

(1951), 416; Alexander Wilder, *History of Medicine: A Brief Outline of Medical History and Sects of Physicians, from the Earliest Historic Period, with an Extended Account of the New Schools of the Healing Art in the Nineteenth Century, and Especially a History of the American Eclectic Practice of Medicine, Never Before Published* (New Sharon, Maine: New England Publishing Co., 1901), 463.

14. Ronald L. Numbers, "Do-It-Yourself the Sectarian Way," in Guenter B. Risse, Ronald L. Numbers, and Judith W. Leavitt (eds.), *Medicine Without Doctors; Home Health Care in American History* (New York: Science History Publications, 1977), 50; Daniel J. Wallace, "Thomsonians: The People's Doctors," *Clio Medica*, XIV (1980), 170; Madge E. Pickard and R. Carlyle Buley, *The Midwest Pioneer; His Ills, Cures, and Doctors* (New York: Henry Schuman, 1946), 173–74.

15. Thomson, *New Guide to Health*, 43.

16. Thomson, *New Guide to Health*, 10–11, 18.

17. Jordan, "The Secret Six," 351.

18. Wallace, "Thomsonians: The People's Doctors," 172; Lester S. King, "Medical Sects and Their Influence," *Journal of the American Medical Association*, CCXLVIII (1982), 1221; Guenter B. Risse, "Calomel and the American Medical Sects during the Nineteenth Century," *Mayo Clinic Proceedings*, XLVIII (1973), 57–64.

19. J. B. Spiers, "Calomel," *New England Botanic Medical and Surgical Journal*, III (1849), 272–73. See also John S. Haller, Jr., "Samson of the Materia Medica: Medical Theory and the Use and Abuse of Calomel in 19th-Century America," *Pharmacy in History*, XII (1971), 27–34; 67–76.

20. John S. Haller, Jr., "Therapeutic Mule: The Use of Arsenic in the 19th-Century Materia Medica," *Pharmacy in History*, XVII (1975), 87–100; John S. Haller, Jr., "The History of Tartar Emetic in the 19th-Century Materia Medica," *Bulletin of the History of Medicine*, XLIV (1975), 235–57.

21. John H. Warner, *The Therapeutic Perspective: Medical Practice, Knowledge, and Identity in America, 1820–1880* (Cambridge: Harvard University Press, 1986), 12.

22. Thomson, *New Guide to Health*, 25.

23. Thomson, *New Guide to Health*, 40–66; Wallace, "Thomsonians: The People's Doctors," 171–72; Jordan, "The Secret Six," 350; Frank G. Halstead, "A First-Hand Account of a Treatment by Thomsonian Medicine in the 1830s," *Bulletin of the History of Medicine*, X (1941), 681–85.

24. Thomson, *New Guide to Health*, 88; John Uri Lloyd, *Origin and History of All the Pharmacopoeial Vegetable Drugs, Chemicals and Preparations* (Cincinnati: Caxton Press, 1921), 48.

25. Thomson, *New Guide to Health*, 65–72.

26. Thomson, *New Guide to Health*, 38.

27. Thomson, *New Guide to Health*, 151–52.

28. Wilder, *History of Medicine . . . Never Before Published*, 452, 455, 462.

29. Samuel Thomson, *Learned Quackery Exposed: Or, Theory According to Art* (Boston: Adams, 1836), 17–19; John Thomson, *A Philosophical Theory of an "Empiric," Proved Practically: Compared with the Doubtful Science Known as Quackery and Practiced by the Regular Physicians during the Prevalence of Cholera in This City* (Albany, N.Y.: Published for the Author, 1833), 5; Charles E. Rosenberg, *The Cholera Years: The United States in 1832, 1849 and 1866* (Chicago: University of Chicago Press, 1962), 162; Wallace, "Thomsonians: The People's Doctors," 172.

30. Ralph Waldo Emerson, "Self-Reliance," October 9, 1832, in Brooks Atkinson (ed.), *The Complete Essays and Other Writings of Ralph Waldo Emerson* (New York: Modern Library, 1950), 815.

31. Wallace, "Thomsonians: The People's Doctors," 173.

32. Thomson, *New Guide to Health*, 7.

33. Numbers, "Do-It-Yourself the Sectarian Way," in Risse et al., *Medicine Without Doctors*, 57.

34. James O. Breeden, "Thomsonianism in Virginia," *Virginia Magazine of History and Biography*, LXXXII (1974), 150–80.

35. Daniel Drake, *The People's Doctors* (Cincinnati: n.p., 1830), 14.

36. King, "Medical Sects and Their Influence," 1222.

37. Berman, "The Thomsonian Movement and Its Relation to American Pharmacy and Medicine," 417, 420; Risse, "Calomel and the American Medical Sects," 60; Philip D. Jordan, "Botanic Medicine in the Western Country," *Ohio State Medical Journal*, XL (1944), 143–46, 240–42.

38. Wallace, "Thomsonians: The People's Doctors," 173.

39. Wallace, "Thomsonians: The People's Doctors," 173.

40. Numbers, "Do-It-Yourself the Sectarian Way," in Risse et al., *Medicine Without Doctors*, 50; Frederick C. Waite, "Thomsonianism in Ohio," *Ohio State Archaeological and Historical Quarterly*, XLIX (1940), 323.

41. Thomson, *New Guide to Health*, 48.

42. Thomson, *New Guide to Health*, 48–49; Numbers, "Do-It-Yourself the Sectarian Way," in Risse et al., *Medicine Without Doctors*, 50; Kebler, "United States Patents Granted for Medicines," 485–89.

43. J. Worth Estes, "The Shakers and Their Proprietary Medicines," *Bulletin of the History of Medicine*, LXV (1991), 164–65, 169.

44. Wallace, "Thomsonians: The People's Doctors," 177.

45. Alex Berman, "A Striving for Scientific Respectability: Some American Botanics and the Nineteenth-Century Plant Materia Medica," *Bulletin of the History of Medicine*, XXX (1956), 11–12; Thomson, *New Guide to Health*, 52. The famous Cholera Syrup, employed by both Thomsonians and eclectics, consisted of nervine, bayberry, goldenseal, and capsicum, which were pulverized and boiled together until their strength was exhausted in a quantity of water to make one gallon of decoction. Then the mixture was strained, and one gallon of brandy, loaf sugar, and tincture of myrrh were added. See [Anonymous], "Cholera Syrup," *New England Botanic Medical and Surgical Journal*, III (1849), 343.

46. Philip D. Jordan, "Samuel Robinson: Champion of the Thomson-

ian System," *Ohio State Archaeological and Historical Quarterly*, LI (1942), 263–70; Samuel Robinson, *A Course of Fifteen Lectures, on Medical Botany, Denominated Thomson's New Theory of Medical Practice; In Which the Various Theories That Have Preceded It Are Reviewed and Compared; Delivered in Cincinnati, Ohio* (Columbus, Ohio: Horton Howard, 1829).

47. Wallace, "Thomsonians: The People's Doctors," 177; Waite, "Thomsonianism in Ohio," 325–26.

48. [Editor], "Literary and Botanico-Medical College of Ohio," *Western Medical Reformer*, II (1837), 14; Wallace, "Thomsonians: The People's Doctors," 178; Wilder, *History of Medicine . . . Never Before Published*, 523; [Anonymous], "The Botanico-Medical College, Its History," *Botanico-Medical Recorder*, II (1844), 59–60; Francis R. Packard, *History of Medicine in the United States* (2 vols. New York: Hafner Publishing Co., 1963), II, 1238; Pickard and Buley, *The Midwest Pioneer; His Ills, Cures, and Doctors*, 186.

49. Wilder, *History of Medicine . . . Never Before Published*, 496; Berman, "A Striving for Scientific Respectability," 14, 16.

50. Harris L. Coulter, *Divided Legacy: A History of the Schism in Medical Thought*. Vol. III, *Science and Ethics in American Medicine: 1800–1914* (3 vols. Washington, D.C.: Wehawken Book Co., 1973), 94–95.

51. Quoted in H. E. Firth, "The Origin of the American Eclectic Practice of Medicine, and Its Early History in the State of New York," *Transactions*, Eclectic Medical Society of New York, X (1878), 176–77.

52. Drake, *The People's Doctors*, 29; Wilder, *History of Medicine . . . Never Before Published*, 470–72.

53. Quoted in Wilder, *History of Medicine . . . Never Before Published*, 477.

54. Wilder, *History of Medicine . . . Never Before Published*, 480; [Editor], "Speech of Mr. Haskell," *Western Medical Reformer*, I (1836), 44–48.

55. Wilder, *History of Medicine . . . Never Before Published*, 508–9; Firth, "The Origin of the American Eclectic Practice of Medicine," 179.

56. Quoted in Berman, "The Thomsonian Movement and Its Relation to American Pharmacy and Medicine," 426.

57. Wilder, *History of Medicine . . . Never Before Published*, 488–91. One popular treatment for cholera consisted of immersing the feet in hot water, applying mustard plasters to the abdomen, and taking copious drafts of stimulating drinks, including the Sudorific Tincture, or Cholera Syrup, prepared by the Thomsonian Laboratories. If this was not at hand, a strong decoction of ginger or cayenne pepper and even a hot-brandy punch was highly recommended. This method compared favorably with the allopathic choice of large doses of calomel. See [Anonymous], "Treatment of Cholera," *New England Botanic Medical and Surgical Journal*, III (1849), 259.

58. Pickard and Buley, *The Midwest Pioneer; His Ills, Cures, and Doctors*, 182.

59. Wilder, *History of Medicine . . . Never Before Published*, 491.

60. Wilder, *History of Medicine . . . Never Before Published*, 492–94.

61. Wallace, "Thomsonians: The People's Doctors," 178; Frederick C. Waite, "American Sectarian Medical Colleges before the Civil War," *Bulletin of the History of Medicine*, XIX (1946), 153.

62. Alex Berman, "Neo-Thomsonianism in the United States," *Journal of the History of Medicine*, XI (1956), 133.

63. Wallace, "Thomsonians: The People's Doctors," 176.

64. Wallace, "Thomsonians: The People's Doctors," 179.

65. Berman, "A Striving for Scientific Respectability," 8.

66. Berman, "Neo-Thomsonianism in the United States," 133; Worthington Hooker, *Dissertation on the Respect Due to the Medical Profession, and the Reasons Why It Is Not Awarded by the Community* (Norwich: J.G. Cooley, 1844), 15.

67. Wilder, *History of Medicine . . . Never Before Published*, 498.

68. L. Reuben, "Our Wants," *New England Botanic Medical and Surgical Journal*, III (1849), 160.

69. [Editor], "Miscellaneous," *Western Medical Reformer*, II (1837), 334.

70. Berman, "Neo-Thomsonianism in the United States," 138.

71. Berman, "Neo-Thomsonianism in the United States," 135–38.

72. Firth, "The Origin of the American Eclectic Practice of Medicine," 194–95.

73. Firth, "The Origin of the American Eclectic Practice of Medicine," 199.

74. Berman, "Neo-Thomsonianism in the United States," 139.

75. Joseph Kett, *The Formation of the American Medical Profession: The Role of Institutions, 1780–1860* (New Haven, Conn.: Yale University Press, 1968), 131, 178.

76. Wallace, "Thomsonians: The People's Doctors," 176.

77. William G. Rothstein, "The Botanical Movements and Orthodox Medicine," in Norman Gevitz (ed.), *Other Healers: Unorthodox Medicine in America* (Baltimore: Johns Hopkins University Press, 1988), 46.

78. Alexander Wilder, "Some of the Reformers," *Eclectic Medical Journal*, LXIV (1904), 132.

3. Reformed Medicine, 1825–1856

1. Alexander Wilder, "Eclectic Medicine; Its History and Scientific Basis," *Transactions*, National Eclectic Medical Association, XXI (1894), 58; Alexander Wilder, *History of Medicine: A Brief Outline of Medical History and Sects of Physicians, from the Earliest Historic Period, with an Extended Account of the New Schools of the Healing Art in the Nineteenth Century, and Especially a History of the American Eclectic Practice of Medicine, Never Before Published* (New Sharon, Maine: New England Eclectic Publishing Co., 1901), 422; Frederick C. Waite, "The First Sectarian Medical School in New England, at Worcester (1846–1859), and Its Relation to Thomsonian-

ism," *New England Journal of Medicine,* CCVII (1932), 985. The term *macrotys* was made popular by Rafinesque and adopted by the eclectic school as the proper name for the plant known to botanists as *Cimicifuga racemosa.* See [Editor], "Established Drug Names," *Eclectic Medical Journal,* LXXXIV (1924), 559–60.

2. Alexander Wilder, *History of Medicine: A Brief Outline of Medical History from the Earliest Historic Period with an Extended Account of the Various Sects of Physicians and New Schools of Medicines in Later Centuries* (Augusta, Maine: Maine Farmer Publishing Co., 1904), 424–25.

3. Francis R. Packard, *History of Medicine in the United States* (2 vols. New York: Hafner Publishing Co., 1963), II, 1229.

4. Wilder, *History of Medicine . . . with an Extended Account of the Various Sects,* 427–28.

5. Wilder, "Eclectic Medicine; Its History and Scientific Basis," 59.

6. Quoted in Wilder, "Eclectic Medicine; Its History and Scientific Basis," 59.

7. Quoted in Wilder, "Eclectic Medicine; Its History and Scientific Basis," 59.

8. Wilder, *History of Medicine . . . with an Extended Account of the Various Sects,* 429, 432; A. H. Barkley, "Constantine Samuel Rafinesque," *Annals of Medical History,* X (1928), 67.

9. Benjamin Smith Barton, *Collections for an Essay Towards a Materia Medica of the United States* (Philadelphia: Way and Groff, 1804), 21–32.

10. Harris L. Coulter, *Divided Legacy: A History of the Schism in Medical Thought.* Vol. III, *Science and Ethics in American Medicine: 1800–1914* (3 vols. Washington, D.C.: Wehawken Book Co., 1973), 88; Morris Fishbein, *The Medical Follies; An Analysis of the Foibles of Some Healing Cults, Including Osteopathy, Homeopathy, Chiropractic, and the Electronic Reactions of Abrams, with Essays on the Anti-Vivisectionists, Health Legislation, Physical Culture, Birth Control, and Rejuvenation* (New York: Boni and Liveright, 1925), 143; Harvey W. Felter, "A Little-Known Pioneer in American Medicine," *Eclectic Medical Journal,* LXXXIV (1924), 576–84.

11. [Anonymous], "Reports on Status of Eclectic Medicine," *Transactions,* National Eclectic Medical Association, V (1877), 291.

12. Wooster Beach, *The American Practice Condensed; Or, The Family Physician: Being the Scientific System of Medicine; On Vegetable Principles, Designed for All Classes* (New York: James M'Alister, 1847), viii.

13. Wooster Beach, *Rise, Progress, and Present State of the New-York Medical Institution, and Reformed Medical Society of the United States* (New York: Mitchell and Davis, 1830), 1–11; Harvey W. Felter, *History of the Eclectic Medical Institute, Cincinnati, Ohio, 1845–1902* (Cincinnati: Alumni Association, 1902), 5–6; Frederick C. Waite, "American Sectarian Medical Colleges before the Civil War," *Bulletin of the History of Medicine,* XIX (1946), 151.

14. Quoted in H. E. Firth, "The Origin of the American Eclectic

Practice of Medicine, and Its Early History in the State of New York," *Transactions*, Eclectic Medical Society of New York, X (1878), 173; Wilder, "Eclectic Medicine; Its History and Scientific Basis," 72; Wilder, *History of Medicine . . . with an Extended Account of the Various Sects*, 436; Norman Howard-Jones, "Cholera Therapy in the Nineteenth Century," *Journal of the History of Medicine*, XXVII (1972), 373–95; Joseph Kett, *The Formation of the American Medical Profession: The Role of Institutions, 1780–1860* (New Haven, Conn.: Yale University Press, 1968), 40–41.

15. Felter, *History of the Eclectic Medical Institute*, 7.

16. Quoted in Firth, "The Origin of the American Eclectic Practice of Medicine," 171; George Washington Lafayette Bickley, "History of the Eclectic Medical Institute of Cincinnati and Its Ethical Peculiarities," *Eclectic Medical Journal*, I (1857), 59–60.

17. Frank Stewart, "Reform and Reformers," *Eclectic Medical Journal*, I (1853), 154.

18. G. Price Smith, "A Few Chapters on Medical Reform," *Eclectic Medical Journal*, I (1855), 541.

19. Smith, "A Few Chapters on Medical Reform," 542.

20. Firth, "The Origin of the American Eclectic Practice of Medicine," 174; Wilder, *History of Medicine . . . Never Before Published*, 437; [Anonymous], "Beach's Practice," *Western Medical Reformer*, I (1836), 41–43; Beach, *The American Practice Condensed*, xxiii-xxxi.

21. Beach, *The American Practice Condensed*, 108.

22. Beach, *The American Practice Condensed*, 152.

23. Beach, *The American Practice Condensed*, 797–800.

24. Beach, *The American Practice Condensed*, 76.

25. Alex Berman, "A Striving for Scientific Respectability: Some American Botanics and the Nineteenth-Century Plant Materia Medica," *Bulletin of the History of Medicine*, XXX (1956), 13.

26. Quoted in [Editor], "Comments," *Boston Medical and Surgical Journal*, XXVIII (1843), 304; Berman, "A Striving for Scientific Respectability," 13.

27. Quoted in Beach, *Rise, Progress, and Present State of the New-York Medical Institution*, 26–27; Harvey W. Felter, "Worthington College, Ohio; Reformed Medical Department," *Eclectic Medical Journal*, LXIV (1904), 10.

28. Felter, *History of the Eclectic Medical Institute*, 9; Jonathan Forman, "The Worthington Medical College," *Ohio State Archaeological and Historical Quarterly*, L (1941), 375–76.

29. Forman, "The Worthington Medical College," 377; Felter, "Worthington College, Ohio; Reformed Medical Department," 12–13; Wilder, *History of Medicine . . . with an Extended Account of the Various Sects*, 484; Waite, "American Sectarian Medical Colleges before the Civil War," 151; Felter, *History of the Eclectic Medical Institute*, 13, 86.

30. Jonathan R. Paddock, "Remarks on the Nature of Mercurial Com-

binations and Their Effects on the Human System," *Western Medical Reformer*, I (1836), 17–21; Richard Jebb, "Rules for the Preservation of Health and Longevity," *Western Medical Reformer*, I (1836), 25–26; Jonathan R. Paddock, "On the Pernicious Effects of Bloodletting," *Western Medical Reformer*, I (1836), 27–29.

31. See Charles Caldwell, *Thoughts on Schools of Medicine, Their Means of Instruction and Modes of Administration* (Louisville, Ky.: Prentice and Wassinger, 1837).

32. Paddock, "On the Pernicious Effects of Bloodletting," 35.

33. Felter, *History of the Eclectic Medical Institute*, 12–13; Jonathan Forman, "The Worthington School and Thomsonianism," *Bulletin of the History of Medicine*, XXI (1947), 772–87. The cost for boarding at the infirmary, including lodging, washing, lights, and fuel, was two dollars per week. An additional charge was assessed for medical service, medicine, and extra nursing. See [Editor], "Worthington Infirmary," *Western Medical Reformer*, II (1837), 302.

34. [Editor], "The Reformer," *Western Medical Reformer*, I (1836), 5.

35. [Editor], "Worthington College," *Western Medical Reformer*, III (1838), 144.

36. [Editor], "Thomsonism—The Term Reform, etc.," *Western Medical Reformer*, II (1837), 43.

37. Alex Berman, "The Thomsonian Movement and Its Relation to American Pharmacy and Medicine," *Bulletin of the History of Medicine*, XXV (1951), 427; [Editor], "Literary and Botanical-Medical College of Ohio, *Western Medical Reformer*, III (1838), 14–15.

38. Quoted in Wilder, *History of Medicine . . . Never Before Published*, 562; [Editor], "Physio-Medical Thunder," *Eclectic Medical Journal*, I (1853), 401.

39. Felter, "Worthington College, Ohio; Reformed Medical Department," 14; Wilder, *History of Medicine . . . with an Extended Account of the Various Sects*, 516; [Editor], "The Reformer," 5.

40. Alexander Wilder, "Eclectic Medicine in the Eastern States," *Transactions*, National Eclectic Medical Association, XX (1892–93), 478; John Uri Lloyd, "A Review of the Principle Events in American Medicine," *Eclectic Medical Journal*, LXXXVI (1926), 262–69.

41. Samuel Thomson, *New Guide to Health; Or, Botanic Family Physician, Containing a Complete System of Practice, upon a Plan Entirely New: With a Description of the Vegetables Made Use of, and Directions for Preparing and Administering Them to Cure Disease* (Boston: J. Howe, 1831), 53.

42. Felter, *History of the Eclectic Medical Institute*, 15; Felter, "Worthington College, Ohio; Reformed Medical Department," 17.

43. [Editor], "To Our Patrons," *Western Medical Reformer*, III (1838), 190.

44. Felter, "Worthington College, Ohio; Reformed Medical Department," 18; Felter, *History of the Eclectic Medical Institute*, 16.

45. Linden F. Edwards, "Resurrection Riots during the Heroic Age of Anatomy in America," *Bulletin of the History of Medicine*, XXV (1951), 178.

46. James Tait Goodrich, "The Colonial American Medical Student: 1750–1776," *Connecticut Medicine*, XL (1976), 841; Julia B. Frank, "Body Snatching: A Grave Medical Problem," *Yale Journal of Biology and Medicine*, XLIX (1976), 399–410; James O. Breeden, "Body Snatchers and Anatomy Professors; Medical Education in Nineteenth-Century Virginia," *Virginia Magazine of History and Biography*, LXXXIII (1975), 321–45.

47. Edwards, "Resurrection Riots during the Heroic Age of Anatomy in America," 180–83; Whitfield J. Bell, Jr., "Body-Snatching in Philadelphia," *Journal of the History of Medicine*, XXIII (1968), 108–10; Whitfield J. Bell, Jr., "Doctors' Riot, New York, 1788," *Bulletin of the New York Academy of Medicine*, XLVII (1971), 1501–3.

48. Felter, "Worthington College, Ohio; Reformed Medical Department," 20; Felter, *History of the Eclectic Medical Institute*, 16–17.

49. Bickley, "History of the Eclectic Medical Institute of Cincinnati and Its Ethical Peculiarities," 61.

50. [Editor], "Free Medical Schools," *Eclectic Medical Journal*, I (1853), 204.

51. [Editor], "Editorial," *Journal of Eclectic Medicine*, I (1854), 44–45.

52. [Anonymous], "Results of the Eclectic and Old School Practice Compared," *New England Botanic Medical and Surgical Journal*, III (1849), 247.

53. Alexander Wilder, "Eclecticism in Medicine Defined by Eclectic Writers," *Transactions*, National Eclectic Medical Association, XXVIII (1901), 98.

54. Quoted in Wilder, "Eclecticism in Medicine Defined by Eclectic Writers," 98; Wilder, *History of Medicine . . . Never Before Published*, 433, 573.

55. Vincent Millasich, "Eclecticism and Its Origin," *California Eclectic Medical Journal*, XXXIV (1913), 299–300; Wilder, *History of Medicine . . . Never Before Published*, 89–92.

56. Fishbein, *The Medical Follies*, 139; Wilder, *History of Medicine . . . Never Before Published*, 212.

57. E. H. Ackerknecht, *Medicine at the Paris Hospital, 1794–1848* (Baltimore: Johns Hopkins University Press, 1967), 5–12, 101; George Rosen, "The Philosophy of Ideology and the Emergence of Modern Medicine in France," *Bulletin of the History of Medicine*, XX (1946), 328–39; Philippe Pinel, *Nosographie philosophique* (2 vols. Paris: Brosson, 1818).

58. Wilder, *History of Medicine . . . Never Before Published*, 212.

59. Jules Simon, *Victor Cousin* (Chicago: A.C. McClurg and Co., 1888), 82–83.

60. Quoted in Wilder, "Eclecticism in Medicine Defined by Eclectic Writers," 99.

61. Bickley, "History of the Eclectic Medical Institute of Cincinnati and Its Ethical Peculiarities," 9.

62. Felter, *History of the Eclectic Medical Institute*, 5.

63. [Anonymous], "Eclectic Medical Institute—Its Early History and Doctrines," *Eclectic Medical Journal*, II (1856), 191.

64. [Anonymous], "Eclecticism," *Eclectic Medical Journal*, II (1856), 226.

65. Wilder, "Eclectic Medicine; Its History and Scientific Basis," 56–57.

66. Wilder, "Eclectic Medicine; Its History and Scientific Basis," 57; Wilder, *History of Medicine . . . with an Extended Account of the Various Sects*, viii–ix.

67. S. A. Merrill, "Eclecticism," *Eclectic Medical Journal*, II (1856), 109.

68. Wilder, *History of Medicine . . . with an Extended Account of the Various Sects*, 402.

69. Quoted in [Editor], "The World's Medical Congress of Eclectic Physicians and Surgeons," *Transactions*, National Eclectic Medical Association, XXI (1894), 54.

70. Firth, "The Origin of the American Eclectic Practice of Medicine," 214.

71. Firth, "The Origin of the American Eclectic Practice of Medicine," 215.

72. G. W. Churchill, "Address Delivered before the Bay State Medical Reform Association," *New England Botanic Medical and Surgical Journal*, III (1849), 48–49.

73. William Paine, *An Epitome of the American Eclectic Practice of Medicine* (Philadelphia: J. Gladding, 1859), 38–39.

74. Paine, *Epitome of the American Eclectic Practice*, 39–40.

75. Paine, *Epitome of the American Eclectic Practice*, 40.

76. Merrill, "Eclecticism," 109–10.

77. [Anonymous], "What Is the American Eclectic System of Medicine?" *Eclectic Medical Journal*, I (1854), 360.

78. P. John, "Randomings, No. 1," *Eclectic Medical Journal*, I (1853), 14.

4. Buchanan's Feuds and Fads

1. Quoted in [Anonymous], "Periscope: Biographical Sketches," *Eclectic Medical Journal*, XC (1930), 184.

2. Joseph R. Buchanan, *Outlines of Lectures on the Neurological System of Anthropology* (Cincinnati: Buchanan's *Journal of Man*, 1854), 1, 17.

3. [Anonymous], "Periscope: Joseph Rodes Buchanan, M.D.," *Eclectic Medical Journal*, XC (1930), 524; Joseph R. Buchanan, "The First Number," *Journal of Man*, I (1849), 3–4.

4. [Anonymous], "Periscope: Joseph Rodes Buchanan, M.D.," 549.

5. [Editor], "Pierpont's Poem—Psychometry," *Journal of Man*, II (1850), 121.

6. Joseph R. Buchanan, "Address to the Eclectic Physicians of the State of Ohio, by the Committee of Eclectic State Associations," *Eclectic Medical Journal*, I (1853), 53–54.

7. Buchanan, "Address to the Eclectic Physicians of the State of Ohio," 55, 57; James H. Cassedy, *American Medical and Statistical Thinking, 1800–1860* (Cambridge: Harvard University Press, 1984), 137.

8. Joseph R. Buchanan, "Introductory Lecture," *Eclectic Medical Journal*, II (1854), 527.

9. Buchanan, "Introductory Lecture" (1854), 534.

10. Joseph R. Buchanan, "Introductory Lecture," *Eclectic Medical Journal*, I (1853), 1.

11. Buchanan, "Introductory Lecture" (1853), 2–3. The American Medical Association was established in 1847.

12. Buchanan, "Introductory Lecture" (1853), 4–5.

13. [Anonymous], "New Year's Night in the Eclectic," *Western Medical Reformer*, VII (1847), 167–68.

14. George Washington Lafayette Bickley, "History of the Eclectic Medical Institute of Cincinnati and Its Ethical Peculiarities," *Eclectic Medical Journal*, I (1857), 105–7; Harvey W. Felter, *History of the Eclectic Medical Institute, Cincinnati, Ohio, 1845–1902* (Cincinnati: Alumni Association, 1902), 28.

15. Joseph R. Buchanan, "Prosperity and Progress of the Institute," *Eclectic Medical Journal*, I (1853), 82; Alexander Wilder, *History of Medicine: A Brief Outline of Medical History and Sects of Physicians, from the Earliest Historic Period, with an Extended Account of the New Schools of the Healing Art in the Nineteenth Century, and Especially a History of the American Eclectic Practice of Medicine, Never Before Published* (New Sharon, Maine: New England Eclectic Publishing Co., 1901), 601.

16. Quoted in [Anonymous], "Eclecticism and Homeopathy," *American Eclectic Medical Review*, IV (1869), 526.

17. Felter, *History of the Eclectic Medical Institute*, 28–30.

18. [Anonymous], "W. Byrd Powell, M.D.," *American Eclectic Medical Review*, III (1867), 94–96; Bickley, "History of the Eclectic Medical Institute of Cincinnati and Its Ethical Peculiarities," 110; Wilder, *History of Medicine . . . Never Before Published*, 600–601.

19. Harvey W. Felter, "The Eclectic Medical Institute, of Cincinnati, Ohio," *Eclectic Medical Journal*, LXII (1902), 360.

20. Joseph R. Buchanan, *Free Collegiate Education* (Cincinnati: W.M. Naudain, 1852), 7.

21. Buchanan, "Introductory Lecture" (1853), 4–5; Joseph R. Buchanan, "Medical Colleges—The Medical Profession and the People," *Eclectic Medical Journal*, I (1854), 287.

22. Buchanan, *Free Collegiate Education*, 8–11.

23. Buchanan, "Introductory Lecture" (1853), 7.

24. Buchanan, *Free Collegiate Education*, 16; Felter, *History of the Eclectic Medical Institute*, 27.

25. George Washington Lafayette Bickley, "Medical Teaching," *Eclectic Medical Journal*, I (1857), 19; Wilder, *History of Medicine . . . Never Before Published*, 604.

26. Bickley, "History of the Eclectic Medical Institute of Cincinnati and Its Ethical Peculiarities," 110.

27. [Editor], "Free Medical Schools," *Worcester Journal of Medicine*, VIII (1853), 69.

28. Bickley, "Medical Teaching," 17.

29. Felter, *History of the Eclectic Medical Institute*, 38.

30. Buchanan, "Prosperity and Progress of the Institute," 82.

31. Quoted in Felter, *History of the Eclectic Medical Institute*, 34.

32. [Editor], "Note—The Spring Session," *Eclectic Medical Journal*, I (1853), 90.

33. George Washington Lafayette Bickley, "Review of Report of Eclectic Physicians," *Eclectic Medical Journal*, I (1853), 12.

34. Bickley, "History of the Eclectic Medical Institute of Cincinnati and Its Ethical Peculiarities," 111; Felter, *History of the Eclectic Medical Institute*, 35.

35. Felter, *History of the Eclectic Medical Institute*, 36.

36. [Editor], "Present State of Medical Science," *Journal of Man*, I (1849), 446.

37. G. N. Cantor, "The Edinburgh Phrenology Debate: 1803–1828," *Annals of Science*, XXXII (1975), 197.

38. Buchanan, *Outlines of Lectures on the Neurological System of Anthropology*, 1.

39. David de Guistino, *Conquest of Mind: Phrenology and Victorian Social Thought* (London: Croom Helm, 1975), 74.

40. Cantor, "The Edinburgh Phrenology Debate: 1803–1828," 202.

41. Steven Shapin, "Phrenological Knowledge and the Social Structure of Early-Nineteenth-Century Edinburgh," *Annals of Science*, XXXII (1975), 231–32.

42. David Bakan, "The Influence of Phrenology on American Psychology," *Journal of the History of the Behavioral Sciences*, II (1966), 200–203; Anthony A. Walsh, "The American Tour of Dr. Spurzheim," *Journal of the History of Medicine*, XXVII (1972), 187–205; Anthony A. Walsh, "Phrenology and the Boston Medical Community in the 1830s," *Bulletin of the History of Medicine*, L (1976), 261–73.

43. William H. Cook, "Connection between Phrenology and Physic," *American Medical and Surgical Journal*, I (1851), 13, 16.

44. Michael H. Stone, "Mesmer and His Followers: The Beginnings of Sympathetic Treatment of Childhood Emotional Disorders," *History of Childhood Quarterly*, I (1974), 663.

45. Ilza Veith, "From Mesmerism to Hypnotism," *Modern Medicine* (1959), 195–203; Fred Kaplan, "The Mesmeric Mania: The Early Victorians and Animal Magnetism," *Journal of the History of Ideas*, XXXV (1974), 697; C. D. T. James, "Mesmerism: A Prelude to Anaesthesia," *Proceedings of the Royal Society of Medicine*, LXVIII (1975), 446; John Elliotson, *Human Physiology* (5th ed. London: Longman, Orme, Brown, Green and Longmans, 1840), 680–81.

46. Kaplan, "The Mesmeric Mania," 697.

47. Joseph R. Buchanan, *Therapeutic Sarcognomy. The Application of Sarcognomy, the Science of the Soul, Brain and Body, to the Therapeutic Philosophy and Treatment of Bodily and Mental Diseases by Means of Electricity, Nervaura, Medicine and Haemospasia, with a Review of Authors on Animal Magnetism and Massage, and Presentation of New Instruments for Electro-Therapeutics* (Boston: J.G. Cupples Co., 1891), 84, 87; Buchanan, "The First Number," 3–4.

48. Buchanan, *Therapeutic Sarcognomy*, 307.

49. Buchanan, *Therapeutic Sarcognomy*, 66–72.

50. Buchanan, *Therapeutic Sarcognomy*, 55, 19.

51. Buchanan, *Therapeutic Sarcognomy*, 54.

52. Joseph R. Buchanan, "Notices," *Journal of Man*, II (1850), 620.

53. Quoted in Alexander Wilder, *History of Medicine: A Brief Outline of Medical History from the Earliest Historic Period with an Extended Account of the Various Sects of Physicians and New Schools of Medicines in Later Centuries* (Augusta, Maine: Maine Farmer Publishing Co., 1904), 387–89.

54. Wilder, *History of Medicine . . . with an Extended Account of the Various Sects*, 306.

55. Wilder, *History of Medicine . . . with an Extended Account of the Various Sects*, 308.

56. Buchanan, *Therapeutic Sarcognomy*, 74.

57. Buchanan, *Therapeutic Sarcognomy*, 133–34.

58. Isaac Miller Comings, "Alchemist Cure—Singular Facts," *Eclectic Medical Journal*, I (1853), 36.

59. William Byrd Powell and Robert S. Newton, *The Eclectic Practice of Medicine: Diseases of Children* (Cincinnati: Rickey, Mallory and Co., 1858), chapters 1–7.

60. John H. Warner, "Physiology," in Ronald L. Numbers (ed.), *The Education of American Physicians: Historical Essays* (Berkeley: University of California Press, 1980), 54–55.

61. Joseph R. Buchanan, *Manual of Psychometry: The Dawn of a New Civilization* (Boston: Holman Brothers, 1885), 3, 4, 8–10.

62. Joseph R. Buchanan, "Psychometry," *Journal of Man*, I (1849), 53–54.

63. Buchanan, *Manual of Psychometry*, 21.

64. Buchanan, *Manual of Psychometry*, 21–23. An interesting view of eclecticism's early fascination with mesmerism and phrenology is found in John King, "Dr. John King's Mesmeric Neurology, 1842," unpublished manuscript, Lloyd Library and Museum, Cincinnati.

65. Buchanan, *Manual of Psychometry*, 48–49.

66. Joseph R. Buchanan, "Science and Her Votaries," *Journal of Man*, III (1851), 365.

67. Buchanan, *Manual of Psychometry*, 43–44; Wilder, *History of Medicine . . . with an Extended Account of the Various Sects*, 386.

68. Buchanan, *Therapeutic Sarcognomy*, 7–8.

69. Buchanan, *Therapeutic Sarcognomy*, 2.

70. Quoted in Wilder, *History of Medicine . . . Never Before Published*, 385. See also S. E. D. Short, "Physicians and Psychics: The Anglo-American Medical Response to Spiritualism, 1870–1890," *Journal of the History of Medicine*, XXXIX (1984), 339–55.

71. Wilder, *History of Medicine . . . Never Before Published*, 624; Wade Boyle, *Herb Doctors: Pioneers in Nineteenth-Century American Botanical Medicine and a History of the Eclectic Medical Institute of Cincinnati* (East Palestine, Ohio: Buckeye Naturopathic Press, 1988), 55–56.

72. [Editor], "Ex-Professor Buchanan an Enemy to Eclecticism," *Eclectic Medical Journal*, II (1856), 281.

73. Minutes of Board of Trustees, April 5, 1856, in Records, Eclectic Medical Institute, Lloyd Library and Museum, Cincinnati; [Editor], "Facts in Regard to the College Difficulty," *Eclectic Medical Journal*, II (1856), 279.

74. [Editor], "Facts in Regard to the College Difficulty," 280.

75. [Anonymous], "Eclectic Medical Institute," *Eclectic Medical Journal*, II (1856), 229–30.

76. Records of Stockholders, Trustees, and Faculty of the Eclectic Medical Institute, p. 8, Lloyd Library and Museum, Cincinnati; [Anonymous], "Eclectic Medical Institute," 231; [Editor], "Facts in Regard to the College Difficulty," 280.

77. [Editor], "Ex-Professor Buchanan an Enemy to Eclecticism," 281; [Editor], "Then and Now—Dr. Joseph R. Buchanan vs. Himself," *Eclectic Medical Journal*, II (1856), 287.

78. [Anonymous], "Eclectic Medical Institute," *Eclectic Medical Journal*, II (1856), 510–12.

79. Felter, *History of the Eclectic Medical Institute*, 45–46; Felter, "The Eclectic Medical Institute of Cincinnati, Ohio," 360.

80. Lorenzo E. Jones, "Ex-Professor J. R. Buchanan, and His Intrigues Against Professors Morrow and Beach," *Eclectic Medical Journal*, II (1856), 283–84.

81. [Editor], "The College Difficulty," *Eclectic Medical Journal*, II (1856), 228–29.

82. Buchanan, *Therapeutic Sarcognomy*, 10.

83. Joseph R. Buchanan, *A Comprehensive View of Restrictive Medical Legislation: An Address* (Boston: Massachusetts Medical Liberty League, 1888), 24; Joseph R. Buchanan, *Defense of the People Against Medical Monopoly* (Boston: National Constitutional Liberty League, 1889), 6; Joseph R. Buchanan, *Legalized Murder: The Treatment of Cancer by the Regular Profession*

Compared with Its Treatment by Irregular Physicians (Boston: National Constitutional Liberty League, 1889), 6–7; John S. Haller, Jr., "Trends in American Gynecology, 1800–1910: A Short History," *New York State Journal of Medicine*, LXXXIX (1989), 278–82.

84. Joseph R. Buchanan, *Primitive Christianity* (2 vols. San Jose, Calif.: J.R. Buchanan, 1897–98), I, 5.

85. Buchanan, *Primitive Christianity*, II, 333–36.

86. Gail T. Parker, *Mind Cure in New England: From the Civil War to World War I* (Hanover, N.H.: University Press of New England, 1973), 41–56.

87. Undated letter from Joseph R. Buchanan to John Uri Lloyd, Box 6, Folder 80, John Uri Lloyd Papers, 1849–1936, Lloyd Library and Museum, Cincinnati.

5. Consolidation, 1856–1875

1. Harvey W. Felter, *History of the Eclectic Medical Institute, Cincinnati, Ohio, 1845–1902* (Cincinnati: Alumni Association, 1902), 48–49.

2. Harvey W. Felter, *Biographies of John King, M.D., Andrew Jackson Howe, A.B., M.D., and John Milton Scudder, M.D., Accompanied by Many Valuable and Historical Portraits and Other Illustrations* (Cincinnati: J.U. and C.G. Lloyd, 1912), 238–39.

3. Madge E. Pickard and R. Carlyle Buley, *The Midwest Pioneer; His Ills, Cures, and Doctors* (New York: Henry Schuman, 1946), 196.

4. Ichabod Gibson Jones and Thomas Vaughan Morrow, *The American Eclectic Practice of Medicine* (2 vols. Cincinnati: Moore, Anderson, Wilstach and Keys, 1854), I, 13.

5. William Byrd Powell and Robert S. Newton, *The Eclectic Practice of Medicine: Diseases of Children* (Cincinnati: Rickey, Mallory and Co., 1858), v–vii, 37.

6. Felter, *Biographies*, 3–5, 10.

7. Felter, *History of the Eclectic Medical Institute*, 57.

8. [Anonymous], "Eclectic Colleges," *Eclectic Medical Journal*, I (1853), 45.

9. H. E. Firth, "The Origin of the American Eclectic Practice of Medicine, and Its Early History in the State of New York," *Transactions*, Eclectic Medical Society of New York, X (1878), 199.

10. Firth, "The Origin of the American Eclectic Practice of Medicine," 200–201, 212.

11. William W. Hadley, "Eclectic Medical Institute, Rochester, New York," *New England Botanic Medical and Surgical Journal*, III (1849), 230, 232.

12. Alexander Wilder, "Outline History of Eclectic Medicine," *Transactions*, National Eclectic Medical Association, V (1877), 45, 47; Frederick C. Waite, "American Sectarian Medical Colleges before the Civil War," *Bulletin of the History of Medicine*, XIX (1946), 159.

13. [Editor], "The Eclectic Medical College of the City of New York," *New York Eclectic Medical Review*, I (1866), 276–78.

14. [Editor], "Object and Plan of the Review," *New York Eclectic Medical Review*, I (1866), 33.

15. Horace Greeley, "Mr. Greeley's Address," *American Eclectic Medical Review*, III (1868), 105–11.

16. Waite, "American Sectarian Medical Colleges before the Civil War," 149, 153; Alexander Wilder, *History of Medicine: A Brief Outline of Medical History from the Earliest Period with an Extended Account of the Various Sects of Physicians and New Schools of Medicines in Later Centuries* (Augusta, Maine: Maine Farmer Publishing Co., 1904), 527.

17. Waite, "American Sectarian Medical Colleges before the Civil War," 155; Frederick C. Waite, "The First Sectarian Medical School in New England, at Worcester (1846–1859), and Its Relation to Thomsonianism," *New England Journal of Medicine*, CCVII (1932), 987; William F. Norwood, *Medical Education in the United States before the Civil War* (Philadelphia: University of Pennsylvania Press, 1944), 420–21; Isaac Miller Comings, "Medical Liberality," *New England Botanic Medical and Surgical Journal*, III (1849), 362.

18. Calvin Newton, "An Address Delivered before the Worcester Medical Institution," *New England Botanic Medical and Surgical Journal*, III (1849), 187–89.

19. [Editor], "The Journal," *American Medical and Surgical Journal*, I (1851), 17–18.

20. [Editor], "Eclectic Students," *Philadelphia University Journal of Medicine and Surgery*, XIII (1869–70), 225.

21. [Advertisement], *Philadelphia University Journal of Medicine and Surgery*, XII (1868–69), frontispiece.

22. [Editor], "Surgeon General Barnes and the Philadelphia University," *Philadelphia University Journal of Medicine and Surgery*, XIII (1869–70), 321.

23. [Editor], "Selling Diplomas," *Philadelphia University Journal of Medicine and Surgery*, XIII (1869–70), 180.

24. [Editor], "Bogus Diplomas," *Philadelphia University Journal of Medicine and Surgery*, XIII (1869–70), 277–78; Harold J. Abrahams, *Extinct Medical Schools of Nineteenth-Century Philadelphia* (Philadelphia: University of Pennsylvania Press, 1966), 426–31; John Uri Lloyd, "Will Our People Ever Learn to Exercise Common Sense?" *Eclectic Medical Journal*, LXXXIV (1924), 1–2.

25. Abrahams, *Extinct Medical Schools of Nineteenth-Century Philadelphia*, 179–81, 454; Martin Kaufman, "American Medical Diploma Mills," *Medical Faculty Bulletin*, Tulane University, XXVI (1967), 53–54; Waite, "American Sectarian Medical Colleges before the Civil War," 159–60; Alexander Wilder, "Eclectic Medicine in the Eastern States," *Transactions*, National Eclectic Medical Association, XX (1892–93), 483; Wilder, "Outline History of Eclectic Medicine," 48; Alexander Wilder, *History of Medicine: A Brief*

Outline of Medical History and Sects of Physicians, from the Earliest Historic Period, with an Extended Account of the New Schools of the Healing Art in the Nineteenth Century, and Especially a History of the American Eclectic Practice of Medicine, Never Before Published (New Sharon, Maine; New England Eclectic Publishing Co., 1901), 597; [Editor], "American University of Philadelphia," *Philadelphia University Journal of Medicine and Surgery*, XIII (1869–70), 282; Aron Wahrman, "The Philadelphia Physician-Factory," *Journal of the History of Medicine*, XXXVIII (1983), 334–35.

26. See John Hughes Bennett, *Researches into the Action of Mercury, Podophyllin, and Taraxacum on the Biliary Secretion* (Chicago: H.D. Garrison, 1874); John Hughes Bennett, *Researches into the Antagonism of Medicines* (London: Churchill, 1875).

27. Luke H. Stoddard, "Eclecticism in Illinois," *Transactions*, National Eclectic Medical Association, V (1877), 88; George H. Field, "Reports on the Status of Eclectic Medicine," *Transactions*, National Eclectic Medical Association, V (1877), 281–83; Wilder, *History of Medicine . . . Never Before Published*, 707; David J. Davis (ed.), *History of Medical Practice in Illinois*. Vol. II, *1850–1900* (Chicago: Illinois State Medical Society, 1955), 451–52, 483.

28. [Editor], "Are we Progressing?" *Eclectic Medical Journal of Pennsylvania*, XII (1874), 280.

29. [Editor], "Rotten Foundations," *Eclectic Medical Journal of Pennsylvania*, XII (1874), 91.

30. Marquis E. Daniel, "Suggestions to Young Physicians," *Eclectic Medical Journal*, LXXVIII (1918), 65–67.

31. Elizabeth Blackwell to Harvey W. Felter, December 11, 1903, Eclectic Medical Institute Records, 1845–1938, Box 27, Folder 724, Lloyd Library and Museum, Cincinnati; [Editor], "Syracuse Medical College," *American Medical and Surgical Journal*, I (1851), 19–20; [Anonymous], "Women Graduates of the Eclectic Medical College," *Eclectic Medical Journal*, XC (1930), 639–40; Elizabeth Blackwell, *Pioneer Work in Opening the Medical Profession to Women: Autobiographical Sketches* (London: Longmans, Green and Co., 1895), 86–91; Thomas N. Bonner, *To the Ends of the Earth: Women's Search for Education in Medicine* (Cambridge: Harvard University Press, 1992), 13.

32. James H. Cassedy, *Medicine and American Growth, 1800–1860* (Madison: University of Wisconsin Press, 1986), 172, 256; [Anonymous], "Female Medical Schools," *Boston Medical and Surgical Journal*, LI (1854–55), 263–64; Richard H. Shryock, "Women in American Medicine," *Journal of the American Medical Women's Association*, V (1950), 375; Wilder, *History of Medicine . . . Never Before Published*, 570–71. Many regular physicians refused to join the faculty of the Female Medical College of Pennsylvania because of the prevailing prejudices against women's education. As a result, several irregular physicians were appointed, and the college carried the title of "irregular" during the first two years, when seventeen women

received the degree of M.D. See Waite, "American Sectarian Medical Colleges before the Civil War," 158–59.

33. Quoted in [Editor], "The World's Medical Congress of Eclectic Physicians and Surgeons," *Transactions*, National Eclectic Medical Association, XXI (1894), 54; John B. Blake, "Women and Medicine in Ante-Bellum America," *Bulletin of the History of Medicine*, XXXIX (1965), 99–123.

34. George Washington Lafayette Bickley, "Female Medical Education," *Eclectic Medical Journal*, I (1857), 117, 119, 120.

35. [Editor], "Female Medical Students," *Eclectic Medical Journal*, I (1857), 369.

36. [Editor], "Prospects of the Institute," *Eclectic Medical Journal*, I (1857), 471. There is also evidence that the E. M. Institute graduated the first black physician in the United States. In a letter from Booker T. Washington to John Uri Lloyd, dated May 2, 1900, Washington thanked Lloyd for sharing the information. Although not clearly identifiable through alumni records, the individual appears to have been William R. Reynolds of Illinois who graduated in the class of 1868. See Box 13, Folder 276, John Uri Lloyd Papers, 1849–1936, Lloyd Library and Museum, Cincinnati.

37. Mary B. Morey, "Women's Advantage and Disadvantage in the Practice of Medicine," *Eclectic Medical Journal*, LXIV (1904), 54.

38. Martin Kaufman, "The Admission of Women to Nineteenth-Century American Medical Societies," *Bulletin of the History of Medicine*, L (1976), 251–60; Shryock, "Women in American Medicine," 375–76; William Barlow, "A Case for Medical Co-Education in the 1870s," *Journal of the American Medical Women's Association*, XXXV (1980), 285–88; Felter, *History of the Eclectic Medical Institute*, 53–54; Thomas N. Bonner, "Medical Women Abroad: A New Dimension of Women's Push for Opportunity in Medicine," 1850–1914, *Bulletin of the History of Medicine*, LXII (1988), 58–73.

39. [Editor], "Women Doctors," *Eclectic Medical Journal*, LXXVIII (1918), 256.

40. James G. Burrow, *AMA: Voice of American Medicine* (Baltimore: Johns Hopkins University Press, 1963), 1; Nathan Smith Davis, *History of the American Medical Association from Its Organization up to January, 1855* (Philadelphia: Lippincott, Grambo and Co., 1855), 31–39; Nathan Smith Davis, *History of Medical Education and Medical Institutions in the United States from the First Settlement of the British Colonies to the Year 1850* (Chicago: S.C. Griggs and Co., 1851), 124–25.

41. Committee on Education, "Report of the Committee on Education," *Transactions*, American Medical Association, I (1848), 236.

42. Committee on Education, "Report of the Committee on Education," 237–38.

43. Lester S. King, "The Painfully Slow Progress in Medical Education," *Journal of the American Medical Association*, CCLXIX (1983), 273.

44. [Editor], "New Plan of Medical Education," *Eclectic Medical Journal*, I (1855), 431; Waite, "American Sectarian Medical Colleges before the Civil War," 161.

45. Committee on Medical Education, "Report," *Transactions*, American Medical Association, XVIII (1867), 365.

46. King, "The Painfully Slow Progress in Medical Education," 273.

47. Samuel D. Gross, *History of American Medical Literature: From 1776 to the Present Time* (New York: B. Franklin, 1972), 55–57.

48. Quoted in Fielding H. Garrison, *John Shaw Billings: A Memoir* (New York: G.P. Putnam's Sons, 1915), 256.

49. Wilder, *History of Medicine . . . Never Before Published*, 540–41.

50. Quoted in Alexander Wilder, "Eclecticism in Medicine Defined by Eclectic Writers," *Transactions*, National Eclectic Medical Association, XXVIII (1901), 100; Alexander Wilder, "Eclectic Medicine; Its History and Scientific Basis," *Transactions*, National Eclectic Medical Association, XXI (1894), 65; Felter, *History of the Eclectic Medical Institute*, 27; Thomas W. Petrisko, "Schism and Suppression: The Elimination of Medical Protest Schools, 1846–1939," *Chiropractic History*, II (1982), 37.

51. [Editor], "A National Convention," *American Medical and Surgical Journal*, I (1851), 127.

52. [Editor], "National Eclectic Medical Association," *American Medical and Surgical Reporter*, I (1851), 97–98; James H. Cassedy, *American Medical and Statistical Thinking, 1800–1860* (Cambridge: Harvard University Press, 1984), 137.

53. Wilder, *History of Medicine . . . Never Before Published*, 589–92.

54. Wilder, *History of Medicine . . . Never Before Published*, 609.

55. Quoted in Wilder, "Eclecticism in Medicine Defined by Eclectic Writers," 100–101.

56. Wilder, "Outline History of Eclectic Medicine," 50.

57. [Editor], "Progress of Eclectic Practice," *New York Eclectic Medical Review*, I (1866), 232; Paul W. Allen, *Eclectic Medicine: The Lessons of Its Past and the Duties of Its Future. Annual Address Before the Eclectic Medical Society of the State of New York, January 15, 1868* (New York: n.p., 1868), 1–6.

58. J. M. Toner, "Statistical Sketch of the Medical Profession of the United States," *Indiana Journal of Medicine*, IV (1873), 4–5. See also Jan Coombs, "Rural Medical Practice in the 1880s: A View from Central Wisconsin," *Bulletin of the History of Medicine*, LXIV (1990), 35–62.

59. Wilder, "Eclectic Medicine; Its History and Scientific Basis," 68–69.

60. Wilder, *History of Medicine . . . Never Before Published*, 766.

61. [Anonymous], "The Eclectic Medical Association of Great Britain," *American Eclectic Medical Review*, VI (1871), 329; H. L. Griffin, "Vaccination," *St. Louis Eclectic Medical Journal*, I (1874), 97–104; Wilder, *History of Medicine . . . Never Before Published*, 676.

62. J. T. H. Connor, " 'A Sort of Felo-de-se': Eclecticism, Related Medical Sects, and Their Decline in Victorian Ontario," *Bulletin of the History of Medicine*, LXV (1991), 503–27.

6. Eclectic Materia Medica

1. Alexander Wilder, "Outline History of Eclectic Medicine," *Transactions*, National Eclectic Medical Association, V (1877), 41.

2. J. H. Beal, "Some Aspects of Eclecticism as They Appear to a Majority of Pharmacists," *Eclectic Medical Journal*, XCI (1931), 433–34.

3. [Anonymous], "Eclectic Perception," *Eclectic Medical Journal*, LXII (1902), 677; William Paine, *An Epitome of the American Eclectic Practice of Medicine* (Philadelphia: J. Gladding, 1859), 36.

4. [Anonymous], "Why American Eclectic Physicians Refuse to Bleed," *American Eclectic Medical Review*, II (1867), 90–92.

5. Texas Eclectic Medical Association, "Proceedings of the Texas Eclectic Medical Association," *Eclectic Medical Journal*, LXII (1903), 644; George Washington Lafayette Bickley, "Prof. Bickley to R. W. Rawlinson," *Eclectic Medical Journal*, I (1857), 139; Rolla L. Thomas, "Local Applications," *Eclectic Medical Journal*, LXIV (1904), 131; Isaac Miller Comings, "Drugs and Water Cure," *American Medical and Surgical Journal*, I (1851), 229–30.

6. [Anonymous], "The Electrolysis of Metals," *American Eclectic Medical Review*, I (1867), 81–82; [Editor], "The Electrolytic Institution of New York," *American Eclectic Medical Review*, III (1867), 73–74.

7. J. Milton Sanders, "Sanders' Magneto-Voltaic Battery," *Eclectic Medical Journal*, I (1857), 112.

8. Richard E. Kunze, "Origin of Medium, or Specific Medication," *Medical Eclectic*, VI (1879), 425–26. See also Johann Martin Honigberger, *Cholera; Its Causes and Infallible Cure, and on Epidemics in General* (Calcutta: R.C. Lepage and Co., 1857); Johann Martin Honigberger, *Thirty-Five Years in the East* (2 vols. London: H. Bailliere, 1852).

9. Kunze, "Origin of Medium, or Specific Medication," 428.

10. R. Stephens, "Who Is to Blame?" *Eclectic Medical Journal*, LXV (1905), 105–6.

11. Pitts E. Howes, "The Dispensing Physician," *Eclectic Medical Journal*, LXV (1905), 303–5.

12. Harvey W. Felter, *The Eclectic Materia Medica, Pharmacology and Therapeutics* (Cincinnati: John K. Scudder, 1922), 50.

13. Alex Berman, "The Eclectic 'Concentrations' and American Pharmacy," *Pharmacy in History*, XXII (1890), 93.

14. Alex Berman, "A Striving for Scientific Respectability: Some American Botanics and the Nineteenth-Century Plant Materia Medica," *Bulletin of the History of Medicine*, XXX (1956), 19.

15. Caswell A. Mayo, "The Lloyd Library and Its Makers," *Bulletin*

of the Lloyd Library of Botany, Pharmacy and Materia Medica, No. 28 (1928), 14.

16. Harvey W. Felter, *Biographies of John King, M.D., Andrew Jackson Howe, A.B., M.D., and John Milton Scudder, M.D., Accompanied by Many Valuable and Historical Portraits and Other Illustrations* (Cincinnati: J.U. and C.G. Lloyd, 1912), 14–15.

17. John Uri Lloyd, *The Eclectic Alkaloids, Resins, Resinoids, Oleo-Resins and Concentrated Principles* (Cincinnati: J.U. and C.G. Lloyd, 1910), 9.

18. Lloyd, *The Eclectic Alkaloids, Resins, Resinoids, Oleo-Resins and Concentrated Principles*, 28–29.

19. Lloyd, *The Eclectic Alkaloids, Resins, Resinoids, Oleo-Resins and Concentrated Principles*, 11.

20. Quoted in Lloyd, *The Eclectic Alkaloids, Resins, Resinoids, Oleo-Resins and Concentrated Principles*, 11, 13.

21. Lloyd, *The Eclectic Alkaloids, Resins, Resinoids, Oleo-Resins and Concentrated Principles*, 12.

22. Alexander Wilder, *History of Medicine: A Brief Outline of Medical History and Sects of Physicians, from the Earliest Historic Period, with an Extended Account of the New Schools of the Healing Art in the Nineteenth Century, and Especially a History of the American Eclectic Practice of Medicine, Never Before Published* (New Sharon, Maine: New England Eclectic Publishing Co., 1901), 659–60.

23. Wilder, *History of Medicine . . . Never Before Published*, 661.

24. H. Wohlgemuth, "Fifty Years of Eclecticism," *Eclectic Medical Journal*, LVI (1896), 350–51; Madge E. Pickard and R. Carlyle Buley, *The Midwest Pioneer; His Ills, Cures, and Doctors* (New York: Henry Schuman, 1946), 190.

25. Lloyd, *The Eclectic Alkaloids, Resins, Resinoids, Oleo-Resins and Concentrated Principles*, 23–24; Alex Berman, *The Impact of the Nineteenth-Century Botanical-Medical Movement on American Pharmacy and Medicine* (Ph.D. Dissertation, Madison: University of Wisconsin, 1954), 276.

26. William Elmer, "American College of Medicine," *American Medical and Surgical Journal*, I (1851), 43.

27. Elmer, "American College of Medicine," 21, 34, 37.

28. Elmer, "American College of Medicine," 96; Edwin S. Wayne, "Examination of the Preparations Made by the American Chemical Institute, New York," *American Journal of Pharmacy*, XXVII (1855), 388–91.

29. Herbert T. Webster, "Podophyllum and Podophyllin," *California Eclectic Medical Journal*, XXXVI (1915), 301.

30. Felter, *History of the Eclectic Medical Institute*, 41–42.

31. Lloyd, *The Eclectic Alkaloids, Resins, Resinoids, Oleo-Resins and Concentrated Principles*, 16, 19, 22.

32. John King, "Concentrated Medicines Adulterated," *Worcester Journal of Medicine*, X (1855), 225–27.

33. Quoted in Lloyd, *The Eclectic Alkaloids, Resins, Resinoids, Oleo-Resins*

and Concentrated Principles, 34, 37; Wayne, "Examination of the Preparations Made by the American Chemical Institute, New York," 388; J. M. Abernathy, "On the Resinoids," *American Journal of Pharmacy*, XXXIII (1861), 299–303.

34. Quoted in Lloyd, *The Eclectic Alkaloids, Resins, Resinoids, Oleo-Resins and Concentrated Principles*, 39.

35. Quoted in Felter, *Biographies*, 332.

36. [Editor], "National Eclectic Pharmacopoeia," *American Eclectic Medical Review*, III (1867), 274–76.

37. Lloyd, *The Eclectic Alkaloids, Resins, Resinoids, Oleo-Resins and Concentrated Principles*, 30–32.

38. John H. Warner, *The Therapeutic Perspective: Medical Practice, Knowledge, and Identity in America, 1820–1880* (Cambridge: Harvard University Press, 1986), 58–63.

39. Iago Galdston, "The Concept of the Specific in Medicine," *Transactions and Studies*, College of Physicians of Philadelphia, IX (1941), 26, 28–29.

40. Richard H. Shryock, "The Concept of the Specific in American Medicine," *Pagine di storia della medicina*, XIII (1969), 8.

41. Quoted in Alexander Wilder, *History of Medicine: A Brief Outline of Medical History from the Earliest Historic Period with an Extended Account of the Various Sects of Physicians and New Schools of Medicines in Later Centuries* (Augusta, Maine: Maine Farmer Publishing Co., 1904), 329.

42. Wilder, *History of Medicine . . . with an Extended Account of the Various Sects*, 335.

43. Wilder, *History of Medicine . . . with an Extended Account of the Various Sects*, 329–31, 338.

44. Quoted in Wilder, *History of Medicine . . . with an Extended Account of the Various Sects*, 338.

45. Beal, "Some Aspects of Eclecticism as They Appear to a Majority of Pharmacists," 434–35.

46. Kunze, "Origin of Medium, or Specific Medication," 435.

47. Felter, *The Eclectic Materia Medica, Pharmacology and Therapeutics*, 54, 58.

48. Herbert T. Webster, "Not the Name, But the Game," *California Eclectic Medical Journal*, XXXIV (1913), 36.

49. W. S. Turner, "Specific Medication a Distinctive Feature of the Eclectic System of Practice," *Eclectic Medical Journal*, LXIII (1903), 12–13.

50. Turner, "Specific Medication a Distinctive Feature of the Eclectic System of Practice," 15.

51. Quoted in Wilder, *History of Medicine . . . with an Extended Account of the Various Sects*, 681.

52. H. C. Smith, "Some Native Remedies Worth Trying," *California Eclectic Medical Journal*, XXXVII (1916), 12, 14.

53. Lloyd, *The Eclectic Alkaloids, Resins, Resinoids, Oleo-Resins and Concentrated Principles*, 42.

54. Turner, "Specific Medication a Distinctive Feature of the Eclectic System of Practice," 9, 11; Felter, *Biographies*, 325.

55. John Thomas Lloyd, *Specific Medicines* (Cincinnati: Lloyd Brothers, Pharmacists, Inc., n.d.), 6.

56. Webster, "Not the Name, But the Game," 35.

57. Otto Juettner, *Daniel Drake and His Followers; Historical and Biographical Sketches* (Cincinnati: Harvey Publishing Co., 1909), 371; Wade Boyle, *Herb Doctors: Pioneers in Nineteenth-Century American Botanical Medicine and a History of the Eclectic Medical Institute of Cincinnati* (East Palestine, Ohio: Buckeye Naturopathic Press, 1988), 28.

58. John Buchanan, "Specific Medication," *Eclectic Medical Journal of Pennsylvania*, XII (1874), 90.

59. E. Younkin, "Eclecticism Is Free," *American Medical Journal*, XXIII (1895), 483.

60. Quoted in Felter, *Biographies*, 116–17, 181.

61. Quoted in Felter, *Biographies*, 204–5.

62. Beal, "Some Aspects of Eclecticism as They Appear to a Majority of Pharmacists," 435–36.

63. John Uri Lloyd, "The Present Trend in Materia Medica," *Eclectic Medical Journal*, LXIII (1903), 673–74.

64. John Uri Lloyd, "Address," *Eclectic Medical Journal*, LVI (1896), 18.

65. Mayo, "The Lloyd Library and Its Makers," 1–10; Margaret Stewart [John Uri's Secretary], "Recollections of Eunice Lloyd, July 14, 1909," John Uri Lloyd Papers, Box 3, Folder 40, Lloyd Library and Museum, Cincinnati, Ohio.

66. Mayo, "The Lloyd Library and Its Makers," 12–13; Corinne Miller Simons, *John Uri Lloyd, His Life and Works, 1849–1936; With a History of the Lloyd Library* (Cincinnati: Privately Printed, 1972), 21–42.

67. Mayo, "The Lloyd Library and Its Makers," 15, 17.

68. Mayo, "The Lloyd Library and Its Makers," 17. Curtis's collections became the basis of the Lloyd Library and Museum in Cincinnati and was enhanced by a generous gift of thirty thousand dollars by Surgeon General James Pattison of England for the study of specific medicines. See M. F. Bettencourt, "The Medical Chameleon," *California Eclectic Medical Journal*, XXXIV (1913), 46.

69. Lloyd, *The Eclectic Alkaloids, Resins, Resinoids, Oleo-Resins and Concentrated Principles*, 5; H. B. Arny, "Seven Glimpses of John Uri Lloyd," *Journal of the American Pharmaceutical Association*, XXV (1936), 885.

70. Lloyd, "Address," 18.

71. John Uri Lloyd, "War Prices of Medicines," *Eclectic Medical Journal*, LXXVIII (1918), 444.

72. John Uri Lloyd, "Made Anywhere But in America," *California*

Eclectic Medical Journal, XXXV (1914), 283, 285; Lloyd, "War Prices of Medicines," 444–45.

73. Rolla L. Thomas, "The Present War and Medicine," *California Eclectic Medical Journal*, XXXVI (1915), 67.

74. [Anonymous], "Most Important and Most Used Drugs," *Eclectic Medical Journal*, LXXVIII (1918), 396.

75. Lloyd, "War Prices of Medicines," 444.

76. John Uri Lloyd, "Informal Remarks Before the California Eclectic Medical College," *California Eclectic Medical Journal*, XXXIV (1913), 64.

77. John Uri Lloyd, "The Mercurials," *Eclectic Medical Journal*, XC (1930), 593–94; John Uri Lloyd, "Drug Discoverers," *Eclectic Medical Journal*, XCIII (1933), 171–76.

78. Harry W. Powers, "A Therapeutic Friend," *Eclectic Medical Journal*, XC (1930), 37–38; Albert F. Stephens, "Lobelia," *The Gleaner*, XXVI (1925), 863–65; Finley Ellingwood, "How Does Subculoyd Lobelia Act?" *The Gleaner*, XXVI (1925), 870–73; Finley Ellingwood, "Lobelia Hypodermically Administered, Its Medical Influence and Physiological Action," *Eclectic Review*, XIV (1911), 298–303.

79. Morris Fishbein, *The Medical Follies; An Analysis of the Foibles of Some Healing Cults, Including Osteopathy, Homeopathy, Chiropractic, and the Electronic Reactions of Abrams, with Essays on the Anti-Vivisectionists, Health Legislation, Physical Culture, Birth Control, and Rejuvenation* (New York: Boni and Liveright, 1925), 150.

80. Lester S. King, "Germ Theory and Its Influence," *Journal of the American Medical Association*, CCXLIX (1983), 794–95.

81. Edmund D. Pellegrino, "The Sociocultural Impact of Twentieth-Century Therapeutics," in Morris J. Vogel and Charles E. Rosenberg (eds.), *The Therapeutic Revolution: Essays in the Social History of American Medicine* (Philadelphia: University of Pennsylvania Press, 1979), 252–53; K. Codell Carter, "The Development of Pasteurs Concept of Disease Causation and the Emergence of Specific Causes in Nineteenth-Century Medicine," *Bulletin of the History of Medicine*, LXV (1991), 528–48.

82. Wilder, *History of Medicine . . . Never Before Published*, 382.

83. King, "Germ Theory and Its Influence," 796.

84. Wilder, *History of Medicine . . . Never Before Published*, 381–83.

85. Russell C. Maulitz, "Physician Versus Bacteriologist: The Ideology of Science in Clinical Medicine," in Vogel and Rosenberg, *The Therapeutic Revolution*, 92.

86. E. P. Herd, "On the Germ Theory of Disease," *Boston Medical and Surgical Journal*, CI (1874), 97–110.

87. The articles were later published in book form. See William T. Belfield, *On the Relation of Micro-organisms to Disease* (Chicago: W.T. Keener, 1884).

88. James T. Whittaker, "Some Points in Bacteriology," *Journal of the American Medical Association*, VI (1886), 533–44.

89. King, "Germ Theory and Its Influence," 797–98; [Editor], "The Early Diagnosis of Diphtheria," *Journal of the American Medical Association,* XXV (1895), 118–19.

90. Robert A. Buerki, "Reception of the Germ Theory of Disease in the *American Journal of Pharmacy,*" *Pharmacy in History,* XIII (1971), 161–63.

91. Younkin, "Eclecticism Is Free," 482.

92. William E. Bloyer, "Annual Address," *Transactions,* National Eclectic Medical Association, XXIV (1896–97), 30.

93. J. W. Hodge, "Bacteriophobia and Medical Fads," *Eclectic Medical Journal,* LXV (1905), 605–7.

94. [Anonymous], "Parisian Medical Chit-Chat," *Eclectic Medical Journal,* LXV (1905), 135.

95. Vincent A. Baker, "Address," *Transactions,* National Eclectic Medical Association, XXIII (1895–96), 49.

96. [Editor], "Hold Fast to Eclectic Principles," *Eclectic Medical Journal,* LVI (1896), 487–88.

97. [Editor], "Practical Teaching," *Eclectic Medical Journal,* LVI (1896), 149; Merriley Borell, "Brown-Séquard's Organotherapy and Its Appearance in America at the End of the Nineteenth Century," *Bulletin of the History of Medicine,* L (1976), 739–46.

98. George H. Knapp, "The Relation of Bacteriology to the Specific Medicationist," *Eclectic Medical Journal,* LXIV (1904), 541.

99. Knapp, "The Relation of Bacteriology to the Specific Medicationist," 547.

100. Charles Clark, "Why Not Use Vaccines and Serums?" *California Eclectic Medical Journal,* XXXVII (1916), 147.

101. J. C. Kilgour, "My Medicine Bag," *Eclectic Medical Journal,* LXIII (1903), 91; [Anonymous], "Eclectic Vegetable Remedies," *Eclectic Medical Gleaner,* VIII (1912), 8–10.

102. [Anonymous], "The Remedies Now Commonly Used by Eclectics," *Eclectic Medical Journal,* LXIV (1904), 398.

103. Harris L. Coulter, *Divided Legacy: A History of the Schism in Medical Thought.* Vol. III, *Science and Ethics in American Medicine: 1800–1914* (3 vols. Washington, D.C.: Wehawken Book Co., 1973), 262–63.

104. [Anonymous], "Fads in Medicine," *Eclectic Medical Journal,* LVI (1896), 340–41.

105. W. R. Fowler, "Psychology in Medicine," *Eclectic Medical Journal,* LXIII (1903), 652–53.

106. H. M. Campbell, "Annual Address," *Eclectic Medical Journal,* LVI (1896), 354–55.

107. [Editor], "The World's Medical Congress of Eclectic Physicians and Surgeons," *Transactions,* National Eclectic Medical Association, XXI (1894), 47–48.

108. [Editor], The World's Medical Congress of Eclectic Physicians and Surgeons, 483.

7. Challenges, 1875–1910

1. Lester S. King, "The Painfully Slow Progress in Medical Education," *Journal of the American Medical Association*, CCXLIX (1983), 270.

2. Kenneth M. Ludmerer, *Learning to Heal: The Development of American Medical Education* (New York: Basic Books, 1985), 72–149.

3. Martin Kaufman, *American Medical Education: The Formative Years, 1765–1910* (Westport, Conn.: Greenwood Press, 1976), 127–28.

4. King, "The Painfully Slow Progress in Medical Education," 271; William F. Norwood, "The Mainstream of American Medical Education, 1765–1965," *Annals of the New York Academy of Sciences*, CXXVIII (1965), 468; Leslie B. Arey, "The Origin of the Graded Medical Curriculum," *Journal of Medical Education*, LI (1976), 1010–12; Ludmerer, *Learning to Heal*, 12, 48–51; Hugh Hawkins, *Between Harvard and America: The Educational Leadership of Charles W. Eliot* (New York: Oxford University Press, 1972); Kenneth M. Ludmerer, "Reform at Harvard Medical School, 1869–1909," *Bulletin of the History of Medicine*, LV (1981), 343–70; John H. Warner, "Remembering Paris: Memory and the American Disciples of French Medicine in the Nineteenth Century," *Bulletin of the History of Medicine*, LXV (1991), 332–33, 335; Thomas S. Huddle, "Looking Backward: The 1871 Reforms at Harvard Medical School Reconsidered," *Bulletin of the History of Medicine*, LXV (1991), 340–65.

5. John M. Dodson, "The Modern University School—Its Purposes and Methods," *Journal of the American Medical Association*, XXXIX (1902), 521.

6. Dodson, "The Modern University School—Its Purposes and Methods," 522–23.

7. Thomas N. Bonner, "The German Model of Training Physicians in the United States, 1870–1914: How Closely Was It Followed?" *Bulletin of the History of Medicine*, LXIV (1990), 31. For background on this transformation, see Ronald L. Numbers (ed.), *The Education of American Physicians: Historical Essays* (Berkeley: University of California Press, 1980); Ludmerer, *Learning to Heal*; and William G. Rothstein, *American Medical Schools and the Practice of Medicine: A History* (Oxford: Oxford University Press, 1987).

8. Richard H. Shryock, *Medical Licensing in America, 1650–1965* (Baltimore: Johns Hopkins University Press, 1967), 55–56; Kaufman, *American Medical Education*, 154–55.

9. Robert P. Hudson, "Abraham Flexner in Perspective: American Medical Education 1865–1910," *Bulletin of the History of Medicine*, XLVI (1972), 554; Thomas N. Bonner, *American Doctors and German Universities: A Chapter in International Intellectual Relations, 1870–1914* (Lincoln: University of Nebraska Press, 1963), 23. See also James H. Means, *The Association of American Physicians: Its First 75 Years* (New York: McGraw Hill, 1961). When the American Academy of Medicine asked fifty medical colleges whether they believed that a college education was desirable for physicians,

twenty-four answered yes and nineteen answered no. See George H. Simmons, "Medical Education and Preliminary Requirements," *Journal of the American Medical Association*, XLII (1904), 1208.

10. Alexander Wilder, *History of Medicine: A Brief Outline of Medical History and Sects of Physicians, from the Earliest Historic Period, with an Extended Account of the New Schools of the Healing Art in the Nineteenth Century, and Especially a History of the American Eclectic Practice of Medicine, Never Before Published* (New Sharon, Maine: New England Eclectic Publishing Co., 1901), 883.

11. [Editor], "Let Them Go," *Eclectic Medical Journal*, LVI (1896), 54–55.

12. J. E. Emerson, "The Requirements for Preliminary Education in the Medical Colleges of the United States and Canada," *Journal of the American Medical Association*, XIV (1890), 271.

13. [Anonymous], "Medical Education in the United States," *Journal of the American Medical Association*, XXII (1894), 394.

14. Quoted in [Anonymous], "Medical Education in the United States," 393.

15. Dodson, "The Modern University School—Its Purposes and Methods," 521.

16. Emerson, "The Requirements for Preliminary Education," 272.

17. Shryock, *Medical Licensing in America*, 53–55.

18. [Anonymous], "Medical Education in the United States," 394.

19. Quoted in Harvey W. Felter, *History of the Eclectic Medical Institute, Cincinnati, Ohio, 1845–1902* (Cincinnati: Alumni Association, 1902), 55–56, 59, 61; Dean F. Smiley, "History of the Association of American Medical Colleges," *Journal of Medical Education*, XXXII (1957), 513, 516.

20. [Anonymous], "The Organization of the Medical Profession," *Journal of the American Medical Association*, XXXIX (1902), 325.

21. [Anonymous], "The Organization of the Medical Profession," 177.

22. [Anonymous], "The Organization of the Medical Profession," 400.

23. [Anonymous], "The Organization of the Medical Profession," 460.

24. Rolla L. Thomas, "Eclecticism," *Eclectic Medical Journal*, LXIV (1904), 228.

25. Herbert T. Webster, "The Merger Proposition," *Eclectic Medical Journal*, LXVI (1906), 323; James G. Burrow, *Organized Medicine in the Progressive Era: The Move Toward Monopoly* (Baltimore: Johns Hopkins University Press, 1977), 84.

26. [Editor], "The American Medical Trust," *California Eclectic Medical Journal*, XXXIV (1913), 48.

27. J. R. Goodale, "Reports on Status of Eclectic Medicine," *Transactions*, National Eclectic Medical Association, V (1877), 296.

28. [Anonymous], "A Fraudulent and Oppressive Medical Statute," *Transactions*, National Eclectic Medical Association, XVII (1889–90), 61–62.

29. Martin Kaufman, "American Medical Diploma Mills," *Medical Faculty Bulletin*, Tulane University, XXVI (1967), 56.

30. Luke H. Stoddard, "Eclecticism in Illinois," *Transactions*, National Eclectic Medical Association, V (1877), 87.

31. H. S. McMaster, "Reports on Status of Eclectic Medicine," *Transactions*, National Eclectic Medical Association, V (1877), 284–85.

32. J. W. Marmon, "Reports on Status of Eclectic Medicine," *Transactions*, National Eclectic Medical Association, V (1877), 277, 280–81.

33. J. R. Borland, "Report on Status of Eclectic Medicine," *Transactions*, National Eclectic Medical Association, V (1877), 287–89.

34. [Anonymous], "A Fraudulent and Oppressive Medical Statute," 60.

35. [Anonymous], "A Fraudulent and Oppressive Medical Statute," 56–57.

36. Quoted in Texas State Medical Association, "Texas Allopaths," *Eclectic Medical Journal*, LVI (1896), 519.

37. Quoted in [Anonymous], "A Fraudulent and Oppressive Medical Statute," 58.

38. Statute quoted in [Anonymous], "A Fraudulent and Oppressive Medical Statute," 46.

39. [Anonymous], "A Fraudulent and Oppressive Medical Statute," 47–48.

40. Quoted in [Anonymous], "A Fraudulent and Oppressive Medical Statute," 51–52.

41. Burrow, *Organized Medicine in the Progressive Era*, 82.

42. D. Maclean, "Come West," *Eclectic Medical Journal*, LVI (1896), 190.

43. Alexander Wilder, "Outline History of Eclectic Medicine," *Transactions*, National Eclectic Medical Association, V (1877), 51–52. Rothstein estimated a much smaller number of 4,752. See William G. Rothstein, *American Physicians in the Nineteenth Century: From Sects to Science* (Baltimore: Johns Hopkins University Press, 1972), 226.

44. Finley Ellingwood, "Eclecticism and the Present Duty of the Eclectic Physician," *Eclectic Medical Journal*, LXII (1902), 167–68.

45. Finley Ellingwood, "Eclectic Statistics," *Eclectic Medical Journal*, LXII (1902), 457.

46. [Editor], "Medical Colleges," *Eclectic Medical Journal*, LXII (1902), 622.

47. Flyer dated March 10, 1905, in Eclectic Medical College Scrapbook, 1904–1922, Lloyd Library and Museum, Cincinnati; [Anonymous], "Medical Schools of the United States," *Journal of the American Medical Association*, XLIII (1904), 503.

48. [Editor], "Eclectics, Homeopaths and Regulars in Chicago and Their Official Recognition," *Journal of the American Medical Association*, XXXV (1900), 1559–60.

49. J. D. McCann, "Address of the President," *Transactions*, National Eclectic Medical Association, XXXI (1903), 15.

50. [Editor], "The American Medical Trust," 83.

51. [Editor], "What Shall Eclectic Colleges Teach?" *Eclectic Medical Journal*, LVI (1896), 339; Corinne Miller Simons, "Lloyd Library," *Cincinnati Journal of Medicine*, LIII (1972), 185–88.

52. Harvey W. Felter, "The Eclectic Medical Institute, of Cincinnati, Ohio," *Eclectic Medical Journal*, LXII (1902), 361; Felter, *History of the Eclectic Medical Institute*, 146.

53. "Announcement," *Eclectic Medical Journal*, LXII (1902), 325–29.

54. Kenneth M. Ludmerer, "The Rise of the Teaching Hospital in America," *Journal of the History of Medicine*, XXXVIII (1983), 389–414.

55. [Editor], "Medical Education," *Eclectic Medical Journal*, LVI (1896), 474–75.

56. Walter A. Wells, "Medical Education and the State," *Journal of the American Medical Association*, XXXVIII (1902), 864. See also Samuel L. Baker, "Physician Licensure Laws in the United States, 1865–1915," *Journal of the History of Medicine*, XXXIX (1984), 173–97; Samuel L. Baker, "A Strange Case: The Physician Licensure Campaign in Massachusetts in 1880," *Journal of the History of Medicine*, XL (1985), 286–308; Robert C. Derbyshire, *Medical Licensure and Discipline in the United States* (Baltimore: Johns Hopkins University Press, 1969).

57. [Editor], "A National Examining Board," *Eclectic Medical Journal*, LVI (1896), 519.

58. [Editor], "The College," *Eclectic Medical Journal*, LVI (1896), 488; [Editor], "No Practitioners' Course," *Eclectic Medical Journal*, LVI (1896), 527.

59. Quoted in Ellingwood, "Eclectic Statistics," 457–58.

60. Nathan Smith Davis, "Requirements for Admission to Medical Schools," *Journal of the American Medical Association*, XLI (1903), 409–10.

61. Simmons, "Medical Education and Preliminary Requirements," 1206.

62. Simmons, "Medical Education and Preliminary Requirements," 1208.

63. T. B. Turner, "History of Medical Education at Johns Hopkins," *Johns Hopkins Medical Journal*, CXXXIX (1976), 27–36; Ludmerer, *Learning to Heal*, 170.

64. [Anonymous], "Medical Education in the United States," *Journal of the American Medical Association*, LXIII (1914), 684–85. With the publication of the council's first classification, ten schools closed in 1907; thirteen closed in 1910, when the council published its second classification; and fourteen closed in 1913, with the publication of the third classification. Of the eighty-five closures, forty-four had been rated in "Classes A" and "B"; forty-one, "Class C." Of the forty-four in "Classes A" and "B," forty-one closed through merger; while of the "Class C" colleges, only six closed through merger.

65. Eclectic Medical Institute 1909 and Eclectic Medical College 1910 Records, pp. 1, 7, Lloyd Library and Museum, Cincinnati.

66. Howard S. Berliner, "A Larger Perspective on the Flexner Report," *International Journal of Health*, V (1975), 573–92; Shryock, *Medical Licensing in America*, 61–62; Richard H. Shryock, *The Unique Influence of the Johns Hopkins University on American Medicine* (Copenhagen: Munksgaard, 1954); Hudson, "Abraham Flexner in Perspective," 545–61; Abraham Flexner, *Abraham Flexner: An Autobiography* (New York: Simon and Schuster, 1960), 74; Abraham Flexner, *Henry S. Pritchett: A Biography* (New York: Columbia University Press, 1943), 70–71.

67. Abraham Flexner, *Medical Education in the United States and Canada; A Report to the Carnegie Foundation on the Advancement of Teaching* (New York: Carnegie Foundation, 1910), vii.

68. Flexner, *Medical Education in the United States and Canada*, ix.

69. Flexner, *Medical Education in the United States and Canada*, x.

70. Flexner, *Medical Education in the United States and Canada*, 28, 46.

71. Flexner, *Medical Education in the United States and Canada*, x–xi.

72. Flexner, *Medical Education in the United States and Canada*, 157.

73. Flexner, *Medical Education in the United States and Canada*, 156.

74. Flexner, *Medical Education in the United States and Canada*, 159.

75. Flexner, *Medical Education in the United States and Canada*, 161.

76. [Editor], "The Pedagogues Rebel," *California Eclectic Medical Journal*, XXXV (1914), 198.

77. Flexner, *Medical Education in the United States and Canada*, 163.

78. Shryock, *Medical Licensing in America*, 62–64.

79. Board of Trustees Meeting, December 19, 1908, Records of the Stockholders, Eclectic Medical College, Lloyd Library and Museum, Cincinnati; [Editor], "College Activities," *Eclectic Medical Journal*, XCIII (1933), 45.

8. Malaise, 1910–1939

1. The same held true for the College of Medical Evangelists in Loma Linda, California, where students studied hygiene and sanitation in a biblical context, enrolling for 540 hours of the practice of medicine, 900 hours of Bible, and 250 hours of general evangelistic fieldwork. See Henry S. Pritchett, "Medical Progress," *Journal of the American Medical Association*, LX (1913), 743; John B. Nichols, "Medical Sectarianism," *Journal of the American Medical Association*, LX (1913), 331–37.

2. G. W. Johnson, "The Medical Profession," *Eclectic Medical Journal*, LXIII (1903), 636, 638.

3. Rolla L. Thomas, "Shall or Will All Medical Schools Merge?" *Eclectic Medical Journal*, LXIII (1903), 564–66.

4. H. C. Smith, "The Practice of Medicine," *California Eclectic Medical Journal*, XXXIV (1913), 261.

5. H. C. Smith, "Concerning a Coalition of Homeopathists and Eclectics," *California Eclectic Medical Journal*, XXXVI (1915), 281–82.

6. [Editor], "A Mutual Recognition," *California Eclectic Medical Journal*, XXXVII (1916), 288.

7. [Editor], "The Unity of the Profession," *Eclectic Medical Journal*, LXIII (1903), 91.

8. O. S. Coffin, "Letter to Editor," *Eclectic Medical Journal*, LXXVIII (1918), 315–16.

9. [Editor], "Responsibility in Medicine," *Eclectic Medical Journal*, XCI (1931), 80–81.

10. John Uri Lloyd, "Love Me, Love My Dog," *Eclectic Medical Journal*, XC (1930), 524.

11. Nichols, "Medical Sectarianism," 334.

12. William E. Bloyer, "The 'Standard' and Other Dictionary Definitions of Eclectic Medicine," *Transactions*, National Eclectic Medical Association, XXIII (1895–96), 217–18.

13. [Editor], "A Declaration of Fundamental Principles of Rational Eclectic Medicine," *St. Louis Eclectic Medical Journal*, X (1883), 522–23; A. S. Tuchler, "Specific Medication—A Review of Thirty-One Years' Experience," *Eclectic Medical Journal*, LXXXIV (1924), 65–66.

14. [Editor], "Laymen in Medical Practice," *Eclectic Medical Journal*, LXV (1905), 151–52; Homer I. Ostrom, "Conservatism in Gynecology," *Eclectic Medical Gleaner*, VIII (1912), 388–92.

15. Wade Boyle, *Herb Doctors: Pioneers in Nineteenth-Century American Botanical Medicine and a History of the Eclectic Medical Institute of Cincinnati* (East Palestine, Ohio: Buckeye Naturopathic Press, 1988), 61.

16. Glenn Sonnedecker, *Kremers and Urdang's History of Pharmacy* (3d ed. Philadelphia: J.B. Lippincott Co., 1963), 249.

17. Samuel L. Baker, "Physician Licensure Laws in the United States, 1865–1915," *Journal of the History of Medicine*, XXXIX (1984), 173–97. See also Samuel L. Baker, *Medical Licensing in America: An Early Liberal Reform* (Ph.D. Dissertation, Cambridge: Harvard University, 1977).

18. Henry Ford Scudder, "An Appeal to the California Legislature to Amend the Present Medical Law," *California Eclectic Medical Journal*, XXXIV (1913), 31–32.

19. Scudder, "An Apeal to the California Legislature," 32–33.

20. Henry Ford Scudder, "A Résumé of California's Medical Law," *California Eclectic Medical Journal*, XXXIV (1913), 160.

21. [Editor], "Our Recent Legislature," *California Eclectic Medical Journal*, XXXIV (1913), 172.

22. [Editor], "Unfortunate Missouri," *Journal of the American Medical Association*, LXXVI (1921), 1251; [Editor], "Medical Licensure in Missouri," *Journal of the American Medical Association*, LXXX (1923), 923.

23. [Editor], "Connecticut Investigation of Medical Diploma Scandal,"

Journal of the American Medical Association, LXXXI (1923), 2054. See also Eclectic Medical College Scrapbook, I, 1919–25, Lloyd Library and Museum, Cincinnati.

24. [Editor], "Connecticut Investigation of Medical Diploma Scandal," *Journal of the American Medical Association*, LXXXI (1923), 1631; [Editor], "Further Diploma Mill Investigations in Connecticut," *Journal of the American Medical Association*, LXXXI (1923), 1714; [Editor], "Medical News," *Journal of the American Medical Association*, LXXXI (1923), 1794; [Editor], "Connecticut's Bogus Diploma Investigation," *Journal of the American Medical Association*, LXXXI (1923), 1810.

25. See Eclectic Medical College Scrapbook, 1910–1927, pp. 21, 82, Lloyd Library and Museum, Cincinnati. See also Norman Gevitz, " 'A Coarse Sieve': Basic Science Boards and Medical Licensure in the United States," *Journal of the History of Medicine*, XLIII (1988), 36–63.

26. Thomas, "Shall or Will All Medical Schools Merge?" 566.

27. M. F. Bettencourt, "The Medical Chameleon," *California Eclectic Medical Journal*, XXXIV (1913), 46.

28. Abraham Flexner, *Medical Education in the United States and Canada; A Report to the Carnegie Foundation on the Advancement of Teaching* (New York: Carnegie Foundation, 1910), 210.

29. David J. Davis (ed.), *History of Medical Practice in Illinois*. Vol. II, *1850–1900* (Chicago: Illinois State Medical Society, 1955), 452; Thomas N. Bonner, *Medicine in Chicago: A Chapter in the Social and Scientific Development of a City, 1850–1950* (Madison, Wis.: American History Research Center, 1957), 116.

30. [Editor], "State Board Statistics for 1912," *Journal of the American Medical Association*, LX (1913), 1639.

31. [Anonymous], "Medical Colleges of the United States," *Journal of the American Medical Association*, LXI (1913), 586–87.

32. "Announcement," *California Eclectic Medical Journal*, XXXIV (1913), 241.

33. "Announcement," 243–44.

34. Flexner, *Medical Education in the United States and Canada*, 190.

35. [Anonymous], "Medical Education in the United States," *Journal of the American Medical Association*, LXV (1916), 687, 691.

36. Flexner, *Medical Education in the United States and Canada*, 257.

37. Flexner, *Medical Education in the United States and Canada*, 205.

38. Flexner, *Medical Education in the United States and Canada*, 227.

39. See letter dated February 5, 1923, from John King Scudder, in Eclectic Medical College Scrapbook, I (1910–1929), 9, Lloyd Library and Museum, Cincinnati.

40. [Editor], "Eclectic Medical Colleges," *Eclectic Medical Journal*, XC (1930), 349.

41. [Editor], "The Present Crisis," *Eclectic Medical Journal*, XCII (1931), 39.

42. [Editor], "College Activities," *Eclectic Medical Journal*, XCIII (1933), 45.

43. Letter of December 12, 1931, from Byron H. Nellans to John Uri Lloyd, Dr. Byron H. Nellans Papers, 1925–37, Box 1, Folder 1, Lloyd Library and Museum, Cincinnati; Ernest V. Hollis, *Philanthropic Foundations and Higher Education* (New York: Columbia University Press, 1938), 217.

44. Meeting of the Board of Trustees, March 28, 1931, Records, Eclectic Medical College, p. 131, Lloyd Library and Museum, Cincinnati.

45. [Editor], "The Eclectic Medical College," *Eclectic Medical Journal*, XCIII (1933), 83–84; [Editor], "Eclectic Medical College," *Eclectic Medical Journal*, XCI (1931), 442.

46. Byron H. Nellans, "The Eclectic Medical College," *National Eclectic Medical Association Quarterly*, XXV (1933), 57–58.

47. Meeting of the Board of Trustees, May 24, 1932, Records, p. 164, Lloyd Library and Museum, Cincinnati. See also earlier discussion in C. L. Bonifield, "The Question of Full-Time Clinical Teachers in Medical Education," *Eclectic Medical Journal*, LXXXVI (1926), 243–48.

48. Meeting of the Board of Trustees, June 22, 1933, Records, Lloyd Library and Museum, Cincinnati.

49. Report of Council on Education of the National Eclectic Medical Association, in Board Meeting, June 26, 1934, Eclectic Medical College, Lloyd Library and Museum, Cincinnati.

50. Flyer entitled "The Eclectic Medical College and Eclecticism," in Eclectic Medical College Scrapbook, II, Lloyd Library and Museum, Cincinnati.

51. [Editor], "Eclectic Assets," *Eclectic Medical Journal*, LXXXIV (1924), 195–200. See also Eclectic Medical College, Miscellaneous Materials, Lloyd Library and Museum, Cincinnati; Eclectic Medical College Scrapbook (newspaper clippings), 1927–34, II, p. 11, Lloyd Library and Museum, Cincinnati.

52. Quoted from Meeting of the Board of Trustees, January 14, 1936, Dean's Report, Lloyd Library and Museum, Cincinnati.

53. Meeting of the Board of Trustees, January 14, 1936, Dean's Report, Lloyd Library and Museum, Cincinnati.

54. [Editor], "An Old Firm under New Management," *National Eclectic Medical Association Quarterly*, XXIX (1938), 198.

55. R. O. Hoffman, "The Future of Eclecticism," *National Eclectic Medical Association Quarterly*, XXIX (1938), 201.

56. Meeting of the Board of Trustees, January 14, 1936, Dean's Report, Lloyd Library and Museum, Cincinnati.

57. Byran H. Nellans, "Dean's Report," Minutes of the Board of Trustees, May 20, 1939, Lloyd Library and Museum, Cincinnati.

58. Minutes of Annual Meeting of the Board of Trustees, June 19, 1941, Lloyd Library and Museum, Cincinnati.

59. [Editor], "An Old Firm under New Management," 198.

60. [Advertisement], *National Eclectic Medical Association Quarterly*, XLI (1949), 5; Corinne Miller Simons, *John Uri Lloyd, His Life and His Works, 1849–1936; With a History of the Lloyd Library* (Cincinnati: Privately Printed, 1972), 119; [Advertisement], *John T. Lloyd, Dealers Now Carrying Complete Stock of Lloydson Preparations* (Cincinnati: John T. Lloyd Laboratories, 1939); John Bird Cook, "John Uri Lloyd, Pharmacist, Philosopher, Author, Man," *Journal of the American Pharmaceutical Association*, X (1949), 543; Interview with William C. Black, archivist and conservator of the Lloyd Library and Museum, and with Mr. Edward K. Alstat, proprietor of the Eclectic Institute Incorporated of Portland, Oregon.

61. June 10, 1939, *Cincinnati Times Star*.

62. [Editor], "Approved Eclectic Medical Colleges," *National Eclectic Medical Association Quarterly*, XLVII (1955), 4.

63. George C. Porter, "Our Great Need," *National Eclectic Medical Association Quarterly*, XXX (1939), 19.

64. George C. Porter, "President Speaks," *National Eclectic Medical Association Quarterly*, XXX (1939), 21.

65. June 10, 1939, *Cincinnati Times Star*.

66. January 15, 1943, *Cincinnati Times Star*.

67. Letter from John Thomas Lloyd to Louis G. Hoeck, May 19, 1938, Lloyd Library and Museum, Cincinnati.

68. Ralph B. Taylor, "The President's Message," *National Eclectic Medical Association Quarterly*, XLI (1949), 8.

69. Laura Z. Clavio, "Comments," *Herbs!*, II, 41–43; Francis Brinker, "Lyophilization of Fresh Medicinal Plants," *Townsend Letter for Doctors* (August/September 1989), 425–28; Georg Thieme Verlag, "Randomized, Double-Blind Study of Freeze-Dried *Urtica dioica* in the Treatment of Allergic Rhinitis," *Planta Medica*, LVI (1990), 44–47.

Selected Bibliography

This book has been researched chiefly from books, pamphlets, and journal articles. To assist the interested reader, I have included a complete list of books, pamphlets, and journals cited in the text, as well as certain general works that afford insight into the period and the subject as a whole.

Journals

American Eclectic Medical Review
American Journal of Cardiology
American Journal of Clinical Medicine
American Journal of Hospital Pharmacy
American Journal of Medical Sciences
American Journal of Pharmacy
American Medical Journal
American Medical Review
American Medical and Surgical Journal
American Medical and Surgical Reporter
Annals of Eclectic Medicine and Surgery
Annals of Medical History
Annals of the New York Academy of Science
Annals of Science
Annual of Eclectic Medicine and Surgery
Boston Medical and Surgical Journal
Botanic Medical Reformer and Home Physician
Botanical Record
Botanico-Medical Recorder
British Journal of Medical Education
British Medical Journal

Selected Bibliography

Bulletin, Eclectic Medical College
Bulletin of the History of Medicine
Bulletin of the Lloyd Library of Botany, Pharmacy and Materia Medica
Bulletin of the New York Academy of Medicine
California Eclectic Medical Journal
California State Journal of Medicine
Chicago Medical Times
Chiropractic History
Cincinnati Journal of Medicine
Clinical Medicine and Surgery
Clio Medica
College Journal of Medical Sciences
Connecticut Medicine
Eclectic
Eclectic Medical and College Journal
Eclectic Medical Gleaner
Eclectic Medical Journal, Cincinnati
Eclectic Medical Journal, St. Louis
Eclectic Medical Journal of Pennsylvania
Eclectic Review
Ellingwood's Therapeutics
Family Journal of Health
Gaillards's Medical Journal
Georgia Eclectic Medical Journal
The Gleaner
Herbs!
History of Childhood Quarterly
Indiana Journal of Medicine
International Journal of Health
Johns Hopkins Medical Journal
Journal of the American Medical Association
Journal of the American Medical Women's Association
Journal of the American Pharmaceutical Association
Journal of Eclectic Medicine
Journal of Foreign Medical Science
Journal of the History of the Behavioral Sciences
Journal of the History of Ideas
Journal of the History of Medicine
Journal of Man
Journal of Medical Education
Journal of Practical Medicine
Journal of Social Philosophy
London Medical and Physiological Journal
Mayo Clinic Proceedings
Medical Communications, Massachusetts Medical Society

Medical Eclectic
Medical Faculty Bulletin, Tulane University
Medical History
Medical Hypotheses
Medical News
Medical Record
Medical and Surgical Reporter
Modern Medicine
National Eclectic Medical Association Quarterly
New England Botanic Medical and Surgical Journal
New England Journal of Medicine
New Era of Eclecticism
New Jersey Eclectic Medical and Surgical Journal
New York Eclectic Medical Review
New York Journal of Medicine
New York State Journal of Medicine
Newton's Express
North Carolina Medical Journal
Ohio State Archaeological and Historical Quarterly
Ohio State Medical Journal
Pagine di storia della medicina
Pennsylvania Magazine of History and Biography
Perspectives in Biology and Medicine
Pharmacy in History
Pharmacy Times
Philadelphia University Journal of Medicine and Surgery
Phrenological Journal
Planta Medica
Popular Science Monthly
Proceedings, Institute of Medicine of Chicago
Proceedings of the American Philosophical Society
Proceedings of the Royal Society of Medicine
Psychological Medicine
Publications, Massachusetts Medical Society
Reformed Medical Journal
Reports on Biology and Medicine
Republican Rush-Light
Social Science and Medicine
Southern Folklore Quarterly
Southern Medical Reformer
St. Louis Eclectic Medical Journal
The Thomsonian Recorder
Townsend Letter for Doctors
Transactions, American Climatological Association
Transactions, American Medical Association

Selected Bibliography

Transactions, American Philosophical Society
Transactions, Eclectic Medical Society of New York
Transactions, National Eclectic Medical Association
Transactions, Ohio Medical Society
Transactions and Studies, College of Physicians of Philadelphia
True Thomsonian
Tufts Folia Medica
Virginia Magazine of History and Biography
Western Druggist
Western Medical Reformer
Worcester Journal of Medicine
Yale Journal of Biology and Medicine
Zoist

Books and Pamphlets

Abbott, Simon B. *The Southern Botanic Physician; Being a Treatise on the Character, Causes, Symptoms and Treatment of the Diseases of Men, Women and Children of All Climates, on Vegetable or Botanical Principles, as Taught at the Reformed Medical Colleges in the United States.* Charleston: Published for the Author, 1844.

Abrahams, Harold J. *The Extinct Medical Schools of Baltimore, Maryland.* Baltimore: Maryland Historical Society, 1969.

Abrahams, Harold J. *Extinct Medical Schools of Nineteenth-Century Philadelphia.* Philadelphia: University of Pennsylvania Press, 1966.

Absolon, Karel B. *The Study of Medical Sciences.* Rockville, Md.: Kabel Publishers, 1986.

Ackerknecht, E. H. *Medicine at the Paris Hospital, 1794–1848.* Baltimore: Johns Hopkins University Press, 1967.

Allen, Paul W. *An Answer to the Following Inquiries, in Relation to the Eclectic System of Medicine: What Is Its Origin? What Are Its Principles? What Are Its Remedies? What Is Its Popularity and Organization? What Are Its Medical Institutions? What Is Its Literature? What Is the Success of the Eclectic Practice? What Are Its Claims to Public Patronage? Designed for All Persons Seeking the Truth as to the Relative Merits of the Different Systems of Medical Practice.* New York: Published for the Author, 1869.

Allen, Paul W. *Eclectic Medicine: The Lessons of Its Past and the Duties of Its Future. Annual Address Before the Eclectic Medical Society of the State of New York, January 15, 1868.* New York: n.p., 1868.

Allen, Richard L. *The American Farm Book.* New York: C.M. Saxton, 1849.

Alstat, Edward K. (ed.). *Eclectic Dispensatory of Botanical Therapeutics.* Portland, Oreg.: Eclectic Institute, Inc., 198?.

American Chemical Institute. *Positive Medical Agents; Being a Treatise on the New Alkaloid, Resinoid, and Concentrated Preparations of Indigenous and Foreign Medical Plants.* New York: B. Keith and Co., 1855.

Selected Bibliography

American Institute of Homeopathy. *The Homeopathic Pharmacopoeia of the United States.* 3d ed. Boston: Clapp, 1914.

American Pharmaceutical Association. *The National Formulary.* 4th ed. Washington, D.C.: The American Pharmaceutical Association, 1916.

Arber, Agnes. *Herbals, Their Origin and Evolution; A Chapter in the History of Botany, 1470–1670.* Darien: Hafner, 1970.

Atkinson, Brooks (ed.). *The Complete Essays and Other Writings of Ralph Waldo Emerson.* New York: Modern Library, 1950.

Attfield, John. *Chemistry: General, Medical, and Pharmaceutical, Including the Chemistry of the U.S. Pharmacopoeia.* 10th ed. Philadelphia: H.C. Lea's Sons and Co., 1883.

Bacon, Francis. *The Advancement of Learning and New Atlantis.* London: Oxford University Press, 1969.

Bacon, Francis. *The Novum Organum.* London: T. Lee, 1620.

Baird, W. David. *Medical Education in Arkansas, 1879–1978.* Memphis: Memphis State University Press, 1979.

Baker, Samuel L. *Medical Licensing in America: An Early Liberal Reform.* Ph.D. Dissertation. Cambridge: Harvard University, 1977.

Bard, Samuel. *Two Discourses Dealing with Medical Education in Early New York.* New York: Columbia University Press, 1921.

Bartlett, Elisha. *An Essay on the Philosophy of Medical Science.* Philadelphia: Lea and Blanchard, 1844.

Bartlett, Elisha. *The History, Diagnosis, and Treatment of the Fevers of the United States.* Philadelphia: Lea and Blanchard, 1847.

Barton, Benjamin Smith. *Collections for an Essay Towards a Materia Medica of the United States.* Philadelphia: Way and Groff, 1804.

Barton, Benjamin Smith. *Elements of Botany: Or, Outlines of the Natural History of Vegetables.* Philadelphia: Published for the Author, 1803.

Barton, William P. C. *The Vegetable Materia Medica of the United States; Or, Medical Botany.* 4 vols. Philadelphia: H.C. Carey and I. Lea, 1817–18.

Beach, Wooster. *The American Practice Condensed; Or, The Family Physician.* 17th ed. New York: Clark, Austin and Smith, 1857.

Beach, Wooster. *The American Practice Condensed; Or, The Family Physician: Being the Scientific System of Medicine; On Vegetable Principles, Designed for All Classes.* New York: James M'Alister, 1847.

Beach, Wooster. *The American Practice of Medicine; Being a Treatise on the Character, Causes, Symptoms, Morbid Appearances and Treatment of the Diseases of Men, Women and Children, of All Climates, on Vegetable or Botanical Principles.* 3 vols. New York: Betts and Anstice, 1833.

Beach, Wooster. *The British and American Reformed Practice of Medicine: Embracing a Treatise on the Causes, Symptoms and Treatment of Diseases Generally, on Eclectic Principles: Including a Synopsis of Physiology and Midwifery.* Birmingham, Great Britain: Thomas Simmons, 1859.

Beach, Wooster. *The Family Physician; Or, The Reformed System of Medicine:*

On Vegetable or Botanical Principles, Being a Compendium of the American Practice of Medicine. New York: Published for the Author, 1844.

Beach, Wooster. *Medical and Botanical Dictionary: Giving a Definition of the Terms Used in the Various Branches of Medical Science.* New York: Baker and Scriber, 1848.

Beach, Wooster. *Rise, Progress, and Present State of the New-York Medical Institution, and Reformed Medical Society of the United States.* New York: Mitchell and Davis, 1830.

Beal, Otto T., Jr., and Richard H. Shryock. *Cotton Mather: First Significant Figure in American Medicine.* Baltimore: Johns Hopkins University Press, 1954.

Beck, John B. *An Historical Sketch of the State of Medicine in the American Colonies from Their First Settlement to the Period of the Revolution.* Albuquerque, N. Mex.: Horn and Wallace, 1966.

Beecher, Henry K., and Mark D. Attschule. *Medicine at Harvard: The First Three Hundred Years.* Hanover, N.H.: University Press of New England, 1977.

Belfield, William T. *On the Relation of Micro-organisms to Disease.* Chicago: W.T. Keener, 1884.

Bell, Whitfield J., Jr. *The Colonial Physician and Other Essays.* New York: Science History Publications, 1975.

Bell, Whitfield J., Jr. *John Morgan, Continental Doctor.* Philadelphia: University of Pennsylvania Press, 1965.

Bennett, John Hughes. *Clinical Lectures on the Principles and Practice of Medicine.* 3d ed. New York: W. Wood and Co., 1866.

Bennett, John Hughes. *Researches into the Action of Mercury, Podophyllin, and Taraxacum on the Biliary Secretion.* Chicago: H.D. Garrison, 1874.

Bennett, John Hughes. *Researches into the Antagonism of Medicines.* London: Ghurchill, 1875.

Berman, Alex. *The Impact of the Nineteenth-Century Botanico-Medical Movement on American Pharmacy and Medicine.* Ph.D. Dissertation. Madison: University of Wisconsin, 1954.

Berman, Alex. *A Striving for Scientific Respectability: Some American Botanics and the Nineteenth-Century Plant Materia Medica.* Madison, Wis.: American Institute of the History of Pharmacy, 1956.

Bichat, Marie-François-Xavier. *Anatomie générale, appliquée à la physiologie et à la medécine.* 4 vols. Paris: Brosson, Gabon, 1801.

Bigelow, Henry J. *Medical Education in America.* Cambridge: Welch, Bigelow and Co., 1871.

Bigelow, Jacob. *American Medical Botany, Being a Collection of the Native Medicinal Plants of the United States.* 3 vols. Boston: Hilliard and Metcaff, 1817–20.

Bigelow, Jacob. *Discourse on Self-Limited Diseases.* Boston: N. Hale, 1835.

Bigelow, Jacob. *Nature in Disease, Illustrated in Various Discourses and Essays, to Which Are Added Miscellaneous Writings.* Boston: Tichnor and Fields, 1854.

Selected Bibliography

Bigelow, Jacob. *A Treatise on the Materia Medica: Intended as a Sequel to the Pharmacopoeia of the United States.* Boston: C. Ewer, 1822.

Billroth, Theodor. *The Medical Sciences in the German Universities.* New York: Macmillan, 1924.

Blackwell, Elizabeth. *Pioneer Work in Opening the Medical Profession to Women: Autobiographical Sketches.* London: Longmans, Green and Co., 1895.

Blanton, Wyndham B. *Medicine in Virginia in the Eighteenth Century.* Richmond: Garrett and Massie, 1931.

Blanton, Wyndham B. *Medicine in Virginia in the Nineteenth Century.* Richmond: Garrett and Massie, 1933.

Blanton, Wyndham B. *Medicine in Virginia in the Seventeenth Century.* Richmond: William Byrd Press, 1930.

Boardman, Andrew. *An Essay on the Means of Improving Medical Education and Elevating Medical Character.* Philadelphia: Haswell, Barrington and Haswell, 1840.

Boerhaave, Hermann. *Institutiones medicae.* London: n.p., 1721.

Boericke, William. *Pocket Manual of Homeopathic Materia Medica.* 9th ed. Philadelphia: Boericke and Runyon, 1927.

Bond, Raymond T. *The Man Who Was Chesterton.* Garden City, N.Y.: Doubleday Image Books, 1960.

Bonner, Thomas N. *American Doctors and German Universities: A Chapter in International Intellectual Relations, 1870–1914.* Lincoln: University of Nebraska Press, 1963.

Bonner, Thomas N. *Educating Physicians in the Nineteenth Century: Selected Titles Bearing on the Subject in the Collections of the National Library of Medicine.* Bethesda, Md.: Department of Health and Human Services, 1988.

Bonner, Thomas N. *Medicine in Chicago. A Chapter in the Social and Scientific Development of a City, 1850–1950.* Madison, Wis.: American History Research Center, 1957.

Bonner, Thomas N. *To the Ends of the Earth: Women's Search for Education in Medicine.* Cambridge: Harvard University Press, 1992.

Boorstin, Daniel J. *The Americans: The Colonial Experience.* New York: Vintage Books, 1964.

Boorstin, Daniel J. *The Lost World of Thomas Jefferson.* Boston: Beacon Press, 1960.

Bower, Alexander. *History of the University of Edinburgh.* 3 vols. Edinburgh: Oliphant, Waugh and Innes, 1817–30.

Boyle, Wade. *Herb Doctors: Pioneers in Nineteenth-Century American Botanical Medicine and a History of the Eclectic Medical Institute of Cincinnati.* East Palestine, Ohio: Buckeye Naturopathic Press, 1988.

Braid, James. *Neurypnology; Or, The Rationale of Nervous Sleep, Considered in Relation with Animal Magnetism. Illustrated by Numerous Cases of Its Successful Application in the Relief and Cure of Disease.* London: Churchill, 1843.

Branch, E. Douglas. *The Sentimental Years, 1836–1860.* New York: Hill and Wang, 1934.

Bridenbaugh, Carl. *Cities in the Wilderness: The First Century of Urban Life in America, 1625–1742.* New York: Ronald Press Co., 1938.

Brieger, Gert H. (ed.). *Medical America in the Nineteenth Century.* Baltimore: Johns Hopkins University Press, 1972.

Brinker, Francis J. *The Toxicology of Common Botanical Medicinal Substances.* Portland, Oreg.: Eclectic Institute, Inc., 1986.

Brooke, Humphrey. *A Conservatory of Health.* London: R.W. for G. Whittington, 1650.

Brooks, Chandler M., and Paul E. Cranefield (eds.). *The Historical Development of Physiological Thought.* New York: Hafner Publishing Co., 1959.

Brown, E. Richard. *Rockefeller Medicine Men: Medicine and Capitalism in America.* Berkeley: University of California Press, 1979.

Brown, John. *The Elements of Medicine.* 2 vols. London: J. Johnson, 1795.

Brown, Oliver Phelps. *The Complete Herbalist; Or, The People Their Own Physicians by the Use of Nature's Remedies.* Jersey City, N.J.: Published for the Author, 1867.

Brown, William Cullen. *The Works of Dr. John Brown.* 3 vols. London: J. Johnson, 1804.

Buchan, William. *Domestic Medicine; Or, A Treatise on the Prevention and Cure of Diseases by Regimen and Simple Medicine.* Edinburgh: Balfour, Auld and Smellie, 1797.

Buchanan, John. *The American Practice of Medicine.* Philadelphia: John Buchanan, 1868.

Buchanan, John. *The Eclectic Practice of Medicine and Surgery.* 3d ed. Philadelphia: John Buchanan, 1867.

Buchanan, Joseph R. *A Comprehensive View of Restrictive Medical Legislation: An Address.* Boston: Massachusetts Medical Liberty League, 1888.

Buchanan, Joseph R. *Defense of the People Against Medical Monopoly.* Boston: National Constitutional Liberty League, 1889.

Buchanan, Joseph R. *Free Collegiate Education.* Cincinnati: W.M. Naudain, 1852.

Buchanan, Joseph R. *Legalized Murder: The Treatment of Cancer by the Regular Profession Compared with Its Treatment by Irregular Physicians.* Boston: National Constitutional Liberty League, 1889.

Buchanan, Joseph R. *Manual of Psychometry: The Dawn of a New Civilization.* Boston: Holman Brothers, 1885.

Buchanan, Joseph R. *Outlines of Lectures on the Neurological System of Anthropology.* Cincinnati: Buchanan's *Journal of Man*, 1854.

Buchanan, Joseph R. *Periodicity; The Absolute Law of the Entire Universe Long Known to Control All Matter, Now Revealed as the Law of All Life.* San Jose, Calif.: J.R. Buchanan, 1897.

Buchanan, Joseph R. *Primitive Christianity.* 2 vols. San Jose, Calif.: J.R. Buchanan, 1897–98.

Buchanan, Joseph R. *Therapeutic Sarcognomy. The Application of Sarcognomy, the Science of the Soul, Brain and Body, to the Therapeutic Philosophy and Treatment of Bodily and Mental Diseases by Means of Electricity, Nervaura, Medicine and Haemospasia, with a Review of Authors on Animal Magnetism and Massage, and Presentation of New Instruments for Electro-Therapeutics.* Boston: J.G. Cupples Co., 1891.

Bulloch, Vern L. *The Development of Medicine as a Profession: The Contribution of the Medieval University to Modern Medicine.* New York: Hafner Publishing Co., 1966.

Bulloch, William. *The History of Bacteriology.* London: Oxford University Press, 1938.

Burrow, James G. *AMA: Voice of American Medicine.* Baltimore: Johns Hopkins University Press, 1963.

Burrow, James G. *Organized Medicine in the Progressive Era: The Move Toward Monopoly.* Baltimore: Johns Hopkins University Press, 1977.

Bury, J. B. *The Idea of Progress; An Inquiry into Its Origin and Growth.* New York: Macmillan, 1932.

Bush, George. *Mesmer and Swedenborg; Or, The Relation of the Developments of Mesmerism to the Doctrines and Disclosures of Swedenborg.* New York: John Allen, 1847.

Butterfield, Lyman H. (ed.). *Letters of Benjamin Rush.* 2 vols. Princeton, N.J.: Princeton University Press, 1951.

Bynum, W. F., and Roy Porter (eds.). *Medical Fringe and Medical Orthodoxy, 1750–1850.* London: Croom Helm, 1987.

Cadwalader, Thomas. *An Essay on the West-India Dry-Gripes; With the Method of Preventing and Curing That Cruel Distemper.* Philadelphia: B. Franklin, 1745.

Caldwell, Charles. *Autobiography of Charles Caldwell, M.D.* Philadelphia: Lippincott, Grambo and Co., 1855.

Caldwell, Charles. *A Discourse on the Advantages of a National University, Especially in Its Influences on the Union of the States.* Cincinnati: E.H. Flint, 1832.

Caldwell, Charles. *Elements of Phrenology.* Lexington, Ky.: T.T. Skillman, 1824.

Caldwell, Charles. *Thoughts on Schools of Medicine, Their Means of Instruction and Modes of Administration.* Louisville, Ky.: Prentice and Wassinger, 1837.

Cangi, Ellen Corwin. *Principles Before Practice: The Reform of Medical Education in Cincinnati Before and After the Flexner Report, 1870–1930.* Ph.D. Dissertation. Cincinnati: University of Cincinnati, 1983.

Carmer, Carl L. *Listen for a Lonesome Drum: A York State Chronicle.* New York: Farrar and Rinehard, 1936.

Carson, Joseph. *A History of the Medical Department of the University of Pennsylvania, from Its Foundation in 1765.* Philadelphia: Lindsay and Blakistan, 1869.

Selected Bibliography

Cassedy, James H. *American Medical and Statistical Thinking, 1800–1860*. Cambridge: Harvard University Press, 1984.

Cassedy, James H. *Medicine and American Growth, 1800–1860*. Madison: University of Wisconsin Press, 1986.

Chambers, John S. *The Conquest of Cholera: America's Greatest Scourge*. New York: Macmillan, 1938.

Chambers, Reuben. *The Thomsonian Practice of Medicine; Containing the Names, and a Description of the Virtues and Uses of the Medicines Belonging to the System of Practice*. Bethania, Pa.: Published for the Author, 1842.

Chesney, Alan M. *The Johns Hopkins Hospital and the Johns Hopkins University School of Medicine; A Chronicle*. Baltimore: Johns Hopkins University Press, 1943.

Clymer, R. Swinburne. *Nature's Healing Agents; The Medicines of Nature, or the Natural System*. Philadelphia: Dorrance, 1963.

Clymer, R. Swinburne. *The Thomsonian System of Medicine: With Complete Rules for the Treatment of Disease: Also a Short Materia Medica*. Allentown, Pa.: Philosophical Publishing Co., 1906.

Coe, Grover. *Concentrated Organic Medicines: Being a Practical Exposition of the Therapeutic Properties and Clinical Employment of the Combined Proximate Medicinal Constituents of Indigenous and Foreign Plants*. New York: B. Keith and Co., 1864.

Coe, Grover. *Positive Medical Agents*. N.p., 1855.

Cogan, Thomas. *The Haven of Health, Chiefly Gathered for the Comfort of Students*. London: A. Griffin, 1636.

Colby, Benjamin. *A Guide to Health; Being an Exposition of the Principles of the Thomsonian System of Practice and Their Mode of Application in the Cure of Every Form of Disease; Embracing a Concise View of the Various Theories*. Nashua, N.H.: Charles T. Gill, 1844.

Colonial Society of Massachusetts. *Medicine in Colonial Massachusetts, 1620–1820*. Boston: Colonial Society of Massachusetts, 1980.

Combe, George. *The Constitution of Man*. New York: Wells, 1828.

Combe, George. *Lectures on Phrenology, Including Its Application to the Present and Prospective Condition of the United States*. New York: Samuel R. Wells, 1874.

Combe, George. *Moral Philosophy; Or, The Duties of Man Considered in His Individual, Social and Domestic Capacities*. New York: W.H. Colyer, 1842.

Comfort, John W. *The Practice of Medicine on Thomsonian Principles, Adapted as Well to the Use of Families as to That of the Practitioner*. Philadelphia: Lindsay and Blaikston, 1863.

Comrie, John D. *History of Scottish Medicine*. 2 vols. London: Bailliere, Tindall, and Cox, 1932.

Cook, William H. *Physio-Medical Dispensatory: A Treatise on Therapeutics, Materia Medica, and Pharmacy, in Accordance with the Principles of Physiological Medication*. Cincinnati: W.M. Cook, 1869.

Cooter, Roger (ed.). *Studies in the History of Alternative Medicine*. New York: St. Martin's Press, 1988.

Cordasco, Francisco (ed.). *American Medical Imprints, 1820–1910.* 2 vols. Fairview, N.J.: Junius-Vaughn Press, 1990.

Cordasco, Francisco (ed.). *Medical Publishing in 19th-Century America.* Fairview, N.J.: Junius-Vaughn Press, 1990.

Cordell, Eugene F. *Historical Sketch of the University of Maryland, School of Medicine (1807–1890).* Baltimore: I. Friedenwald, 1891.

Corner, George W. *Two Centuries of Medicine: A History of the School of Medicine, University of Pennsylvania.* Philadelphia: J.B. Lippincott, 1965.

Coulter, Harris L. *Divided Legacy: A History of the Schism in Medical Thought.* Vol. III. *Science and Ethics in American Medicine: 1800–1914.* 3 vols. Washington, D.C.: Wehawken Book Co., 1973.

Cowper, William. *The Anatomy of Human Bodies.* London: Samuel Smith, 1698.

Cross, Whitney R. *The Burned-Over District: The Social and Intellectual History of Enthusiastic Religion in Western New York, 1800–1850.* New York: Harper and Row, 1950.

Culbreth, David M. R. *A Manual of Materia Medica and Pharmacology.* Philadelphia: H.C. Lea's Sons and Co., 1896.

Cullen, William. *First Lines of the Practice of Physic.* 4 vols. Edinburgh: T. Cadell, 1786.

Culpeper, Nicholas. *The English Physician—Enlarged; With Three Hundred Sixty and Nine Medicines Made of English Herbs.* London: A. and J. Churchill, 1703.

Currie, William. *A Dissertation on the Autumnal Remitting Fever.* Philadelphia: Peter Stewart, 1789.

Curtis, Alva. *The Provocation and the Reply: Allopathy Versus Physio-Medicalism.* Cincinnati: By the Proprietor, 1870.

Curtis, Alva. *Synopsis of a Course of Lectures on Medical Science.* Cincinnati: E. Shepard, 1846.

Darnton, Robert. *Mesmerism and the End of the Enlightenment in France.* New York: Schocken Books, 1970.

Davenport, Horace W. *Doctor Dock: Teaching and Learning Medicine at the Turn of the Century.* New Brunswick, N.J.: Rutgers University Press, 1987.

Davis, David J. (ed.). *History of Medical Practice in Illinois.* Vol. II, *1850–1900.* Chicago: Illinois State Medical Society, 1955.

Davis, Emerson. *The Half Century; Or, A History of Changes That Have Taken Place, and Events That Have Transpired, Chiefly in the United States, Between 1800 and 1850.* Boston: Tappan and Whittemore, 1851.

Davis, Loyal E. *Fellowship of Surgeons: A History of the American College of Surgeons.* Springfield, Ill.: Thomas, 1960.

Davis, Nathan Smith. *Contributions to the History of Medical Education and Medical Institutions in the United States of America, 1776–1876.* Washington, D.C.: Government Printing Office, 1877.

Davis, Nathan Smith. *History of the American Medical Association from Its*

Organization up to January, 1855. Philadelphia: Lippincott, Gambo and Co., 1855.

Davis, Nathan Smith. *History of Medical Education and Medical Institutions in the United States from the First Settlement of the British Colonies to the Year 1850*. Chicago: S.C. Griggs and Co., 1851.

Davis, Nathan Smith. *Medical Education and Medical Institutions in the United States of America, 1776–1876*. Washington, D.C.: U.S. Bureau of Education, 1877.

Day, Meeker L. *The Improved American Family Physician; Or, Sick Man's Guide to Health: Concerning a Complete Theory of the Botanic Practice of Medicine on the Thomsonian and Hygeian System, with Alterations and Improvements*. New York: n.p., 1833.

Debus, Allen G. *The Chemical Dream of the Renaissance*. Cambridge: Heffer, 1968.

Debus, Allen G. *The Chemical Philosophy: Paracelsian Science and Medicine in the Sixteenth and Seventeenth Centuries*. New York: Science History Publications, 1977.

Debus, Allen G. *The English Paracelsians*. London: Oldbourne, 1965.

Debus, Allen G. *Man and Nature in the Renaissance*. Cambridge, Great Britain: Cambridge University Press, 1978.

Debus, Allen G. (ed.). *Medicine in Seventeenth-Century England*. Berkeley: University of California Press, 1974.

Debus Allen G. (ed.). *Science, Medicine and Society in the Renaissance: Essays to Honor Walter Pagel*. New York: Science History Publications, 1972.

de Guistino, David. *Conquest of Mind: Phrenology and Victorian Social Thought*. London: Croom Helm, 1975.

Denton, William. *Soul of Things: Or, Psychometric Researches and Discoveries*. Boston: Walker, Wise and Co., 1863.

Derbyshire, Robert C. *Medical Licensure and Discipline in the United States*. Baltimore: Johns Hopkins University Press, 1969.

Dickson, Samuel. *The Fallacy of the Art of Physic, as Taught in the Schools; With the Development of New and Important Principles of Practice*. Edinburgh: Adam Charles Black, 1836.

Dickson, Samuel. *Memorable Events in the Life of a London Physician*. London: Virtue Brothers, 1863.

Dickson, Samuel. *The Principles of the Chrono-Thermal System of Medicine, With Fallacies of the Faculty, in a Series of Lectures*. New York: Long and Brothers, 1850.

Dispensatory of the United States of America. Philadelphia: Grigg, Elliot, and Co., 1833–49.

Dispensatory of the United States of America. 5th to 25th editions. Philadelphia: J.B. Lippincott, 1880–1960.

Donald, David H. *An Excess of Democracy: The American Civil War and the Social Process*. Oxford: Clarendon Press, 1960.

Douglass, William. *The Practical History of a New Epidemical Eruptive Military*

Fever, with Anangina Ulcusculosa, Which Prevailed in Boston New-England in the Years 1735 and 1736. Boston: Thomas Fleet, 1736.

Drachman, Virginia G. *Hospital with a Heart: Women Doctors and the Paradox of Separatism at the New England Hospital, 1862–1969*. Ithaca, N.Y.: Cornell University Press, 1984.

Drake, Daniel. *Discourse on the History, Character, and Prospects of the West*. Gainesville, Fla.: Scholars' Facsimiles and Reprints, 1955.

Drake, Daniel. *The People's Doctors*. Cincinnati: n.p., 1830.

Drake, Daniel. *A Systematic Treatise, Historical, Etiological, and Practical, on the Principal Diseases of the Interior Valley of North America, as They Appear in the Caucasian, African, Indian, and Esquimaux Varieties of Its Population*. Cincinnati: Winthrop B. Smith and Co., 1850.

Duffy, John. *Epidemics in Colonial America*. Baton Rouge: Louisiana State University Press, 1953.

Duffy, John. *The Healers: A History of American Medicine*. Urbana: University of Illinois Press, 1979.

Duffy, John. *The Healers: The Rise of the Medical Establishment*. New York: McGraw-Hill, 1976.

Dyer, D. *The Eclectic Family Physician; A Scientific System of Medicine, on Vegetable Principles*. Hallowell, Maine: Published for the Author, 1855.

Ekirch, Arthur A., Jr. *The Idea of Progress in America, 1815–1860*. New York: Columbia University Press, 1944.

Ellingwood, Finley. *The Eclectic Practice of Medicine*. 2 vols. Chicago: Ellingwood's Therapeutist Publishing Co., 1910.

Ellingwood, Finley. *A Manual of the Eclectic Treatment of Disease*. Chicago: Chicago Medical Times Publishing. Co., 1906–7.

Ellingwood, Finley. *A Treatise on Therapeutics and Materia Medica*. Chicago: Published for the Author, 1898.

Ellingwood, Finley, and John Uri Lloyd. *New American Materia Medica, Therapeutics and Pharmacognosy*. Evanston, Ill.: Ellingwood's Therapeutist Publishing Co., 1919.

Elliotson, John. *Human Physiology*. 5th ed. London: Longman, Orme, Brown, Green and Longmans, 1840.

Elliott, Stephen. *A Sketch of the Botany of South-Carolina and Georgia*. 2 vols. Charleston: J.R. Schenck, 1821–24.

Everitt, Graham. *Doctors and Doctors: Some Curious Chapters in Medical History and Quackery*. London: S. Sonnenschein, Lowrey and Co., 1888.

Faber, Knud. *Nosography: The Evolution of Clinical Medicine in Modern Times*. 2d ed. Rev. New York: Paul B. Hoeber, 1930.

Faber, Knud. *Nosography in Modern Internal Medicine*. New York: Paul B. Hoeber, 1923.

Felter, Harvey W. *Biographies of John King, M.D., Andrew Jackson Howe, A.B., M.D., and John Milton Scudder, M.D., Accompanied by Many Valuable and Historical Portraits and Other Illustrations*. Cincinnati: J.U. and C.G. Lloyd, 1912.

Felter, Harvey W. *The Eclectic Materia Medica, Pharmacology and Therapeutics.* Cincinnati: John K. Scudder, 1922.

Felter, Harvey W. *History of the Eclectic Medical Institute, Cincinnati, Ohio, 1845–1902.* Cincinnati: Alumni Association, 1902.

Felter, Harvey W., and John Uri Lloyd. *King's American Dispensatory.* 2 vols. 18th ed. 3d rev. Cincinnati: Ohio Valley Co., 1898–1900.

Finney, Charles G. *Charles G. Finney; An Autobiography.* Westwood, N.Y.: Fleming H. Revel, 1876.

Fishbein, Morris. *A History of the American Medical Association, 1847–1947.* Philadelphia: Saunders, 1947.

Fishbein, Morris. *The Medical Follies; An Analysis of the Foibles of Some Healing Cults, Including Osteopathy, Homeopathy, Chiropractic, and the Electronic Reactions of Abrams, with Essays on the Anti-Vivisectionists, Health Legislation, Physical Culture, Birth Control, and Rejuvenation.* New York: Boni and Liveright, 1925.

Fleming, Donald. *William H. Welch and the Rise of Modern Medicine.* Baltimore: Johns Hopkins University Press, 1987.

Flexner, Abraham. *Abraham Flexner: An Autobiography.* New York: Simon and Schuster, 1960.

Flexner, Abraham. *Henry S. Pritchett: A Biography.* New York: Columbia University Press, 1943.

Flexner, Abraham. *I Remember; The Autobiography of Abraham Flexner.* New York: Simon and Schuster, 1940.

Flexner, Abraham. *Medical Education in the United States and Canada; A Report to the Carnegie Foundation on the Advancement of Teaching.* New York: Carnegie Foundation, 1910.

Flexner, James T. *Doctors on Horseback: Pioneers of American Medicine.* New York: Viking Press, 1937.

Flexner, Simon. *The Evolution and Organization of the University Clinic.* Oxford: Clarendon Press, 1939.

Foltz, Kent O. *Diseases of the Eye.* Cincinnati: Scudder, 1909.

Foltz, Kent O. *Diseases of the Nose, Throat and Ear.* Cincinnati: Scudder, 1906.

Forbes, Sir John. *Nature and Art in the Cure of Disease.* New York: S.S. and W. Wood, 1858.

Ford, Paul L. (ed.). *The Writings of Thomas Jefferson.* 10 vols. New York: G.P. Putnam's Sons, 1892–99.

Foster, William D. *A History of Medical Bacteriology and Immunology.* London: William Heinemann Medical, 1970.

Fuller, Robert C. *Alternative Medicine and American Religious Life.* New York: Oxford University Press, 1989.

Fyfe, John W. *Specific Diagnosis and Specific Medication.* Cincinnati: John K. Scudder, 1914.

Garrison, Fielding H. *An Introduction to the History of Medicine.* 4th ed. Philadelphia: W.B. Saunders Co., 1929.

Selected Bibliography

Garrison, Fielding H. *John Shaw Billings: A Memoir*. New York: G.P. Putnam's Sons, 1915.

Gevitz, Norman (ed.). *Other Healers: Unorthodox Medicine in America*. Baltimore: Johns Hopkins University Press, 1988.

Goodman, Louis S., and A. Gilman. *The Pharmacological Basis of Therapeutics; A Textbook of Pharmacology, Toxicology and Therapeutics for Physicians and Medical Students*. New York: Macmillan, 1941.

Grainger, Thomas H. *A Guide to the History of Bacteriology*. New York: Ronald Press, 1958.

Griffith, Freda G. *The Swedenborg Society, 1810–1960*. London: Swedenborg Society, 1960.

Griggs, Barbara. *Green Pharmacy, A History of Herbal Medicine*. New York: Viking, 1982.

Gross, Samuel D. *History of American Medical Literature: From 1776 to the Present Time*. New York: B. Franklin, 1972.

Guerra, Francisco. *American Medical Bibliography 1639–1783*. New York: L.C. Harper, 1962.

Hall, Marshall. *Researches Principally Relative to the Morbid and Curative Effects of Loss of Blood*. Philadelphia: E.L. Carey and A. Hart, 1830.

Haller, Albrecht von. *A Dissertation on the Sensible and Irritable Parts of Animals*. London: J. Nourse, 1755.

Haller, John S., Jr. *American Medicine in Transition, 1840–1910*. Urbana: University of Illinois Press, 1981.

Harrington, Thomas F. *The Harvard Medical School; A History, Narrative and Documentary, 1782–1905*. 3 vols. Chicago: Lewis Publishing Co., 1905.

Harris, Seymour E. *The Economics of American Medicine*. New York: Macmillan, 1964.

Hart, James. *Klinekeh; Or, The Diet of the Diseased, Divided into Three Books, Wherein is Set Downe at Length the Whole Matter and Nature of Diet for Those in Health, But Especially for the Sicke*. London: John Beale, 1633.

Harvey, A. McGehee. *For the Welfare of Mankind: The Commonwealth Fund and American Medicine*. Baltimore: Johns Hopkins University Press, 1986.

Harvey, A. McGehee. *Science at the Bedside: Clinical Research in American Medicine, 1905–1945*. Baltimore: Johns Hopkins University Press, 1981.

Harvey, William. *De motu cordis*. London: Geoffrey Keynes, 1628.

Harvey, William. *Exercitationes de generatione animalium*. London: Pulleyn, 1651.

Hawkins, Hugh. *Between Harvard and America: The Educational Leadership of Charles W. Eliot*. New York: Oxford University Press, 1972.

Hempel, Charles J. *Organon of Specific Homeopathy; Or, An Inductive Exposition of the Principles of the Homeopathic Healing Art, Addressed to Physicians and Intelligent Laymen*. Philadelphia: Rademacher and Sheek, 1854.

312

Henry, Frederick P. (ed.). *Standard History of the Medical Profession of Phila-delphia.* [1897]. New York: AMS Press, 1977.

Henry, Samuel. *A New and Complete American Medical Family Herbal.* New York: S. Henry, 1814.

Herrick, J. B. *Memories of Eighty Years.* Chicago: University of Chicago Press, 1947.

Hildreth, Arthur G. *The Lengthening Shadow of Dr. Andrew Taylor Still.* Mason, Mo.: Arthur Grant Hildreth, 1938.

Hill, Benjamin L. *Lectures on the American Eclectic System of Surgery.* Cincinnati: W. Phillips and Co., 1850.

Hobbs, Christopher. *The Echinacea Handbook.* Portland, Oreg.: Eclectic Medical Publications, 1989.

Hollemback, Henry. *The American Eclectic Materia Medica.* Philadelphia: Published for the Author, 1865.

Holling, S. A., John Senior, Betty Clarkson, and Donald A. Smith (eds.). *Medicine for Heroes: A Neglected Part of Pioneer Life.* Mississauga, Ontario: Boston Mills Press, 1981.

Hollis, Ernest V. *Philanthropic Foundations and Higher Education.* New York: Columbia University Press, 1938.

Holmes, Peter. *The Energetics of Western Herbs: Integrating Western and Oriental Herbal Medicine Traditions.* Boulder, Colo.: Artemis Press, 1989.

Holzer, Hans. *Beyond Medicine: The Facts About Unorthodox and Psychic Healing.* Chicago: Regnery, 1973.

Honigberger, Johann Martin. *Cholera; Its Causes and Infallible Cure, and on Epidemics in General.* Calcutta: R.C. Lepage and Co., 1857.

Honigberger, Johann Martin. *Thirty-Five Years in the East.* 2 vols. London: H. Bailliere, 1852.

Hooker, Worthington. *Dissertation on the Respect Due to the Medical Profession, and the Reasons Why It Is Not Awarded by the Community.* Norwich: J.G. Cooley, 1844.

Hooker, Worthington. *The Present Mental Attitude and Tendencies of the Medical Profession.* New Haven, Conn.: T.J. Stafford, 1852.

Horine, Emmet F. *Daniel Drake, 1785–1852: Pioneer Physician of the Midwest.* Philadelphia: University of Pennsylvania Press, 1961.

House, Eleazer G. *The Botanic Family Friend: Being a Complete Guide to the New System of Thomsonian Medical Practice.* Boston: Published for the Author, 1844.

Howard, Horton. *Howard's Domestic Medicine.* Philadelphia: R. Rulison, 1859.

Howard, Horton. *An Improved System of Botanic Medicine, Founded upon Correct Physiological Principles; Embracing a Concise View of Anatomy and Physiology.* Columbus, Ohio: Published for the Author, 1832.

Illinois State Board of Health. *Report on Medical Education and the Regulation of the Practice of Medicine in the United States and Canada.* Springfield, Ill.: State Board of Health, 1883.

Inglis, Brian. *The Case for Unorthodox Medicine*. New York: Putnam, 1965.

Jackson, Samuel. *The Principles of Medicine, Founded on the Structure and Functions of the Animal Organism*. Philadelphia: Carey and Lea, 1832.

James, Henry. *The Secret of Swedenborg: Being the Elucidation of His Doctrine of the Divine Natural Humanity*. New York: AMS Press, 1983.

Johnson, Victor E. *A History of the Council on Medical Education and Hospitals of the American Medical Association, 1904–1959*. Chicago: AMA Press, 1959.

Jones, Billy M. *Health-Seekers in the Southwest, 1817–1900*. Norman: University of Oklahoma Press, 1967.

Jones, Eli G. *Cancer, Its Causes and Treatment*. Boston: Therapeutic Publishing Co., 1911.

Jones, Ichabod Gibson, and Thomas Vaughan Morrow. *The American Eclectic Practice of Medicine*. 2 vols. Cincinnati: Moore, Anderson, Wilstach and Keys, 1854.

Jones, Lorenzo E. *An Exposition of the Character of Prof. J. R. Buchanan, in Reply to His Defamatory Attack Upon L. E. Jones and Others*. Cincinnati: n.p., 1853.

Jones, Lorenzo E., and John M. Scudder. *The American Eclectic Materia Medica and Therapeutics*. Cincinnati: Moore, Wilstach, Keys and Co., 1858.

Juettner, Otto. *Daniel Drake and His Followers; Historical and Biographical Sketches*. Cincinnati: Harvey Publishing Co., 1909.

Kaufman, Martin. *American Medical Education: The Formative Years, 1765–1910*. Westport, Conn.: Greenwood Press, 1976.

Kaufman, Martin. *Homeopathy in America: The Rise and Fall of a Medical Heresy*. Baltimore: Johns Hopkins University Press, 1971.

Kelly, Howard A. *Cyclopedia of American Medical Biography*. 2 vols. Philadelphia: W.B. Saunders and Co., 1912.

Kelly, Howard A., and Walter L. Burrage. *Dictionary of American Medical Biography; Lives of Eminent Physicians of the United States and Canada, From the Earliest Times*. New York: D. Appleton and Co., 1928.

Kennedy, Gail (ed.). *Evolution and Religion; The Conflict Between Science and Theology in Modern America*. Boston: D.C. Heath and Co., 1957.

Kent, Countess Elizabeth. *A Choice Manual of Rare and Select Secrets in Physick and Chyrurgery*. London: G.D., 1653.

Kett, Joseph. *The Formation of the American Medical Profession: The Role of Institutions, 1780–1860*. New Haven, Conn.: Yale University Press, 1968.

King, John. *The American Dispensatory*. Cincinnati: Moore, Wilstach and Baldwin, 1864.

King, John. *The American Eclectic Dispensatory*. Cincinnati: Moore, Wilstach and Keys, 1854.

King, John. *American Eclectic Obstetrics*. Cincinnati: Moore, Wilstach, Keys and Co., 1855.

King, John. *The American Family Physician; Or, Domestic Guide to Health*. Indianapolis: A.D. Streight, 1860.

King, John. *The Causes, Symptoms, Diagnosis, Pathology, and Treatment of Chronic Diseases.* Cincinnati: Moore, Wilstach and Baldwin, 1867.

King, John. *The Coming Freeman; Or, Justice and Equality to All.* Cincinnati: Published for the Author, 1886.

King, John. *The Eclectic Dispensatory of the United States of America.* Cincinnati: H.W. Derby and Co., 1852.

King, John. *The Microscopist's Companion.* Cincinnati: Rickey, Mallory and Co., 1859.

King, John. *Women—Their Diseases and Their Treatment.* Cincinnati: Longley Brothers, 1858.

King, Lester S. *The Medical World of the Eighteenth Century.* Huntington, N.Y.: Robert E. Krieger Publishing Co., 1971.

King, Lester S. *The Philosophy of Medicine: The Early Eighteenth Century.* Cambridge: Harvard University Press, 1978.

Kohlstedt, Sally G. *The Formation of the American Scientific Community: The American Association for the Advancement of Science, 1848–1860.* Urbana: University of Illinois Press, 1976.

Konold, Donald E. *A History of American Medical Ethics, 1847–1912.* Madison: State Historical Society of Wisconsin, 1962.

Kost, John. *The Practice of Medicine According to the Plan Most Approved by the Reformed or Botanic Colleges of the United States, Embracing a Treatise on Materia Medica and Pharmacy.* Mt. Vernon, Ohio: n.p., 1847.

Kremers, Edward, and George Urdang. *History of Pharmacy: A Guide and a Survey.* Philadelphia: J.B. Lippincott Co., 1951.

Lang, William. *Mesmerism; Its History, Phenomena, and Practice.* Edinburgh: Fraser, 1843.

Leavitt, Judith W., and Ronald L. Numbers (eds.). *Sickness and Health in America: Readings in the History of Medicine and Public Health.* Madison: University of Wisconsin Press, 1985.

Lesky, Erna. *The Vienna Medical School of the Nineteenth Century.* Baltimore: Johns Hopkins University Press, 1976.

Lewis, Richard W. B. *The American Adam: Innocence, Tragedy, and Tradition in the Nineteenth Century.* Chicago: University of Chicago Press, 1955.

Lippard, Vernon W. *A Half-Century of American Medical Education, 1920–1970.* New York: Josiah Macy, Jr., Foundation, 1974.

Lloyd, John Thomas. *Specific Medicines.* Cincinnati: Lloyd Brothers, Pharmacists, Inc., n.d.

Lloyd, John Uri. *The Eclectic Alkaloids, Resins, Resinoids, Oleo-Resins and Concentrated Principles.* Cincinnati: J.U. and C.G. Lloyd, 1910.

Lloyd, John Uri. *History of the Vegetable Drugs of the Pharmacopoeia of the United States.* Cincinnati: J.U. and C.G. Lloyd, 1911.

Lloyd, John Uri. *The Life and Medical Discoveries of Samuel Thomson and a History of Thomsonian Materia Medica, as Shown in "The New Guide to Health," (1835), and the Literature of the Day.* Cincinnati: J.U. and C.G. Lloyd, 1909.

Selected Bibliography

Lloyd, John Uri. *Origin and History of All the Pharmacopoeial Vegetable Drugs, Chemicals and Preparations*. Cincinnati: Caxton Press, 1921.

Lloyd, John Uri (comp.). *Drugs and Medicines of North America; A Publication Devoted to the Historical and Scientific Discussion of Botany, Pharmacy, Chemistry and Therapeutics of the Medical Plants of North America*. Cincinnati: J.U. and C.G. Lloyd, 1884–87.

Lloyd, John Uri, and Curtis Gates Lloyd. *Drugs and Medicines of North America*. Cincinnati: J.U. and C.G. Lloyd, 1884–87.

Long, Esmond R. *History of Pathology*. Baltimore: Williams and Wilkins Co., 1928.

Louis, Pierre. *Researches on the Effects of Bloodletting in Some Inflammatory Diseases*. Boston: Hilliard, Gray and Co., 1836.

Ludmerer, Kenneth M. *Learning to Heal: The Development of American Medical Education*. New York: Basic Books, 1985.

MacDermot, Violet. *Emanuel Swedenborg's Philosophy of the Human Organism*. Richmond, Great Britain: New Atlantis Foundation, 1974.

Markham, Gervase. *The English House-Wife. Containing the Inward and Outward Vertues Which Ought to Be in a Compleate Woman*. London: Nicholas Okes, 1613.

Mather, Cotton. *A Letter about a Good Management under the Distemper of the Measles, at This Time Spreading in the Country*. Boston: n.p., 1713.

Mattson, Morris. *The American Vegetable Practice; Or, A New and Improved Guide to Health Designed for the Use of Families*. Boston: Daniel L. Hale, 1841.

Mattson, Morris. *The American Vegetable Practice; Or, A New and Improved Guide to Health Designed for the Use of Families*. 3d ed. Boston: Published for the Author, 1855.

McClurg, James. *Experiments upon the Human Bile*. London: n.p., 1772.

Mead, Sidney E. *The Lively Experiment: The Shaping of Christianity in America*. New York: Harper and Row, 1963.

Mead, Sidney E. *The Nation with the Soul of a Church*. New York: Harper and Row, 1975.

Means, James H. *The Association of American Physicians: Its First 75 Years*. New York: McGraw-Hill, 1961.

Meyer, Clarence. *Vegetarian Medicines*. Glenwood, Ill.: Meyer Books, 1981.

Meyer, Clarence (comp.). *American Folk Medicine*. New York: Crowell, 1973.

Meyer, Joseph E. *The Herbalist*. Glenwood, Ill.: Meyer Books, 1981.

Miller, Amy B. *Shaker Herbs—A History and a Compendium*. New York: C.N. Potter, 1976.

Miller, Genevieve. *Bibliography of the History of Medicine in the United States and Canada, 1939–1960*. Baltimore: Johns Hopkins University Press, 1964.

Miller, Perry. *The Life of the Mind in America from the Revolution to the Civil War*. New York: Harcourt, Brace, and World, 1965.

Selected Bibliography

Moerman, Daniel. *American Medical Ethnobotany: A Reference Dictionary.* New York: Garland, 1977.

Morantz-Sanchez, Regina M. *Sympathy and Science: Women Physicians in American Medicine.* New York: Oxford University Press, 1985.

Mumford, Lewis. *Technics and Civilization.* New York: Harcourt, Brace and Co., 1934.

Myers, Burton D. *The History of Medical Education in Indiana.* Bloomington: Indiana University Press, 1956.

National Formulary. Washington, D.C.: American Pharmaceutical Association, 1888.

Newman, Charles. *The Evolution of Medical Education in the Nineteenth Century.* London: Oxford University Press, 1957.

Newton, Robert S. *Ancient and Modern Eclecticism in Medicine.* Brooklyn: W.C. Wilton, 1864.

Newton, Robert S. *An Eclectic Treatise on the Practice of Medicine; Embracing the Pathology of Inflammation and Fever, with Its Classification and Treatment.* Cincinnati: Published for the Author, 1861.

Nicholls, Phillip A. *Homeopathy and the Medical Profession.* London: Croom Helm, 1988.

Nissenbaum, Stephen. *Sex, Diet, and Debility in Jacksonian America: Sylvester Graham and Health Reform.* Westport, Conn.: Greenwood Press, 1980.

Norwood, William F. *Medical Education in the United States Before the Civil War.* Philadelphia: University of Pennsylvania Press, 1944.

Numbers, Ronald L. (ed.). *The Education of American Physicians: Historical Essays.* Berkeley: University of California Press, 1980.

Numbers, Ronald L., and Darrell W. Amundsen (eds.). *Caring and Curing: Health and Medicine in the Western Religious Tradition.* New York: Macmillan, 1986.

O'Malley, C. D. (ed.). *The History of Medical Education: An International Symposium Held February 5–9, 1968.* Berkeley: University of California Press, 1970.

Osler, William. *An Alabama Student, and Other Biographical Essays.* London: H. Milford, 1908.

Packard, Francis R. *History of Medicine in the United States.* 2 vols. New York: Hafner Publishing Co., 1963.

Paine, Thomas. *Common Sense.* Philadelphia: Edes and Gill, 1776.

Paine, William. *An Epitome of the American Eclectic Practice of Medicine.* Philadelphia: J. Gladding, 1859.

Paine, William. *The Medical Properties and Uses of Concentrated Medicines.* Philadelphia: Rodgers, 1865.

Paine, William. *New School Treatment Reduced to a Science, with Rules and Directions.* Philadelphia: n.p., 1875.

Paine, William. *Pennsylvania Frauds! How State Officials Teach Political Arithmetic.* Philadelphia: n.p., 187?.

Parker, Gail T. *Mind Cure in New England: From the Civil War to World War I.* Hanover, N.H.: University Press of New England, 1973.

Pepper, William. *Higher Medical Education, the True Interest of the Public and the Profession: An Address*. Philadelphia: Collins, 1877.

Pharmacopoeia of the United States of America. Philadelphia: John Grigg, 1831.

Pharmacopoeia of the United States of America. Philadelphia: Grigg, Elliot and Co., 1833–49; J.B. Lippincott Co., 1851–1919.

Pickard, Madge E., and R. Carlyle Buley. *The Midwest Pioneer; His Ills, Cures, and Doctors*. New York: Henry Schuman, 1946.

Pinel, Philippe. *Nosographie philosophique*. 2 vols. Paris: Brosson, 1818.

Platter, Felix. *Praxeos medical tomi tres*. Basileae: Joannis Schroeteri, 1625.

Post, Albert. *Popular Freethought in America, 1825–1850*. New York: Columbia University Press, 1943.

Powell, John H. *Bring Out Your Dead; The Great Plague of Yellow Fever in Philadelphia in 1793*. Philadelphia: University of Pennsylvania Press, 1949.

Powell, William Byrd. *The Natural History of the Human Temperaments*. Cincinnati: H.W. Derby and Co., 1856.

Powell, William Byrd, and Robert S. Newton. *The Eclectic Practice of Medicine: Diseases of Children*. Cincinnati: Rickey, Mallory and Co., 1858.

Professors and Members of the Reformed Medical Colleges in New York and Worthington, Ohio. *The Reformed Practice of Medicine*. Boston: n.p., 1831.

Puschmann, Theodor. *A History of Medical Education*. New York: Hafner Publishing Co., 1966.

Pusey, William Allen. *A Doctor of the 1870's and 80's*. Springfield, Ill.: Charles C. Thomas, 1932.

Rafinesque, Constantine Samuel. *Medical Flora: Or, Manual of the Medical Botany of the United States of North America*. 2 vols. Philadelphia: Atkinson and Alexander, 1828–30.

Rau, Gottlieb M. W. Ludwig. *Organon of the Specific Healing Art*. New York: W. Radde, 1847.

Rau, Gottlieb M. W. Ludwig. *Ueber den werth des homeöopathischen Heilverfahrens*. Heidelberg: Groos, 1824.

Reed, Louis S. *The Healing Cults; A Study of Sectarian Medical Practice: Its Extent, Causes, and Control*. Chicago: University of Chicago Press, 1932.

Risse, Guenter B., Ronald L. Numbers, and Judith W. Leavitt (eds.). *Medicine Without Doctors; Home Health Care in American History*. New York: Science History Publications, 1977.

Robinson, Samuel. *A Course of Fifteen Lectures, on Medical Botany, Denominated Thomson's New Theory of Medical Practice; In Which the Various Theories That Have Preceded It Are Reviewed and Compared; Delivered in Cincinnati, Ohio*. Columbus, Ohio: Horton Howard, 1829.

Roemer, Milton I. (ed.). *Henry E. Sigerist on the Sociology of Medicine*. New York: M.D. Publications, 1960.

Roorbach, Orville A. *Bibliotheca Americana. Catalog of American Publications, Including Reprints and Original Works from 1820 to 1850, Inclusive. To-*

gether with a List of Periodicals Published in the United States. New York: Orville A. Roorbach, 1852.

Rosenberg, Charles E. *The Cholera Years: The United States in 1832, 1849 and 1866.* Chicago: Uniersity of Chicago Press, 1962.

Rothstein, William G. *American Medical Schools and the Practice of Medicine: A History.* New York: Oxford University Press, 1987.

Rothstein, William G. *American Physicians in the Nineteenth Century: From Sects to Science.* Baltimore: Johns Hopkins University Press, 1972.

Rush, Benjamin. *Medical Inquiries and Observations.* 4 vols. 2d ed. Philadelphia: J. Conrad and Co., 1789.

Sauvages de la Croix, François Boissier de. *Nosologia methodica sistens morborum classes juxta Sydendami mentem and botanicorum ordinem.* 2 vols. Amstelodami: Tournes, 1768.

Scarborough, John (ed.). *Folklore and Folk Medicines.* Madison, Wis.: American Institute of the History of Pharmacy, 1987.

Scudder, John King. *Eclectics and Life Insurance.* Cincinnati: n.p., 1898.

Scudder, John M. *Domestic Medicine: Or, Home Book of Health.* Cincinnati: J.R. Hawley, 1865.

Scudder, John M. *Dose Book, Giving Specific Uses, Indications and Doses of Specific Medicines.* 5th ed. Cincinnati: Lloyd Brothers, 1885.

Scudder, John M. *The Eclectic Family Physician.* Cincinnati: J.K. Scudder, 1887.

Scudder, John M. *The Eclectic Practice in Diseases of Children.* Cincinnati: American Publishing Co., 1869.

Scudder, John M. *The Eclectic Practice in Diseases of Children.* Cincinnati: Published for the Author, 1881.

Scudder, John M. *The Eclectic Practice of Medicine.* Cincinnati: Moore, Wilstach, Keys and Co., 1864.

Scudder, John M. *The Eclectic Practice of Medicine.* 8th ed; Cincinnati: Medical Publishing Co., 1877.

Scudder, John M. *The Eclectic Practice of Medicine for Families.* Cincinnati: Wilstach, Baldwin and Co., 1876.

Scudder, John M. *The Essential Differences Between the Three Schools of Medicine: Eclectic, Allopathic and Homeopathic.* Cincinnati: n.p., n.d.

Scudder, John M. *A Practical Treatise on the Diseases of Women.* Cincinnati: Wilstach, Keys and Co., 1857.

Scudder, John M. *The Principles of Medicine.* Cincinnati: Moore, Wilstach and Baldwin, 1867.

Scudder, John M. *On the Reproductive Organs, and the Venereal.* Cincinnati: Wilstach, Baldwin and Co., 1874.

Scudder, John M. *Specific Diagnosis: A Study of Disease with Special Reference to the Administration of Remedies.* Cincinnati: Wilstach, Baldwin and Co., 1874.

Scudder, John M. *Specific Medication and Specific Medicines.* Cincinnati: Wilstach, Baldwin and Co., 1870.

Scudder, John M. *Specific Medication and Specific Medicines*. 16th ed. Cincinnati: John K. Scudder, 1913.

Shafer, Henry B. *The American Medical Profession: 1783–1850*. New York: Columbia University Press, 1936.

Sharp, William. *Essays on Medicine: Being an Investigator of Homeopathy and Other Medical Systems*. London: Leath and Ross, 1874.

Sherwood, Henry H. *The Motive Power of Organic Life, and Magnetic Phenomena of Terrestrial and Planetary Motions, with the Application of the Ever-Active and All-Pervading Agency of Magnetism, to the Nature, Symptoms, and Treatment of Chronic Diseases*. New York: H.A. Chapin and Co., 1841.

Short, Thomas. *Medicina Britannica; Or, A Treatise on Such Physical Plants as Are Generally Found in the Fields or Gardens in Great Britain*. London: n.p., 1747.

Shryock, Richard H. *American Medical Research, Past and Present*. New York: Commonwealth Fund, 1947.

Shryock, Richard H. *The Development of Modern Medicine; An Interpretation of the Social and Scientific Factors Involved*. Philadelphia: University of Pennsylvania Press, 1936.

Shryock, Richard H. *Medical Licensing in America, 1650–1965*. Baltimore: Johns Hopkins University Press, 1967.

Shryock, Richard H. *Medicine and Society in America, 1660–1860*. New York: New York University Press, 1960.

Shryock, Richard H. *The Unique Influence of the Johns Hopkins University on American Medicine*. Copenhagen: Munksgaard, 1954.

Simon, Jules. *Victor Cousin*. Chicago: A.C. McClurg and Co., 1888.

Simons, Corinne Miller. *John Uri Lloyd, His Life and His Works, 1849–1936; With a History of the Lloyd Library*. Cincinnati: Privately Printed, 1972.

Smith, Dale C. *The Emergence of Organized Clinical Instruction in the Nineteenth-Century American Cities of Boston, New York and Philadelphia*. Ph.D. Dissertation. Minneapolis: University of Minnesota, 1979.

Smith, E. *The Compleat Housewife; Or, Accomplished Gentlewoman's Companion*. Williamsburg: W. Parks, 1742.

Smith, Elias. *The American Physician and Family Assistant*. Boston: E. Bellamy, 1826.

Smith, Elias. *The Medical Pocket-Book, Family Physician and Sick Man's Guide to Health*. Boston: Henry Bowen, 1822.

Smith, Elisha. *The Botanic Physician, Being a Compendium of the Practice of Medicine, upon Botanic Principles*. New York: Murphy and Bingham, 1830.

Smith, Peter. *The Indian Doctor's Dispensatory, Being Father Smith's Advice Respecting Diseases and Their Cure*. Cincinnati: Browne and Looker, 1813.

Smith, R. W. Innes. *English-Speaking Students of Medicine at the University of Leyden*. Edinburgh: Uhuer and Boyd, 1932.

Selected Bibliography

Smith, Timothy L. *Revivalism and Social Reform in Mid-Nineteenth-Century America*. New York: Abingdon Press, 1957.
Smith, William. *History of the Province of New York*. London: T. Wilcox, 1757.
Sonnedecker, Glenn. *Kremers and Urdang's History of Pharmacy*. 3rd ed. Philadelphia: J.B. Lippincott Co., 1963.
Stannard, David E. *The Puritan Way of Death: A Study of Religion, Culture, and Social Change*. New York: Oxford University Press, 1977.
Starr, Paul E. *The Social Transformation of American Medicine: The Rise of a Sovereign Profession and the Making of a Vast Industry*. New York: Basic Books, 1982.
Stearns, R. P. *Science in the British Colonies of America*. Urbana: University of Illinois Press, 1970.
Stephens, Albert F. *The Essentials of Medical Gynecology*. Cincinnati: Scudder Brothers, 1907.
Stern, Bernhard J. *American Medical Practice in the Perspectives of a Century*. New York: Commonwealth Fund, 1945.
Stevens, Rosemary. *American Medicine and the Public Interest*. New Haven, Conn.: Yale University Press, 1971.
Stevens, Rosemary. *Medical Practice in Modern England: The Impact of Specialization and State Medicine*. New Haven, Conn.: Yale University Press, 1966.
Stevenson, Lloyd G., and Robert P. Multhauf. *Medicine, Science, and Culture: Historical Essays in Honor of Owsei Temkin*. Baltimore: Johns Hopkins University Press, 1968.
Stone, Eric. *Medicine among the American Indians*. New York: Hafner Publishing Co., 1962.
Stookey, Bryan P. *A History of Colonial Medical Education: In the Province of New York, with Its Subsequent Development, 1767–1830*. Springfield, Ill.: Thomas, 1962.
Stroh, Alfred H. (ed.). *Emanuel Swedenborg as a Scientist: Miscellaneous Contributions*. 3 vols. Stockholm: Aftonbladets Tryckeri, 1908–11.
Sydenham, Thomas. *Opera universa*. London: Walteri Kettilby, 1685.
Taeuber, Conrad, and Irene B. Taeuber. *The Changing Population of the United States*. New York: Wiley, 1958.
Taylor, Norman. *Plant Drugs That Changed the World*. New York: Dodd, Mead, 1965.
Temkin, Owsei. *Galenism: Rise and Decline of a Medical Philosophy*. Ithaca, N.Y.: Cornell University Press, 1973.
Tennant, Abel. *The Vegetable Materia Medica and Practice of Medicine. Containing in Detail His Practical Knowledge of American Remedies, in Curing Diseases*. Batavia, N.Y.: D.D. Wait, 1837.
Tennant, John V. B. *Every Man His Own Doctor; Or, The Poor Planter's Physician*. Philadelphia: B. Franklin, 1734.
Thacher, Thomas. *A Brief Rule to Guide the Common People of New England,*

How to Order Themselves and Theirs in the Small-Pocks, or Measles. Boston: John Foster, 1677.

Theobald, John. *Every Man His Own Physician.* Boston: Cox and Berry, 1767.

Thomas, Rolla L. *The Eclectic Practice of Medicine.* Cincinnati: J.K. Scudder, 1922.

Thoms, H. *The Doctors of Yale College, 1702–1815, and the Foundation of the Medical Institution.* Hamden, Conn.: Shoe String Press, 1960.

Thomson, John. *A Historical Sketch of the Thomsonian System of the Practice of Medicine on Botanical Principles.* Albany, N.Y.: B.D. Packard and Co., 1830.

Thomson, John. *A Philosophical Theory of an "Empiric," Proved Practically: Compared with the Doubtful Science Known as Quackery and Practiced by the Regular Physicians during the Prevalence of the Cholera in This City.* Albany, N.Y.: Published for the Author, 1833.

Thomson, John. *A View of Science and Quackery Compared Theoretically and Practically; Or, The Difference Between Vegetable and Mineral Medicines in Restoring the Sick to Health.* Albany, N.Y.: S. Southwick, 1831.

Thomson, Samuel. *Learned Quackery Exposed: Or, Theory According to Art.* Boston: Adams, 1836.

Thomson, Samuel. *A Narrative of the Life and Medical Discoveries of Samuel Thomson; Containing an Account of His System of Practice, and the Manner of Curing Disease with Vegetable Medicine, upon a Plan Entirely New, to Which Is Added an Introduction to His Guide to Health, or, Botanic Family Physician, Containing the Principles upon Which the System Is Founded, with Remarks on Fevers, Steaming, Poison, etc.* Boston: E.G. House, 1825.

Thomson, Samuel. *New Guide to Health; Or, Botanic Family Physician, Containing a Complete System of Practice, upon a Plan Entirely New: With a Description of the Vegetables Made Use of, and Directions for Preparing and Administering Them to Cure Disease.* Boston: E.G. House, 1825.

Thomson, Samuel. *New Guide to Health; Or, Botanic Family Physician, Containing a Complete System of Practice, upon a Plan Entirely New: With a Description of the Vegetables Made Use of, and Directions for Preparing and Administering Them to Cure Disease.* Boston: J. Howe, 1831.

Thomson, Samuel [with John Thomson]. *The Thomsonian Materia Medica; Or, Botanic Family Physician: Comprising a Philosophical Theory, the Natural Organization and Assumed Principles of Animal and Vegetable Life: To Which Are Added the Description of Plants.* 12th ed. Albany, N.Y.: J. Munsell, 1841.

Tocqueville, Alexis de. *Democracy in America.* London: Longman, Green, Longman, and Roberts, 1862.

United States, National Library of Medicine. *Early American Medical Imprints: A Guide to Works Printed in the United States, 1668–1820.* Compiled by Robert B. Austin. Washington, D.C.: National Library of Medicine, 1961.

Selected Bibliography

Vesalius, Andreas. *De humani corporis fabrica libri septem.* Basileae: I.O. Oporini, 1543.

Vogel, Morris J., and Charles E. Rosenberg (eds.). *The Therapeutic Revolution: Essays in the Social History of American Medicine.* Philadelphia: University of Pennsylvania Press, 1979.

Vogel, Virgil J. *American Indian Medicine.* Norman: University of Oklahomá Press, 1970.

Wallis, Roy, and Peter Morley (eds.). *Marginal Medicine.* London: Peter Owen, 1976.

Wallis, Wilson D. *Culture and Progress.* New York: McGraw-Hill, 1930.

Walsh, James J. *History of Medicine in New York.* 5 vols. New York: National Americana Society, 1919.

Waring, Joseph A. *A Brief History of the South Carolina Medical Association.* Charleston: South Carolina Medical Association, 1967.

Waring, Joseph A. *A History of Medicine in South Carolina, 1670–1825.* Charleston: South Carolina Medical Association, 1964.

Warner, John H. *The Therapeutic Perspective: Medical Practice, Knowledge, and Identity in America, 1820–1880.* Cambridge: Harvard University Press, 1986.

Warren, Sidney. *American Freethought, 1860–1914.* New York: Columbia University Press, 1943.

Weaver, George H. *Beginnings of Medical Education in and near Chicago; The Institutions and the Men.* Chicago: AMA, 1925.

Weil, Andrew. *Natural Health, Natural Medicine: A Comprehensive Manual for Wellness and Self-Care.* New York: Houghton Mifflin Co., 1990.

Weiss, Rudolf F. *Herbal Medicine.* Gothenburg: A.B. Arcanum, 1988.

Wesley, John. *Primitive Physick; Or, An Easy and Natural Method of Curing Most Diseases.* London: R. Hawes, 1776.

Wheatley, Steven C. *The Politics of Philanthropy: Abraham Flexner and Medical Education.* Madison: University of Wisconsin Press, 1988.

Wheelwright, Edith G. *Physick Garden: Medicinal Plants and Their History.* New York: Dover, 1974.

Wilde, Arthur H. (ed.). *Northwestern University: A History, 1855–1905.* 4 vols. New York: The University Publishing Co., 1905.

Wilder, Alexander. *History of Medicine: A Brief Outline of Medical History from the Earliest Historic Period with an Extended Account of the Various Sects of Physicians and New Schools of Medicines in Later Centuries.* Augusta, Maine: Maine Farmer Publishing Co., 1904.

Wilder, Alexander. *History of Medicine: A Brief Outline of Medical History and Sects of Physicians, from the Earliest Historic Period, with an Extended Account of the New Schools of the Healing Art in the Nineteenth Century, and Especially a History of American Eclectic Practice of Medicine, Never Before Published.* New Sharon, Maine: New England Eclectic Publishing Co., 1901.

Wilder, Alexander. *Plea for Collegiate Education for Women.* New York: n.p., 1874.

Selected Bibliography

Wilkinson, G. E. *Wilkinson's Botanico-Medical Practice*. Cincinnati: M. Swank, 1845.

Willis, Thomas. *The London Practice of Physick*. London: T. Bassel, 1685.

Winslow, Charles-Edward A. *The Conquest of Epidemic Disease: A Chapter in the History of Ideas*. Princeton, N.J.: Princeton University Press, 1943.

Wood, George B., and Franklin Bache. *The Dispensatory of the United States of America*. 14th ed. Philadelphia: J.B. Lippincott, 1877.

Woodward, Charles. *Pathological Alkalinity*. Chicago: Charles Woodward, 1926.

Woodward, John. *The State of Physick and of Disease*. London: n.p., 1718.

Worthy, Alfred N. *A Treatise on the Botanic Theory and Practice of Medicine, Compiled from Various Sources, with Revisions and Additions*. Forsyth, Ga.: C.R. Hanleiter, 1842.

Wrobel, Arthur (ed.). *Pseudo-Science and Society in Nineteenth-Century America*. Lexington: University Press of Kentucky, 1987.

Yonge, James. *Currus Triumphalis, e Terebintho; Or, An Account of the Many Admirable Virtues of Oleum Terebinthinae*. London: J. Martyn, 1679.

Young, James H. *The Toadstool Millionaires: A Social History of Patent Medicines in America before Federal Regulation*. Princeton, N.J.: Princeton University Press, 1961.

Zeuch, Lucius H. (comp.). *History of Medical Practice in Illinois*. Chicago: Book Press, 1926.

Index

Academy of Arts and Sciences, 118
Ackerknecht, E. H., 85
Advice literature, 73–74
Agassiz, Louis, 72, 118
Alabama, licensing in, 211–12
Alkaloids, 176, 188
Allegheny County Eclectic Medical Society, 210
Allopathy. *See* Regulars
Alstat, Edward K., 247, 248
American Academy of Medicine, 203
American Association for the Advancement of Science, 118
American Association of Anatomists, 202
American Association of Pathologists and Bacteriologists, 202–3
American Association of Physicians and Surgeons, 203
American Association of Physio-Medical Physicians and Surgeons, 63
American College of Medicine (Philadelphia), 148
American College of Medicine and Surgery (Macon, GA), 146, 151
American College of Pharmacy (New York City), 173

American Dispensatory, The (King), 142–43, 233
American Eclectic Dispensatory (Newton), 119–20
American Eclectic Medical Association, 160
American Eclectic Medical College of Cincinnati, 210
American Institute of Homeopathy, 229, 240
American Medical Association, xvii; absorbs sectarians, 207, 229–30; college classification of, 221, 237, 239–40; on eclecticism, 118, 207, 243–44, 245; eclectics on, 123, 207–8, 221, 229–30; ethical code of, 211; on homeopathy, 207; on hospital access, 157, 217; journal of, 190, 213–14, 215, 237; on licensing, 221, 234–36; on medical education, 157, 158–59, 202, 204, 205, 206, 217, 220, 221, 233, 237, 239–40, 243–44, 245; on preceptorship, 157; on proprietary schools, 220; women in, 155
American Medical College (Indianapolis), 203, 237
American Medical College Association, 202, 205–6

breaks with Thomson, 54, 59,
62; as independent Thom-
sonian, 62, 78, 160; schools
founded by, 54, 60, 78

Davidge, John B., 14, 81
Davis, Nathan Smith, 199, 202,
219–20
Degree, medical, 2, 5; sold, 201;
states regulate, 70
Democracy: in medicine, xvi, 31–
32; sectarianism based on, 32,
35, 40, 41–42, 47–48, 86–87
Depletion, 21, 26; eclectics question, 69–70, 73, 88, 161, 167–
68, 231; regulars use, 89–90,
169
Diagnosis, 25, 179, 228; pathology
aids, 26, 27; specific (see Disease:
as specific entity)
Dickson, Samuel, 150
Dietl, Joseph, 168
Diploma: as license, 14; mills, 148,
149–50, 209, 236
Disease: antigerm theory of, 190–
91; causes of, 20, 21, 41, 177–
78, 188–89; as condition, 17; as
contagious, 188; eclectics on, 91,
113, 167, 181; homeopaths on,
72, 177–78; identified, 8, 21,
26; as imbalance, 19, 20, 187–
88; self-limited, 26, 72; as
specific entity, 85, 176–77, 179–
81, 188–89, 231; symptoms of,
20, 187–88; treatment of, 8, 91,
113, 167, 177–78, 181, 188–89
Doctors' Riot, 81
Dodson, John M., 201
Douglass, William, 2, 5
Drake, Daniel, 50, 56, 102
Drug manufacture. See Pharmaceuticals
Drug potencies, 101, 117, 178
Drugs, mineral: eclectics on, 69–
70, 73, 87, 88, 91, 143, 164,
167, 171–72, 195–96, 231; regulars use, 18, 45, 89–90. See also

Arsenic; Calomel; Mercury;
Tarter emetic
Drugs, plant. See Botanic medi-
cine; Eclectics: plant materia
medica of; Herbal medicine
Dynamization, 72, 101, 117

Eclectic Botanic Medical Associa-
tion of Pennsylvania, 82, 84, 159
Eclectic College of Medicine
(Buchanan's) (Cincinnati), 122,
174
Eclectic Institute Incorporated
(Portland, OR), 247
Eclectic Medical Association of the
State of Pennsylvania, 210
Eclectic Medical College (Cincin-
nati). See Eclectic Medical
Institute
Eclectic Medical College (Kansas
City), 214
Eclectic Medical College (New
York City), 123
Eclectic Medical College of
Indiana (Indianapolis); 237
Eclectic Medical College of Penn-
sylvania (Philadelphia), 62, 148,
151
Eclectic Medical College of Phila-
delphia, 90, 148, 149, 150
Eclectic Medical College of the
City of New York, 145–46, 152,
214, 224, 237, 239
Eclectic Medical Institute (Cincinnati), xvii, 82–84, 86, 151, 209,
214, 216–19; AMA on, 243–44,
245; on AMA classification, 221;
Beach at, 82; black students at,
279n.36; Buchanan at, 96–97,
101, 103–6, 115–16, 119–22,
124, 141, 242; in Civil War,
140; closes, 241, 245–47;
compared to regulars' schools,
140; educational reform at,
103–6, 205, 206, 217, 219;
enrollment of, 83, 105, 140,
216, 219, 225, 226; entry

JOHN S. HALLER, JR., holds a dual appointment as professor of history at Southern Illinois University, Carbondale, and professor of medical humanities at the SIU School of Medicine, Springfield. He is the author of *Outcasts from Evolution: Scientific Attitudes of Racial Inferiority, 1859–1900* (winner of the Anisfield-Wolf Prize in Race Relations); *The Physician and Sexuality in Victorian America* (with Robin M. Haller); *American Medicine in Transition, 1840–1910*; and *Farmcarts to Fords: A History of the Military Ambulance, 1790–1925*, as well as numerous articles on the history of nineteenth-century sexuality, anthropology, medicine, and pharmacy.